Contents

Treatment of Cerebral Palsy and Motor Delay

Fifth edition

Sophie Levitt

BSc (Physiotherapy) Wits
Fellow of the Chartered Society of Physiotherapy
Consultant Paediatric Physiotherapist
Tutor on Developmental Therapy

With contributions to Chapters 1, 2, 4 and 8 by

Dawn Pickering, MSc, PGCME, MCSP
Lecturer in Physiotherapy
School of Healthcare Studies
Cardiff University
Wales

WILEY-BLACKWELL

A John Wiley & Sons, Ltd., Publication

Blackwell Publishing was acquired by John Wiley & Sons in February 2007. Blackwell's publishing programme has been merged with Wiley's global Scientific, Technical, and Medical business to form Wiley-Blackwell.

Registered office
John Wiley & Sons Ltd, The Atrium, Southern Gate, Chichester, West Sussex, PO19 8SQ, United Kingdom

Editorial offices
9600 Garsington Road, Oxford, OX4 2DQ, United Kingdom
350 Main Street, Malden, MA 02148-5020, USA

For details of our global editorial offices, for customer services and for information about how to apply for permission to reuse the copyright material in this book please see our website at www.wiley.com/wiley-blackwell.

Library of Congress Cataloging-in-Publication Data

Levitt, Sophie.
   Treatment of cerebral palsy and motor delay / Sophie Levitt. – 5th ed.
      p. ; cm.
   Includes bibliographical references and index.
   ISBN 978-1-4051-7616-3 (pbk. : alk. paper)
   1. Cerebral palsied children–Rehabilitation.   2. Physical therapy for children.   3. Movement disorder in children.   4. Cerebral palsied.   I. Title.
   [DNLM: 1. Cerebral Palsy–therapy.   2. Child.   3. Motor Skills Disorders–therapy.   4. Motor Skills.
5. Physical Therapy Modalities.   WS 342 L666t 2010]
   RJ496.C4L43 2010
   618.92′83603–dc22
                                                                                                    2009028120

A catalogue record for this book is available from the British Library.

Set in 9.5/11.5pt Sabon by Aptara® Inc., New Delhi, India
Printed in Singapore by Ho Printing Singapore Pte Ltd

2   2011

Foreword

I greatly welcome the fifth edition of this book which brings together the management of cerebral palsies into a comprehensive but readable form. It builds on the strengths of previous editions including specific methodologies, their conceptual framework and the long and quite tortuous historical pathway of our attempts to help children with early onset motor disorders and their parents and teachers. The developing scientific background is expanded and balanced with the understanding of what can realistically be researched in children who show such wide variations of motor, cognitive and behavioural impairments.

The approach shows recognition of the forces that have driven the subject but produces an account of what a therapist can realistically offer by way of assessment and therapy. There is always the problem of how an inexperienced therapist extracts ideas and practical methodologies from the writings of someone of Sophie Levitt's long experience. This book is in my view an essential part of both a therapist's and doctor's basic understanding of the subject, but requires the practical interplay with experienced practitioners in a multidisciplinary team to set priorities for an individual child.

At one level the 'cerebral palsies' are being reclassified into more precise diagnostic entities, partic-ularly by magnetic resonance imaging. At a more practical level there are a large number of young children with motor delay and disorder whose families need help on how to handle them and help them to achieve their potential. Whether you can show that a varied group of children are better for this or that intervention on a global scale of assessment may mean less than that a family has been able to relax with their disabled daughter and feel that they understand something of her needs and the methods by which they can help her.

It also may well be that setting-agreed aims to be achieved within a defined time is the best way of bridging the gap between different levels of experience. It also provides an auditable target for those who would wish to measure the efficacy of the enterprise in a mechanistic rather than psychological one.

This book remains essential for those managing children with disability.

Brian Neville
Professor of Childhood Epilepsy
Professor of Paediatric Neurology
University College London
Institute of Child Health/Great Ormond
Street Hospital for Children NHS Trust

Preface

The five editions of this book reflect where we have been and where we are now. Ideas from the past are still prevalent today, but we fortunately have studies which confirm the value of some of them. Research on others may not be easy or perhaps possible at this time. In order for this book to reflect both what we did and what we do now, I have learned not only from my physiotherapy colleagues and the questions from my students but also from parents and their children. Listening attentively to parents, I have learned of their fundamental human needs for respect, for support and for a sense of control of their lives. Their practical ideas, their courage and their determination to do the best for their child are inspiring. Parents and their children with disabilities taught me that they needed empathy not sympathy. How does one present physiotherapy in this style? Did I have adequate professional knowledge to warrant the trust of parents and their children?

Fortunately, I had contact with many professionals in medicine, therapy, education, psychology and social work. This was as a member of multidisciplinary and interdisciplinary teams in both clinical work, special schools and in postgraduate education. I am grateful to many different professionals in various countries, who have given me generously of their knowledge and helped me understand their views for the benefit of the whole child and his or her family. It was not always easy to incorporate their essential messages into physiotherapy as there are contradictions in the cultures of different disciplines. However, I have drawn on their fundamental concerns for the whole child and have tried to integrate them into the development of a child's motor function.

As a physiotherapist I simultaneously sought and am still seeking the best ways to treat and manage a child with cerebral palsy. This was challenging as it involved dealing with contradictory views in my own profession. As I was attempting to understand the views of different professions, it was somewhat easier to understand different views in my own profession! I found some common ground between different therapy approaches and recommended that an eclectic approach would be best. To my mind, there were useful contributions from various experts.

The first edition of this book (1977) proposed an eclectic approach drawing on topics in neurology, orthopaedics and normal (typical) and abnormal child development. In addition, there was always the recognition that children 'do not move by neurophysiology alone' but that learning processes enable a child to progress through stages of motor development. The second and third editions continued to elaborate learning principles to develop children's motor function. Since publication of earlier editions of this book it has been rewarding to find an increase in an eclectic viewpoint and in more functional physiotherapy, which were so controversial in the past. In my work, functional therapy grew out of the question: 'How do parents and other adults learn?' I was helped by those studies in adult education which showed that people learn best what has meaning for them in their daily lives. Parents were clearly interested in their child's daily function, which was so limited by cerebral palsy.

The third edition contained a specific chapter on a collaborative learning approach. I had developed this approach over some years for working with parents, carers and others involved with a child with cerebral palsy. This 'client-centred' approach depends on their participation in a learning process. Unlike some learning models, this model also includes the therapist's own participation in learning, as well as the emotional issues affecting learning of parent and therapist in collaborative work. This approach involves consideration of the views and needs of both of them.

This approach develops respect for a family's cultural and social values as I learned in my experience in developing countries and as a tutor/guest lecturer with international students in the Community-Based Rehabilitation Courses, Institute of Child Health, London. The collaborative learning approach depends on daily tasks chosen by people with disabilities and their parents, carers and teachers in different communities. This promotes *inclusion* in mainstream schools and in the specific cultural communities in which a child or older person find themselves. The collaborative approach is a learning process which can allow parents and others involved to learn at their own pace, so adjusting their expectations and attitudes while maintaining hope.

The older person. The fifth edition continues to suggest use of the framework of my collaborative learning approach in Chapter 7 'The older person with cerebral palsy'. Similarly, as with child and parents, it offers mutual respect between individuals and therapists and develops self-esteem and confidence in adolescents and adults. Meaning is given for their daily lives so that the procedures suggested can improve their participation in their daily life. Therapy methods and recreational therapeutic activities are included to add to their quality of life. However, currently there is the growing view among psychologists and social scientists that participation does not necessarily equal a quality of life.

Family-centred approach (care). This is also based on 'client-centred' practice first originated by Carl Rogers in the 1960s which formerly inspired the collaborative learning approach, but has only emerged in family-centred physiotherapy and occupational therapy at the end of the 1990s and in recent years. This approach involves all the members of a cerebral palsy team and is a welcome development. However in some places, this demands reflective learning and re-examination of long-held professional attitudes. 'We are doing this anyway' is often felt by genuinely well-meaning professionals, but given the new measures of what parents and families really experience from a service, there is not necessarily agreement with this statement. References to such measures are given in this edition.

A framework for assessment, therapy and management. This fifth edition crystallises ideas from earlier editions for further development of the col-

laborative learning approach in the following framework:

(1) The task(s) (e.g., a daily activity, self-care, play or social interaction) are chosen by the person with cerebral palsy, together with his parents or other people involved in their familiar environments of home and community.
(2) The motor functions for the chosen task are selected.
(3) The components (abilities, skills, prerequisites) of the motor function are analysed, for example specific postural mechanisms, voluntary movement, perception and understanding (cognitive and emotional).
(4) The motor impairments which constrain motor function are assessed, for example limited joint range, weakness, abnormal postural alignment, limited repertoire of movements, abnormal movement patterns (synergies) or abnormal reflex reactions, as well as general health.
(5) The non-motor impairments which constrain motor function and task are considered, for example problems of vision, perception, understanding and communication.
(6) The residual abilities in all areas of function are identified, so they can be augmented to increase achievement through different strategies.

The individual person and those assisting him or her in home, school or community contribute most to items 1 and 2, while the physiotherapist and her multidisciplinary colleagues contribute most to items 3–6. The clinician will find there are overlaps between items, which are addressed in the practical chapters.

Therapy goals. Therapy goals can be clarified in this framework so that methods can be selected to activate components and minimise impairments *at the same time*. Postural control in the best possible alignments and movements, strengthening and joint ranges and coordination are themselves improved if appropriately used whilst training function. A number of us have found that our previous focus on impairments did not always lead to function. It is dependent on the condition of individuals as to when there is a need to add specific treatment and medical procedures for impairments.

In earlier editions a view was given that spasticity has more relevance to deformities than to direct causation of most of the motor dysfunction. Nevertheless, if a deformity was developing, this acted as a block to function and needed therapy. There were very few studies on spasticity that I could find to support my clinical impression. Today, there are many studies which have questioned the role of spasticity in function. For example, the studies on selective dorsal rhizotomies show that though spasticity was removed, there was little change in overall function. In addition, since the first edition I have found recent studies in support of my long-held view that spasticity and reflex reactions or 'reflex-hunting' were overemphasised. However, typical postural control or the postural mechanisms have been emphasised since the first edition. Many new studies are growing to assert the importance of postural control or balance. More of these studies are included in this edition.

Strengthening procedures. In the past, my inclusion of strengthening methods was considered controversial. This book continues to suggest strengthening methods using manual resistance, selected from proprioceptive neuromuscular facilitation and additional motor functions involving lifting of heavy objects. The methods are selected for use in the context of developmental motor functions. The treatment of deformities also continues to employ strengthening of agonists and antagonists according to the muscle imbalance.

Evidence-based practice. The fifth edition has many revisions in the light of new knowledge, research studies and clinical evidence. Unfortunately, in this complex field and with this heterogeneous population, reliable scientific evidence to support interventions that we make can be difficult to obtain. Therefore, we still rely on long experience and expert opinion. Fortunately, research studies have increased and are becoming more rigorous and we look forward to further clinical progress as a result. This edition contains sections on current 'Assessment measures' and 'Evidence-based practice' which increases information previously given in 'Appraisal of Research Studies' in the fourth edition.

It is worth pointing out that there is a tendency to overrate numerical data, which is the norm in the physical sciences. However, while science may often involve numbers, this is not always necessary but good research must always involve careful systematic observation and detailed analysis, that is a lot of hard thinking.

Again, even when the research is thorough, it is often reported in obscurely written papers where little attempt seems to be made to communicate the findings to clinicians who are seeking to use results to improve their practice. On behalf of therapists, I would plead with researchers to keep their findings clear and reasonably simple, and to realise that most practicing therapists have little training in or aptitude for statistical analysis. Please spell out what your statistical tests are testing and also what assumptions are made. It is well known that medical research can be harmed by poorly applied statistics.

Suggestions not recipes. There remain many methods suggested from long clinical experience which still await research studies as to their value for specific problems, at different ages or developmental stages. This is not a book of 'recipes' but of suggestions for therapy and daily care or management based on assessment of an *individual* person with cerebral palsy and/or motor delay. They are presented with any evidence that exists at this time. The suggestions are not prescriptive and need to be assessed as appropriate for an individual person with cerebral palsy. Therapy methods based on research studies are desirable, but still need assessment with a particular person and with the parents and carers.

Not all methods are given, as some are difficult to describe and need demonstration. However, wherever possible, the principle has been given as to why, when and when not to use methods, which also allows a therapist to use her own methods and invent her own methods besides those suggested in this book. Not all possibilities for each person with cerebral palsy can be covered, so the therapist will also need to solve problems in each case and draw on his or her clinical experience. This book should be used with practical courses, further study and supervision by senior colleagues.

Current theories are given but there remain limitations as well as advantages for clinical workers. Some of the advantages tune in with clinical practice for which outdated theories were used. Clinicians feel well supported by the observations of researchers, and some clinicians are reticent about acknowledging the limitations of a theory. There remains the fact that no one theory or model exists for motor control and for motor learning. There is still controversy and fortunately research continues. For example, Dynamical Systems Theory originated in the field of motor control, where it was hoped that making analogies with the physics of complex systems (a notoriously difficult subject I am told) would lead to advances. The main conclusion seems to be that 'we should be aware that many factors are involved in the development of motor control'. This is an excellent notion. In fact, many thoughtful clinicians, particularly those working in interdisciplinary teams and in the community, have long been aware of this.

Unfortunately, Dynamical Systems Theory does not yet offer much guidance as to which of the varied factors are most important and how they interact in any particular circumstance. In addition, this and other theories relate to able-bodied subjects, to normal cognition and to adults with or without brain damage.

The plan of the book

Chapter 1 gives the clinical picture in direct relationship with principles of management. Chapter 2 discusses a collaborative learning approach for a child or older person and his or her parents and family. This approach is also relevant to work with other disciplines. Chapter 3 reviews the different treatment approaches with some current additions. The historical background shows how we arrived at some of our current good practice and perhaps avoids unnecessary effort to 'reinvent the wheel'. Contemporary theories are also discussed with their usefulness and limitations in clinical practice. Chapter 4 considers the current evidence for the treatment systems and for various new methods. There is discussion on the appraisal of quantitative and qualitative research for clinicians. (Measures used in research and clinical work are given later in Chapter 8 as this is closely linked with assessment.) Chapter 5 discusses and offers a synthesis of different approaches. This eclectic approach has grown out of my studies, discussions and observations or courses with Dr Phelps, Dr and Mrs Bobath, Dr Fay, Dr Vojta, Miss Knott, Mrs Collis, Dr Hari and Mrs Cotton, as well as from my own experience. Chapter 6 integrates the learning principles for an eclectic viewpoint. Chapter 7, on the older person, suggests modifying or selecting methods described for

a child's motor function, as well as other issues of specific relevance to adolescence and adulthood.

Chapter 8 offers practical assessments and measurements with comments on their usefulness. Chapter 9 presents methods of treatment and management. As this book emphasises that equipment need to be associated with motor training and not substituted for it, equipment are discussed and described in Chapters 8, 9 and 10 (Assessment for therapy and daily function; Treatment procedures and management; Motor function and the child's daily life). An appendix (Appendix 2) on equipment is given for reference and useful addresses include organisations which have information on current suppliers.

Swimming, horse riding, skiing, abseiling, angling, wheelchair dancing and other therapeutic and recreational leisure activities are highly recommended and the list of useful addresses include those specialising in these areas.

It is hoped that this book will respond to some extent to the remarks of my postgraduate students and colleagues who suggested I write it – remarks such as:

> 'I agree with your eclectic approach, but how do I go about doing it?'

> 'How is it possible to combine such different viewpoints in our field?'

> 'I have followed one system but would like to extend my repertoire of methods and I am open to hearing other views.'

But especially to the remark:

> 'Teach me how to enable these people and their families.'

Sophie Levitt
London

Note: For the sake of clarity a child will be referred to as 'he' and a therapist as 'she'. There are a small number of exceptions.

Acknowledgements

This fifth edition is updated with acknowledgements to my reviewers and colleagues who have given me constructive criticism and much encouragement.

Dawn Pickering has stimulated me with useful discussions and her contributions. I thank her for her work and support.

I would particularly like to thank Alison Wisbeach, paediatric occupational therapist, for most of the drawings and useful discussions over the years. My special thanks to Dr Richard Lovell, physicist, who has been a great help and support in facing and critically appraising the enormous number of research studies now available for physiotherapists and occupational therapists. I am grateful for useful clinical comments from Lyn Horrocks on Chapter 11, April Winstock on communication and feeding in Chapter 10, as well as helpful discussions with Jeanne Hartley, Gillian Hill, Lesley Carroll-Few, Eva Bower, Helen Stevens, Maria Ash, Katrin Stroh, Elinor Goldschmied and from many of my postgraduate students in both the United Kingdom and overseas.

I feel privileged to have been awarded a Folke Bernadotte Fellowship supported by the paediatric group of the Swedish Physiotherapy Association and their chairperson Elisabeth Price in 1990. Their encouragement of my eclectic approach and work with parents has been an inspiration. My thanks are also due to Dr Patricia Sonksen, the late Dr Joan Reynell, Dr Pam Zinkin, the late Mary Kitzinger and others with whom I worked on severely visually impaired children at the Wolfson Centre, Institute of Child Health.

This book was originally commenced when I was Director of Studies at The Cheyne Centre for Children with Cerebral Palsy, London, where I was given encouraging support from Dr John Foley and the staff. The foundation of this book was the correlation of the neurology of Dr Foley and Dr J. Purdon Martin with the child development studies of the late Dr Mary Sheridan.

I am grateful to the Leverhulme Trust Fund, which kindly awarded me a Research Fellowship for part of my studies on the synthesis of treatment systems in cerebral palsy, which formed the basis of this book in all its editions.

I remain particularly appreciative of the privilege of many observations, discussions or courses in the past with Dr Phelps, Dr Fay, Dr Vojta, Maggie Knott, Eirene Collis, Dr and Mrs Bobath, Professor Guy Tardieu, Ester Cotton and Dr Hari. They have inspired and influenced me, and without them this book would not have been written.

Thanks for the photographs to Cheyne Centre for photographs in Figs 9.62, 9.76, 9.130, 9.132, 9.133 and 12.1; to Alison Wisbeach for photographs in Figs 9.92, 9.93, 9.114 and 9.120–9.124; to the Wolfson Centre for Figs 2.2, 2.6, 9.167 and 9.170; to the Indian Spastics Society for photographs in Figs 2.1, 2.3 and 2.7; to the Foxdenton School, Lancashire for photographs in Figs 9.125 and 9.126. Many recent photographs were taken by David Halpern, with enormous organisation by Helen Stevens, formerly Superintendent Paediatric Physiotherapist, Winchester and Eastleigh Healthcare NHS Trust, and wonderful cooperation of parents and young people. Thanks for Figs 2.8, 7.2, 8.2, 8.3, 9.68, 9.111, 9.154, 9.173, 9.207, 9.210–9.212 and 10.3. Thanks for most of the remaining photographs to Ted Remington, previously Assistant Head of the Richard Cloudsley School, London, who patiently photographed them with help from Christine White, former Head Ms Suckling and staff at the time.

A special thanks to my son David Halpern who as a boy showed much patience and understanding, with skill in supplying numerous cups of coffee, and now is a great help with advice on editing and discussing my manuscripts. Both he and Richard Lovell have amazed me with their computer skills which have helped me enormously.

I am deeply grateful to all the children, adolescents and their parents who cooperated so amazingly with all the long sessions of photography used throughout the book. My special appreciation goes to all the children and older people with cerebral palsy, their parents and families, with whom I have been privileged to work and from whom I have learned so much.

My publishers have been particularly kind, helpful and sensitive and I thank Amy Brown, Katrina Hulme-Cross, James Sowden and their staff at Wiley-Blackwell for all their help and support.

Professor Brian Neville has honoured and encouraged me by writing the Forewords for the last three editions and for having generously shared his ideas.

Disclaimer: New research and experience may lead to changes in practice, use of equipment, treatment and management. The treating practitioner is responsible for selecting the best treatment and management based on his/her expertise and knowledge of an individual patient. Practitioners should take responsibility for safety precautions. Readers should check the most up-to-date information from the literature and from manufacturers of equipment.

The clinical picture for therapy and management

Cerebral palsy is the commonly used name for a group of conditions characterised by motor dysfunction due to non-progressive brain damage early in life. There are usually associated disabilities as well as emotional, social and family difficulties. Cerebral palsies are the most common cause of childhood disability. The range of severity may be from total dependency and immobility to adequate abilities of talking, independent self-care and walking, running and other skills, although with some clumsy actions. A number of people with cerebral palsy are now able to benefit from mainstream education and further education. They participate more in various activities in society. These opportunities are assisted by legislation, advances in technology and changing attitudes in their society. Bax and Brown (2004) have given an overview of the cerebral palsies.

The motor dysfunction

The brain damage results in disorganised and delayed development of the neurological mechanisms of postural control, balance and movement. The muscles activated for these motor aspects are therefore inefficient and uncoordinated. Individuals have specific impairments such as hypertonicity or hypotonicity with weakness, abnormal patterns of muscle activation including excessive co-contractions. There are absent or poor isolated movements (poor selective motor control), abnormal postures and problems with manipulation. Besides neuromuscular impairments, the motor dysfunction has musculoskeletal problems. There are biomechanical difficulties resulting from both the neuromuscular dysfunction and musculoskeletal problems, which add to this complex picture.

The motor dysfunction changes with both growth and a child's development. Change also depends on how an individual uses his body. Physiotherapy positively contributes to body function. However, the brain damage is not progressive, though the motor behaviour changes. Musculoskeletal problems may increase in late childhood and adolescence needing physiotherapy input to minimise this.

What matters most to a child and his family is the overall functional delay and abnormal performance. Therapists need to address these daily functional difficulties together with a child and his parents or directly with an older person with cerebral palsy (see Chapters 2 and 7). Therapists will assess and assume which of the impairments and functional components are responsible for any functional disabilities. The associated impairments and disabilities below also influence the motor function. It is encouraging to know that functional limitations can be minimised even though basic impairments cannot strictly be cured.

There are different views as to which motor impairments are responsible for the total motor dysfunction and what correlation exists between them. Views also differ as to which impairments can be changed, and if not, when to make adaptations, including use of equipment, so that function can still take place. The underlying motor dyscontrol is controversial. This is not surprising, as not all the normal and abnormal neurological mechanisms are fully understood. There are also various ideas on biomechanics. Research continues on the basic dyscontrol and biomechanics.

The first edition of this book (Levitt 1977) presented a synthesis of valuable contributions from different therapy systems, some of which had been regarded as mutually exclusive. This synthesis or eclectic approach was further developed to include ideas from motor control and motor learning systems. The new edition of this book continues to synthesise current contributions from different approaches. As many colleagues are now not wedded to any one system of therapy, selections of their views are presented as well as those from each of the author's own studies and experience.

As a child does not 'move by neurophysiology alone', not only various ideas on learning motor control have been integrated into the general therapy framework, but the influence of the context of a child's function is given special consideration. This takes place in a child's home, school and community. A child learns best in a familiar environment and gains meaning for what is being achieved clinically. It is primarily the motivation of a child by people in these contexts and a child's own intrinsic motivation which have a profound impact on his or her achievement. In addition, consideration needs to be given to any environmental physical constraints and social attitudes which challenge a child and older person with cerebral palsy.

Associated impairments and disabilities

Brain damage in cerebral palsy may also be responsible for special sense defects of vision and hearing, abnormalities of speech and language, and aberrations of perception (Hall 1984; Neville 2000). Included in the perceptual defects are the *agnosias*. The agnosias are difficulties in recognising objects or symbols, even though sensation as such is not impaired, and the patient can prove by other means to know or have known what the object or symbol is. There may also be *dyspraxias*, some of which are also called visuomotor defects. This means that the child is unable to perform certain movements even though there is no paralysis, because the patterns or *engrams* have been lost or have not developed. Dyspraxia can involve movements of the limbs, face, eyes, tongue or be specifically restricted to such acts as writing, drawing and construction or even dressing. In other words, there seems to be a problem in 'motor planning' in those children who are dyspraxic. Some children may also have various behavioural problems such as distractibility and hyperkinesis, which are based on the brain damage. All these defects result in various learning problems and difficulties in communication. In addition, there may be intellectual impairment and various epilepsies (Himmelmann *et al.* 2006).

Not every child has some or all of these associated impairments. Even if the impairment were only motor, the resulting paucity of movement would prevent the child from fully exploring the environment. He is therefore limited in the acquisition of sensations and perceptions of everyday things. A child may then *appear* to have defects of perception, but these may not be due to the brain damage but caused by lack of experience. The same lack of everyday experiences retards the development of language and affects the child's speech. His general understanding may suffer, so he appears to be intellectually retarded. This can go so far that normal intelligence has been camouflaged by severe physical disability. Furthermore, the lack of movement can affect the general behaviour of the child. Thus, some abnormal behaviour may be due to the lack of satisfying emotional and social experiences for which movement is necessary. Motor dysfunction may therefore interact with emotional and social development of a child. However, positive attitudes in a family and child can encourage optimum development.

Teamwork. It is therefore important for any therapist to recognise that motor function cannot be isolated from other functions and that she is treating a child who is not solely physically but multiply disabled. Therapists will also need to consider when the associated physical and behavioural problems constrain motor function (Thylefors *et al.* 2000).

In order to manage the multiple disabilities and lack of related learning experiences which interfere with a child's development, a physiotherapist or occupational therapist needs to be part of a team. The teamwork varies in different places such as community centres, child development centres, units in hospitals or within educational settings. Teamwork is discussed in Chapters 2, 8, 10 and 12.

Aetiology

Premature infants are at greater risk of brain dysfunction. There are many causes of the brain damage, including abnormal development of the brain, anoxia, intracranial bleeding, excessive neonatal asphyxia (hypoxic ischaemic neonatal encephalopathy), trauma, hypoglycaemia, anoxia as in neardrowning, choking, neurotrophic virus and from various infections. These have been extensively discussed in the medical literature (Rosenbloom 1995; Hagberg *et al.* 1996; Stanley *et al.* 2000; Himmelmann *et al.* 2005). The therapist is, however, rarely guided by the aetiology in her treatment planning. In some cases the cause is not certain, and in many cases knowing the cause does not necessarily indicate a specific diagnosis or specific treatment. Nevertheless, the therapist should acquaint herself with the history of the case. Many of these children have been affected from infancy and have been difficult to feed and handle. Many hospitalisations and separations of babies from parents may happen in the early period. This may easily have influenced the parent–child relationships so essential for child development. Furthermore, the history may sometimes give an indication of the prognosis; for example, with marked microcephaly with severe multiple impairments the prognosis would be poor.

Clinical picture and development

It is important to recognise that the causes of cerebral palsy take place in the prenatal, perinatal and postnatal periods. In all cases, it is an immature nervous system which suffers the insult and the nervous system afterwards continues to develop in the presence of the damage. The therapist must therefore not think of herself as treating an upper motor neurone lesion in a 'little adult' nor can she regard

the problem solely as one of retardation in development. What the therapist faces is a complex situation of pathological symptoms within the context of a developing child (Sheridan 1975, 1977; Drillien & Drummond 1977, 1983; Illingworth 1983; McGraw 1989; Sheridan *et al.* 2008). There are six main aspects to the clinical picture:

(1) Retardation in the development of new skills expected at the child's chronological age.
(2) Persistence of infantile behaviour in all functions, including infantile reflex reactions.
(3) Slow rate of progress from one developmental stage to the next.
(4) A smaller variety of skills than in the ablebodied child.
(5) Variations in the normal sequence of skills.
(6) Abnormal and unusual performance of skills.

In order to recognise abnormal motor and general behaviour, the therapist should know what a normal child does and how he does it at the various stages of his development. Information on each individual child's developmental levels should be sought from the consultants and other members of the cerebral palsy team. Reference will have to be made to the extensive literature on the field of child development.

Although normal child development is the basis on which the abnormal development is appreciated, it does not follow that assessment and treatment should rely upon a strict adherence to normal developmental schedules. Even 'normal' children show many variations from the 'normal' developmental sequences and patterns of development which have been derived from the *average* child. Cultural differences exist for normal motor development (Solomons & Solomons 1975; Hopkins & Westra 1989). However, in any culture, the child with cerebral palsy will show additional variations due to neurological and mechanical difficulties. If one considers, say, the normal developmental scales of gross motor development, in cerebral palsy a child has frequently achieved abilities (components) and motor functions at one level of development, omitted abilities at another level and only partially achieved motor abilities and functions at still other levels. There is thus more of a scatter of abilities and whole motor functions than in able-bodied children. The analysis of motor function into components is discussed in Chapters 5, 6, 8 and 9.

If the gross motor development is generally considered to be around a given age, the development of hand function, speech and language, social and emotional and intellectual levels may all be at different ages. None of these ages may necessarily coincide with the child's chronological age.

Therefore, the developmental schedules in normal child development should only be used as *guidelines* in treatment, and adaptation should be made for each child's disabilities and individuality (see Chapter 9).

More attention is usually given to motor development rather than other avenues of development, as it is the motor dysfunction which characterises cerebral palsy. Here again, the therapist should remember that abnormal motor behaviour interacts with other functions. Each area of development – such as gross motor, manipulation, speech and language, perception, social and emotional adjustments, and cognition – interacts as well as has its own pattern or avenue of development. Furthermore, the potential for function is dependent not only on the disabilities present but also on a child, his personality and 'drive' as well as his capacity to learn. Therefore, a total habilitation programme is necessary and should be planned to deal with the whole development of each child.

Whilst aiming at the maximum function possible, the therapists concerned must take account of the *damaged* nervous system and adjust their expectations of achievements by the child. This depends on a therapist's clinical experience as prognosis is difficult in view of the multiple factors involved. There are measures of the severity of a child's disability in Chapter 8, which guide the expectations of a therapist, but overdependence on levels of severity may not always be reliable in individual children.

Change in clinical picture

As the lesion is in a developing nervous system, the clinical picture is clearly not a static set of signs and symptoms for treatment. But whilst the lesion itself is non-progressive, its manifestations change as the nervous and musculoskeletal systems mature. As more is demanded of the child, the degree of the motor disability appears to be greater. For example, a 3-year-old is expected to do more than a baby, and therefore his difficulties are greater for the same pathology.

In addition, the pathological symptoms may develop with the years. Spasticity may increase, involuntary movements may only appear at the age of 2 or 3 years and ataxia may only be diagnosed when the child walks or when grasp is expected to become more accurate. Diagnoses may change as the baby develops to childhood, and especially as the child becomes more active. For example, a monoplegia reveals itself as a hemiplegia. Later a triplegia reveals itself as a tetraplegia. Cerebral palsies have an emerging diagnosis. Later, especially in adolescence, growth and increase in weight contribute to apparent deterioration. Recent research identifies that deterioration is not inevitable in all cases (see Chapter 7).

Treatment and management in infancy. The earlier the treatment is started, the more opportunity is given for whatever potential there may be for developing any normal abilities and for decreasing the abnormal movement patterns and postural difficulties (Kong 1987; de Groot 1993). However, abnormalities detected in infants may be transient as some infants overcome them without intervention. Therapists offer pleasurable and a variety of developmentally appropriate and active motor activities enjoyed by both parent and baby. During intervention, therapists observe if a baby or young child makes his own efforts to move using compensatory or adaptive patterns which can be 'good enough' but block the development of more efficient patterns or result in 'learned disuse' of a body part. Any immobility threatens musculoskeletal growth and development which can lead to deformities. Early physiotherapy minimises such problems.

The value of early developmental intervention is to provide an increase in a baby's sensory-motor and everyday experiences and interaction with his mother and father. The sooner a baby can be helped to move, the sooner he can explore and the sooner he can communicate the information he gains through such exploration. The therapist is in fact contributing to his learning and understanding as well as enabling him to bond with his mother and father.

Although the clinical picture is known to change with the years, it is not yet possible to predict the natural history of the condition in each particular child. Infants and babies with marked early neurological signs may later prove to be only mildly affected, or even normal (Ellenberg & Nelson 1981; Nelson & Ellenberg 1982). On the other hand, apparently mildly affected ones may become progressively worse with the years. It is therefore difficult to prove the value of a number of different early treatment approaches (Vojta 1984; Kong 1987; Katona 1989; Morris 1996). However, research in neonatal physiotherapy continues. Blauw-Hospers and Hadders-Algra (2005) have found positive effects on babies at term, rather than preterm, with specific and general developmental early treatments in their systematic review of 12 studies. The review by Spittle *et al.* (2007) found little evidence of early intervention on motor development. Reviews point out that the studies involve heterogeneous samples.

Nevertheless, until we know more definitely which babies are going to 'come right' on their own, it is better to let them have the benefit of treatment so that any potentials for improvement are not lost. Despite the controversy as to the value of early treatment, there is clearly no doubt about its importance to the parents, who receive a great deal of practical advice and support from the therapists. Among others, Goodman *et al.* (1991) found that if their research could not firmly state that neonatal physiotherapy was responsible for babies' motor developmental progress, all mothers confirmed their great appreciation for the support and practical ideas from their physiotherapists. Olow (1986) emphasises that early intervention reduces the frustration of early rearing of children with disabilities. Whilst medical practitioners are watching the development of the child in order to make a reliable diagnosis, the parents have to live with that child throughout each day of those months and years. Parents need support and practical ideas for feeding, childcare and motor activities for their child throughout the emerging diagnoses. This is an essential part of the therapist's management programme with them. Well-supported parents are most likely to benefit their young children's development (see Chapter 2).

Treatment and management in childhood, adolescence and adulthood. During these changes in the clinical picture, treatment and management programmes need to relate to an individual's wider environments of the playgroup, nursery, preschool, schools, adult day care centres and work places. The persons with cerebral palsy at different ages also change through interaction with the variety of personnel in environments in which they find themselves. Physiotherapy and occupational therapy as well as other therapies are therefore being planned across a lifespan of each person with cerebral palsy.

Management will include working with orthotists, orthopaedic surgeons and other consultants. The therapist will share selected skills and advice on equipment with anybody closely involved with each person having a disability.

Classification

Numerous classifications and subclassifications have been proposed by different authorities, and though clinically helpful, none of these diagnostic labels suffice to formulate adequate treatment plans. The therapist must also have a detailed assessment based primarily on motor functions in order to work out a treatment programme.

Classifications of topography of cerebral palsy

The topographical classifications frequently used are as follows:

Tetraplegia (quadriplegia). Involvement of all limbs and body. Arms are equally or more affected than the legs. Many are asymmetrical (one side more affected).

Diplegia. Involvement of limbs, with arms much less affected than legs. Asymmetry may be present.

Hemiplegia. Limbs and body on one side are affected.

Neville and Goodman (2001) present different authors in a book on congenital hemiplegia. These topographical classifications can be imprecise, as they may change with a child's development. One useful upper limb may convey a triplegia which could become a tetraplegia. Upper limbs may appear unaffected, suggesting a paraplegia but being really a diplegia with only fine-hand use being affected when this is later expected. Hemiplegia may have minor involvement on the unaffected side. A monoplegia is rare, usually becoming a hemiplegia with increased activity.

Classification of types of cerebral palsies

There are spastic types, athetoid (dyskinetic) types and a rare ataxic type. There is a hypotonic type which either becomes a spastic, athetoid or ataxic type. There is a transient dystonic stage in babies before they are diagnosed as a spastic or dyskinetic type of cerebral palsy (Bax & Brown 2004). Tetraplegias usually have either spasticity, dystonia, dyskinesia (athetosis), hypotonia or ataxia. Hemiplegia is usually a spastic type often starting out hypotonic. Hemi-athetoids with or without dystonia are occasionally seen. Once again, classifications are not always clear-cut and the therapist may have to treat impairments of one type in another type. The predominant impairments will contribute to the diagnostic type referred for therapy. Developmental functional training is nevertheless indicated for all types of cerebral palsies.

Spastic cerebral palsy

Main motor characteristics are as follows:

Hypertonus. If spastic muscles are stretched at a particular speed, they respond in an exaggerated fashion. They contract, blocking the movement. If this sudden passive stretch is continued, the spasticity may melt away in some cases. The movement block is the 'catch' and with the subsequent movement this is called a 'clasp-knife' variety of spastic hypertonus. This hyperactive stretch reflex may occur at the beginning, middle or near the end of the range of movement. There are increased tendon jerks, occasional clonus and other signs of upper motor neurone lesion. The velocity-dependent hyperactive stretch reflex is the physiological definition of spasticity. Stiffness is not true spasticity and may or may not accompany the reflex reaction to brisk passive stretch. Viscoelastic muscle and soft tissue changes are also causes of stiffness (Katz & Rymer 1989; Dietz & Berger 1995). However, clinicians usually use 'spasticity' and 'spastic muscles' as an umbrella term for stiffness of limbs and recognise that other motor symptoms are also included under this umbrella. These are discussed below. Current views are that the hyperactive stretch reflex is not as much the cause of abnormal function as weakness (Lin 2004; Ross & Engsberg 2007). Movements are usually slower than the velocity needed to obtain the hyperactive stretch reflex.

Hypertonus may be either spasticity or rigidity (dystonia). The overlap between the two is almost

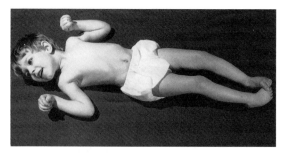

Figure 1.1 Child with spastic quadriplegia. Head preference to right, shoulders protracted, semi-abduction, elbows flexed-pronated, wrists and fingers flexed, thumb adducted. Hips and knees flexed, tendency to internal rotation–adduction with feet in equinovarus, toes flexed.

impossible to differentiate when severe. A mixture of spasticity and rigidity may be diagnosed (Lin 2004). Rigidity is recognised by a *plastic* or continuous resistance to passive stretch throughout the full range of motion. This *lead-pipe* rigidity differs from spasticity as spasticity offers resistance at a point or small part of the passive range of motion. Spasticity is selective affecting specific muscles, for example giving a predominantly flexor pattern in the arm and extensor pattern in the leg. Rigidity (dystonia) affects all muscle groups equally. Drugs such as botulinum toxin A, oral and intrathecal baclofen are used to control spasticity and dystonia (Lin 2004), together with a physiotherapy programme.

Abnormal postures (see Figs 1.1–1.3). These are usually associated with the antigravity muscles which are extensors in the leg and the flexors in the arm. However, the therapist will find *many* variations on this, especially when the child reaches different levels of development (Bobath & Bobath

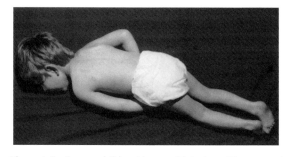

Figure 1.2 Same child with quadriplegia with postural changes in prone. Asymmetry of arms caught under body. Hips and knees flexed, feet in equinovarus. Head preference is now to left.

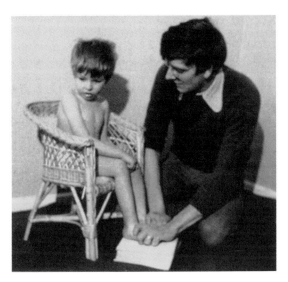

Figure 1.3 Same child being taught to sit by his father. Head preference to right, shoulders protracted, elbows flexed-pronated, hands flexed, knees and feet held symmetrical with hips. Symmetrical trunk.

1972). Children have floppiness of the head and trunk together with stiff spastic limbs. This is associated with delayed development of the mechanisms of postural stabilisation and postural adjustment of the head and trunk as well as delay in stabilisation of pelvic and shoulder girdles (Foley 1977, 1998). The postural mechanisms and the common abnormal postures in supine, prone, sitting, standing and hand positions are described in Chapters 5, 9 and 11.

The abnormal limb postures become held by stiff shorter 'spastic' muscle groups whose lengthened antagonists are weak, or apparently weak, in that they cannot overcome the tight pull of the shortened muscles and so correct the abnormal postures. The short muscle groups are also weak and cannot easily assume a normal alignment of posture. In time, there is transformation of structure of the stiff spastic muscle (see below). Besides spasticity, there are therefore various other causes of abnormal postures of limbs and body including the weakness and especially compensation for absent or poor postural mechanisms of balance control. Spasticity is therefore not overemphasised as a cause in this and previous editions of this book.

Abnormal postures appear as unfixed deformities, which in time may become fixed deformities or contractures with subsequent bony deformities.

Abnormal postures and deformities, particularly in the upright positions, contribute to abnormal gaits.

Changes in spasticity and postures. These changes may occur with excitement, fear or anxiety, and pain, which increases muscle tension. Shifts in spasticity may occur in the same affected parts of the body or from one part of the body to another in, say, stimulation of abnormal reactions such as occasional remnants of tonic reflex activity. Changes in spasticity are seen with changes of position in some children. Position of the head and neck may affect the distribution of spasticity. Sudden or fast movements, rather than slow movements, increase spasticity.

Voluntary movement. Spasticity does not necessarily mean paralysis. Voluntary motion is present and may be laboured. There may be weakness in the initiation of motion or during movement at different parts of its range. If spasticity is decreased or removed by treatment or drugs, the spastic muscles may be found to be weak. For example, the removal of spasticity of the gastrocnemius with botulinum toxin A injection reveals weak plantarflexion. Spastic muscles may have specific structural changes due to adaptability to abnormal use or disuse (Tabary *et al.* 1981). Initially, spastic muscles are, however, *structurally* normal though not normally extensible (Tardieu *et al.* 1982). Therefore, spastic muscles tend to shorten in dynamic deformity and later may become fixed contractures. Once spasticity is decreased the antagonists may also be stronger once they no longer have to overcome the resistance of tight spastic muscles and can work in mid-range or full range. However, in time these antagonists may have become weak with disuse within the muscle imbalance between agonists and antagonists.

The groups of muscles or *chains* of muscles used in the movement patterns (muscle activation patterns) are different from those used in normal children of the same age. Either the muscles which work in association with each other are stereotyped and are occasionally seen in the normal child, usually at an infantile level of movement, or the association of muscles is abnormal. For example, hip extension–adduction–internal rotation is normally used in creeping movements or within the push-off in walking but many other combinations must be used during the full execution of creeping and walking. This may be impossible and a child only uses the same pattern at all times in the motor skill. One example of a normal arm pattern is shoulder flexion–adduction with some external rotation for feeding or combing one's hair. In the case of the child with spasticity, the arm pattern is usually flexion–adduction with *internal* rotation and *pronation* of the elbow. The ability to fractionate movement is very difficult for the child, for example to maintain flexion at the shoulder and extension of the elbow and wrist when reaching for an object. The arm pattern usually tends to persist in flexion at all joints.

Co-contraction of the agonist with the antagonist instead of the normal reciprocal relaxation persists in the spastic type of cerebral palsy. Normal co-contraction is also evident in any person attempting a new and difficult skill in hand function or in the legs. Before the postural control develops in normal infants there is a co-contraction response in weight-bearing and co-contraction features in early stages of walking in children without cerebral palsy. These patterns persist in cerebral palsy (Leonard *et al.* 1991; Foley 1998; Lin 2000). The co-contraction provides some stability but for a more flexible mature gait, postural control training is essential. Voluntary arm and leg movements are also directly affected by poor postural control, as this interferes with their efficiency creating weakness of both postural muscles and voluntary synergies (movement patterns).

Lack of isolated or discrete movements (selective motor control) and fine motor coordination are also delayed in younger able-bodied children as well as in the spastic type, particularly if severe.

Associated impairments

(1) Intelligence varies and is usually more impaired in tetraplegia.
(2) Sensory loss occasionally occurs in hemiplegia with visual field loss and lack of sensation in the hand (Tizard *et al.* 1954). Sensory dysfunction such as sensory discrimination and sensory integration rather more than sensory loss is present in individuals (Lesny *et al.* 1993; Yekutiel *et al.* 1994). Lack of sensory awareness and sensory information for motor actions often relates to poor motor experience rather than loss of sensation. A child may be hyposensitive or hypersensitive to sensory input, so sensory-motor therapy needs to be carefully assessed.
(3) Perceptual problems especially of body and spatial relationships are more common in the spas-

tic type of cerebral palsy. They relate to sensory dysfunction and cognitive problems as well as to poor sensory-motor experiences.
(4) Poor respiration with later rib cage abnormalities may exist.
(5) Feeding problems exist, particularly in tetraplegia.
(6) Growth of hemiplegic limbs or severely affected lower limbs in bilateral cases can be less than the other limbs.
(7) Epilepsies are more common in tetraplegia and hemiplegia but minimal in diplegia (Neville 2000).
(8) A congenital suprabulbar palsy is found in some tetraplegias with mild spasticity (Neville 2000) or severe involvement.

Athetoid (dyskinetic, dystonic) cerebral palsy

Main motor characteristics are as follows:

Involuntary movements – athetosis. These are bizarre, purposeless movements which may be uncontrollable. The involuntary movements may be slow or fast; they may be writhing, jerky, tremor, swiping or rotary patterns or they may be unpatterned. They are present at rest in some children. The involuntary motion is increased by excitement, any form of insecurity and the effort to make a voluntary movement or even to tackle a mental problem. Factors which decrease dyskinesia (athetosis) are fatigue, drowsiness, sleep, fever, prone lying or the child's attention being deeply held. Involuntary motion may be present in all parts of the body including the face and tongue. Dyskinesia may only appear in hands or feet or in proximal joints or in both distal and proximal joints. Generally the child finds great difficulty in being still.

Postural control. The involuntary movements or dystonic spasms may throw a child off balance. However, the well-known instability in children with dyskinesia is often directly connected with the postural mechanisms discussed in Chapter 5 (Foley 1983). Foley (1998) relates involuntary motion with abnormal tilt reactions. Abnormal standing postures usually involve backward lean with hip extension, lordosis and kyphosis with chin jutting well forward. This is a compensation for instability.

Voluntary movements. These are possible but there may be an initial delay before the movement is begun. The involuntary movement may partially or totally disrupt the willed movement, making it uncoordinated. There is a lack of finer movements and weakness. Grasp and release have extreme flexion and extension movements which some older children learn to control for finer grasp or use of large keys on a computer.

Hypertonia or hypotonia. Either they may exist or there may be fluctuations of tone. The hypertonus or dystonia is a 'lead-pipe' or 'cog-wheel' rigidity. There is a continuous resistance to passive stretch throughout full range of motion. Dystonia can be particularly disabling, especially if combined with spasticity. Arousal of emotions increases tone. Sudden flexion or extensor spasms could occur. Sudden wide opening of the mouth with spasm can take place. Sleep decreases spasms or dystonic postures. Deformities are less likely due to the fluctuations in muscle spasms and stiffness.

The athetoid dance. Some athetoids are unable to maintain weight on their feet and continually withdraw their feet either upwards, or upwards and outwards, in an 'athetoid dance'. They may take weight on one foot whilst pawing or scraping the ground in a withdrawal motion with the other leg. This has been attributed to a conflict between grasp and withdrawal reflexes. This conflict of reflexes may also be seen in the hands (Twitchell 1961). A common pattern is a 'run headlong' using momentum as they cannot stand still nor adjust their posture for slower walking. They run before they can walk.

Paralysis of gaze movements may occur, so athetoids may find it difficult to look upwards and sometimes also to close their eyes voluntarily. Poor head control also disrupts use of the eyes.

The dyskinetic types change with time. They may be floppy in babyhood and only exhibit the involuntary movements when they reach 2 or 3 years of age. Adult athetoids do not appear hypotonic but have muscle tension. Muscle tension also seems to be increased in an effort to control involuntary movements. The standing posture of late childhood, adolescence and adulthood is usually with extended hips, bent knees and pronated feet and rounded back with arms and chin held forward to counter the extension backwards (Fig. 1.4).

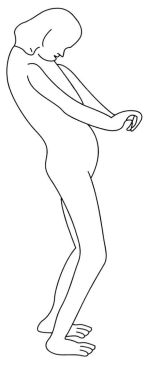

Figure 1.4 Person with dystonia/dyskinesia in standing or walking positions.

Associated impairments

(1) Intelligence is frequently good and may be very high. Intellectual impairment is occasionally present.
(2) Hearing loss of a specific high frequency type is associated with athetoids caused by kernicterus, though it is now a rare cause.
(3) 'Drive' and outgoing personalities are often observed. Emotional lability is more frequent than in other types of cerebral palsies.
(4) Articulatory speech difficulties and breathing problems may be present, and the child's oro-motor problems create feeding difficulties. Poor arm function may adversely affect the development of self-feeding.

Ataxic cerebral palsy

Main motor characteristics are as follows:
Disturbances of balance. There is poor stabilisation of the head, trunk, shoulder and pelvic girdles.

Some ataxics overcompensate for this instability by having excessive balance-saving reactions in the arms. Instability is also found in children with any type of cerebral palsy and may be called ataxia in the dyskinetic or spastic type as pure ataxia is fairly rare. Unsteady gaits arise from the brain lesion affecting motor control (Foley 1998; Neville 2000).

Voluntary movements. They are present but clumsy or uncoordinated. The child overreaches or underreaches for an object and is said to have 'dysmetria'. This inaccurate limb movement in relation to its objective may also be accompanied by intention tremor. Poor fine hand movements occur.

Hypotonia. It is usual. There is excessive flexibility of joints and poor muscle power.

Nystagmus. It may exist.

Associated impairments

(1) Intellectual impairment may exist, especially in the presence of visual and perceptual problems.
(2) 'Clumsy' intelligent children are sometimes diagnosed as having ataxic cerebral palsy.
(3) A 'pure' ataxic is rarely diagnosed except for a group of genetic origin called 'dysequilibrium syndrome' (Neville 2000).

Common features in all types of cerebral palsies

Postural mechanisms

The classification into types of cerebral palsies has tended to obscure the fact that there are important motor features which are common to all types. For instance, all cerebral palsied children are delayed in motor development. However, the symptoms of the different types of cerebral palsies, such as spasticity, sudden spasms and the various involuntary movements, only play a part in this disturbance of development. Delayed or abnormal development of the postural balance mechanisms significantly disturbs the motor development. Postural mechanisms are an intrinsic part of motor skills. When they are absent or abnormal, this leads to absent or abnormal motor skills.

Chapters 5 and 9 discuss these aspects in detail, as they are fundamental to the framework for therapy.

A common feature is also associated weakness of neck, trunk, shoulder and pelvic muscles, which are not activated by undeveloped postural mechanisms.

Classification based on motor function

A classification based on motor function incorporates postural control, which is intrinsic to motor developmental functions. This is not directly based on any diagnostic type of cerebral palsy.

The Gross Motor Function Classification System (GMFCS) for children with cerebral palsy (Palisano *et al.* 1997, updated 2008) classifies children according to what they can do at different ages. There are five levels of classification, giving distinctions in self-initiated motor functions. Level I children function without restriction, only having limitations in advanced motor skills. The motor functions decrease from I to V, with level V representing children with severe motor restrictions. This is a clinical and research classification which is detailed. This classification provides good communication between colleagues internationally rather than 'mild, moderate or severe' classifications.

Abnormal reflexes

Besides the desirable postural mechanisms, there are abnormal reflexes which have no predilection for any specific type of cerebral palsy. These are infantile (primitive) reflexes which are present in the normal newborn and which become integrated or disappear as the baby matures. In cerebral palsied children, infantile reflexes are still present long after the ages when they should have become integrated within the nervous system. As children with cerebral palsy have not been able to develop more mature neurological postural mechanisms, the infantile reflexes can be their only way to function. Whilst there are many infantile reflexes, those of most interest to the therapist are the Moro reflex, the palmar and plantar grasp reflexes, automatic stepping, excessive neck righting reflex, positive supporting, extensor thrust and feeding reflexes (Capute *et al.* 1984; see Table 8.3). These reactions may be stimulated by either peripheral or cortical activations. Some children with severe multiple disabilities activate some of these reflex responses in their efforts to balance, move or communicate non-verbally. A therapist needs to include knowledge of how her peripheral stimulation and handling might cause undesirable reflex responses instead of developing more advanced motor control. Examples of the use of reflexes are as follows: a child may use grasp reflexes to hold a small object, a plantar grasp to grip the floor for stability, automatic stepping when the body is fully supported in a walker and positive supporting reaction for standing in a standing frame. Children use extensor thrusts or Moro reactions to communicate non-verbally.

There are also the tonic reflexes, which are the tonic labyrinthine reflexes, the asymmetrical tonic neck reflex and the symmetrical tonic neck reflexes. Some neurologists group these tonic reflexes amongst the infantile reflexes, whereas others argue that they are not present in the normal infant and are always pathological. Tonic reflexes are only seen in the most severely impaired children (Foley 1977), especially if obligatory. These tonic reflexes are sometimes called *postural reflexes* but they are *abnormal* postural reflexes and should not be confused with the normal postural mechanisms as described by Rushworth (1961), Martin (1967), Foley (1977, 1998), Shumway-Cook and Woollacott (2001) and others.

The principle of treatment which therapists should follow in relation to the complicated collection of reflexes is *not* to go 'reflex hunting'. In the past, some therapists observed that reflexes interfere with motor function and speech. This does *not* always occur. The approach is to examine the function of the child first and, only when abnormality has been detected, to then consider whether *one* of the reasons for this abnormality seems to be a pathological or primitive reflex. However, it is the therapist's work in building a child's function that simultaneously can modify or overcome any reflex reactions in a child. Table 8.3 of primitive and tonic reflex reactions is given so that a therapist recognises any total or remnants of these reflex reactions or infantile (primitive) responses in individual children so that she can assess if children are using these infantile patterns as compensation for lack of motor control.

Recent research calls into question the importance of primitive (infantile) reflexes. They are no longer considered a substrate for motor control and are not reliable predictors of future motor development. New ideas on theoretical bases of motor training disagree with therapy using the 'hierarchical lists' of primitive and tonic reflexes followed by more mature reactions (Cioni *et al.* 1989, 1992; Horak 1992; Prechtl 2001; Einspieler *et al.* 2005). These studies on reflexes lend support to 'avoid reflex hunting' expressed in this book since the first edition in 1977.

Additional impairments

Individual children, particularly with severe cerebral palsy, may have sleep problems, fatigue, feeding problems and poor nutrition, decreased bone mineral density, musculoskeletal pain or pain from severe gastroesophageal reflux, and are less fit than able-bodied children. Most of these problems develop in later childhood and are managed by medical consultants. Nevertheless, a therapist needs to be aware of them as they may impinge on the amount of energy a child has available for therapy programmes. Parents are often short of sleep as they need to comfort, feed or give medicines to their child at night. This impacts on their capacities to carry out a child's home therapy. Fitness is naturally in the realm of therapy and management. Pain and decreased bone mineral density are prevented to some degree by therapists using activities and weight-bearing postures.

Motor delay

Cerebral palsy consists of both motor delay and motor disorder. There are many other conditions which present similar problems of motor delay or of delay and disorder. All these conditions are also called the *developmental disabilities* (Pearson & Williams 1972; Levitt 1984).

They may be due to the following:

Intellectual impairment, which is caused by various metabolic disorders, chromosome anomalies, leucodystrophies, microcephaly and other abnormalities of the skull and brain, endocrine disorders and the causes of brain damage given for the cerebral palsies. Down's syndrome also creates motor delay.

Deprivation of normal stimulation associated with social, economic and emotional problems, including maternal depression.

Malnutrition alone, but usually together with deprived environments. Once malnutrition is treated, lack of normal stimulation may still retard the child's development.

The presence of non-motor impairments, which may lead to motor delay, for example severe visual impairments, severe perceptual defects, apraxias as well as intellectual disabilities mentioned above. Children with delay in any developmental area may have an associated delay in motor development (see the section on motor development and the visually impaired child in Chapter 9).

Presence of motor impairments other than the cerebral palsies. For example, spina bifida, the myopathies, myelopathies and various progressive neurological diseases and congenital deformities may obviously delay development of fine and gross motor function (Holt 1975).

Principles of treatment and organisation of treatment will be similar to those discussed in Chapters 2, 5, 6 and 9. *Specific problems* in the conditions above are considered in other publications (Levitt 1984; Eckersley 1993; Shepherd 1995; Burns & MacDonald 1996; Campbell *et al.* 2006; Tecklin 2008).

Principles of learning and therapy

Broad framework for therapy and management

A broad framework for therapy and management assists interpreting assessments and comprehensive programme planning for intervention. Details of how each aspect is implemented are not given. The World Health Organization's current International Classification of Functioning, Disability and Health (ICF) (WHO 2001) describes a person's functioning in terms of body structures, body functions, activity and participation.

Definitions of components in the ICF

Body functions are physiological functions of body systems (including psychological functions).

Body structures are anatomical parts of the body and limbs.

Impairments are problems in body function or structure such as abnormal balance, and deformity.

Activity is the execution of a task or action by an individual such as standing, walking, grasping. This can include daily living tasks such as eating, dressing, toileting and washing. However, these tasks can also be participation in life situations.

Participation is involvement in a life situation such as participation in an individual's community, as in some school activities, shopping, caring for children, social and sporting activities, and use of playgrounds.

Personal factors influence how disability is experienced by an individual. These include age, coping styles, character and overall behaviour.

Environmental factors affect the individual's function and participation. These include family and social attitudes, architectural barriers, climate and terrain.

Practical application

The components of the ICF model are not sequential. Participation in society may not depend on improving impairments when a person's own functional strategies are used and when special equipment, electric wheelchairs, computers and other technology are chosen. Depending on the severity of cerebral palsy, innovative functional strategies or motor compensations may allow independent function without focusing on impairments, for example MOVE (Bidabe & Lollar 1990) and Conductive Education (Hari & Akos 1988). Research by Charles *et al.* (2006) did not change impairment but improved function in the arm and hand. Quality of life is particularly dependent on participation. Bjornson *et al.* (2008), in their research with people aged 10 and over, found that 'functional level and performance did not influence quality of life'.

There are three points supporting this view confirmed by clinical experience:

- Owing to the brain damage, not all impairments can be minimised.
- When selected impairments have been minimised, this did not always carry over into daily function.
- Participation may not be dependent on impairments nor functional performance.

However, secondary impairments such as contractures and musculoskeletal pain may result from particular motor compensations, and impairments such as specific weakness, poor balance, abnormal coordination and hypertonus may increase with time. These secondary impairments have limited the reliability of daily functions and limited the range of participation in an individual's home and community. Current and future research will clarify these different views for individuals with cerebral palsy. The relationships of impairment, activity and participation are complex. We cannot firmly maintain that treatment of impairment leads to function and that improvement of function leads to participation in the individual's different environments.

Therefore, therapy principles include:

■ Assessment and management based on the perspectives of an individual, the family, teachers and others involved with that individual.
■ Assessment and management of impairments which constrain functions and daily tasks needed.
■ Assessment and prevention of secondary and increasing impairments.
■ Focus on functional therapy and correction of impairments within function.
■ Assess and manage function in the context of a person's home, school and community.
■ Consideration of attitudes in family and society that disable a person.
■ Encouragement of the personal attributes of an individual with disability and of his or her family.

There is increasing research on the relationships between the items in the ICF model, which will be discussed in this book.

Aims of physiotherapy, occupational therapy and speech therapy are:

(1) To develop forms of communication (gesture, speech, typing and alternative forms of communication with signs or electronic aids).
(2) To develop independence in the daily activities of eating, drinking, dressing, washing, toileting and general self-care with and without aids, such as special utensils, toys and special furniture.
(3) To develop abilities to play and achieve hobbies and recreational activities with or without adapted equipment.
(4) To develop some form of locomotion and independent mobility, which may include wheelchairs, playthings, tricycles or driving adapted motor vehicles.

All these aims need to be considered in terms of learning processes interacting with neurological and orthopaedic aspects and environmental constraints. Therefore all therapists draw on the fields of education and psychology and gain much from close teamwork with teachers, psychologists, social workers and psychotherapists. The psychotherapists and social workers are important as learning is intimately involved with emotions. Some learning models do not give adequate attention to this fact. The role of cultural factors in planning the programme needs to be considered by everyone. A collaborative learning approach initially developed by the author in consultation with a psychiatric social worker (Levitt & Goldschmied 1990) carries out the principles of therapy and management, with emphasis on physiotherapy and occupational therapy.

Summary

This chapter provides basic information for planning treatment and management.

(1) The child should be seen as having primarily a motor impairment but may have individual associated impairments due to the brain damage. The motor and other functional disabilities are created by some of the impairments as well as by lack of many everyday learning experiences in various environments.
(2) There is an interaction between the communication, intellectual, sensory, perceptual and motor functions. Physiotherapists therefore consider the influence of associated disabilities on the motor programmes.
(3) Treatment is aimed at impairments and developing gross-motor and fine-motor functions which involve procedures for individual combinations of:
    ■ Postural mechanisms of balance
    ■ Movement patterns (synergies) of voluntary movement, including hand function
    ■ Strengthening for weakness of various kinds
    ■ Minimising hypertonicity, hypotonicity and involuntary movements
    ■ Improving postural alignments and patterns of gait
    ■ Improving ranges of motion of muscles, joints and soft tissues.

Views differ on the significance of specific problems and also on the relationship between them. Therapists need to make careful assessments to clarify the impairment and functional problems of an individual with cerebral palsy, and reflect on their relationships.

(4) Therapy programmes should not have a strict adherence to specific diagnostic classifications, and aetiology may not always influence the treatment used by therapists.

(5) Emphasis needs to be given to the daily functional activities and a participation in life situations, which are priorities of a child or an adult with disabilities and of their families.

(6) The various impairments are preferably treated *in the context of* total daily functions as well as in specific treatments for individuals. The emphasis is therefore less on isolated treatments and more on integrating therapy of impairments within developmental functional training.

(7) The therapist always needs to recognise the emerging functional *abilities and whole functions* within each child's developmental pattern. Normal developmental schedules are only guides and need to be carefully adapted.

(8) Management and therapy are planned from infancy throughout an individual's lifespan to take account of clinical change and different circumstances in an individual's home, schools and community. Management focuses on educating all those primarily involved with a person with cerebral palsy. Chapter 2 discusses this in more detail in a collaborative learning approach. Management also involves working with any other disciplines involved with an individual with cerebral palsy.

(9) Physiotherapists and occupational therapists need to integrate motor learning principles in their therapy programmes. Motor learning models need to encompass emotional, cultural and social issues.

(10) Treatment and management need to commence as early as possible for parental support, parent–child relationships and to promote a child's motor activity as well as minimise any musculoskeletal problems.

(11) The model suggested by the ICF is a general guide to assessment and planning of therapy and management, which matches much that is discussed in this book.

(12) Promoting positive motor experience is key for motivating the best therapy.

A collaborative learning approach 2

Working with parents

Today, therapists recognise the importance of working with the parents of each child and for some time home programmes have been shown to them (Collis l947; Finnie 1997; among others). This chapter emphasises client-centred or person-centred therapy and learning (Rogers 1983), which may not be used by professionals who devise home programmes for parents. A more person-centred view presenting home programmes is given in a book for carers and parents of children with multiple disabilities (Levitt 1994).

King *et al.* (1997) and Rosenbaum (2004), in their many studies of the wishes of parents of children with disabilities, found that parental involvement in decisions about their child lowers stress levels and improves parents' mental health. This was the top priority of the parents' list of what they wanted from a service. This chapter conveys a belief that this also applies to parent participation in therapy programmes.

In the last 21 years, I have been developing a practical style of working which involves a child along with his parents in a collaborative learning experience with a physiotherapist. All share responsibility in assessments, therapy plans, methods and evaluations (Levitt & Goldschmied 1990; Levitt 1991b, 1999: 153–155). Ross and Thomson (1993) have recommended this specific collaborative approach (outlined in Levitt & Goldschmied 1990) following their studies on the evaluation of parents' involvement in physiotherapy. Piggot *et al.* (2003) also find this approach of interest in their qualitative research project on parental adjustment and participation in home therapy.

This collaborative learning approach is a creative learning process, not only for a child and his parents but also for any therapist. The therapist learns what the hopes and expectations of a child and his parents are and what they already know and can do. Using these resources, therapists are better able to draw on their technical expertise for a more relevant programme. The respect and trust given to what parents and child already understand and can manage develops their confidence. More positive relationships grow between parents, child and therapist. There is more motivation as parents and child respond positively to a therapist who appreciates their desires and their ideas for solving some of their own problems.

The idea of joint goal setting and involving the parents and child in the shared decision-making process fits well with the United Kingdom's National Service Framework for disabled children and young people with complex health needs (Department of Health and Department for Education and Skills 2004).

Odman *et al.* (2007) carefully studied parents' perceptions of the service quality of two training programmes for a range of severity in children with cerebral palsy. Most parents were 'influenced by high service quality rather than by perceived functional improvements'. The researchers used a measure (given in the appendix to their volume). This measure, 'Patient Perspective on Care and Rehabilitation Process' (POCR), was slightly adapted and has seven dimensions of the needs of the parent or child. Experience with the collaborative learning approach has shown substantial agreement with many of the findings of Odman *et al.* (2007).

Collaboration with other adults

When considering parents as adult learners, it is useful to draw on the studies of Rogers (1983, 2003, recent books following his many writings since the 1960s), Knowles (1984) and others in adult education. Rogers developed his ideas on human behaviour and the process of learning from studies of adults in psychotherapy. Rogers and Knowles applied 'whole-person' learning, together with other studies, to adult education. Similar concepts underlie the collaborative learning model developed from practical teaching experience not only for parents but also for other adults such as family members, other professionals and carers assisting a child's development. This approach is also relevant to older people with disabilities (Chapter 7). The therapist will grow both professionally and personally as she or he learns and takes into account the knowledge, priorities and preferred learning style of these adults. A therapist becomes better able to select and devise methods to suit individual adults involved with a child. She or he also gains information from adults about various environments and cultures in which a child needs to function.

When family members and carers assist with the therapy programme in the way that parents wish, time needs to be given for them to become familiar with these programmes to maximise the child's potential. This inclusive team approach facilitates both parents' and family's participation and helps them feel of value to their child with cerebral palsy. However, some family members may find working with their child stressful and prefer to give their

personal strength to support the parents and child emotionally.

Family members also need support from therapists whether they participate or not in therapy programmes. The well-being of families positively affects the development of their child. Therapists need to listen respectfully to their views and concerns and promote their education about therapy.

Consideration must also be given to the fact that babies and young children with disabilities prefer being handled by one or two adults as they have to relate to an adult and adapt to different ways of being handled. No two adults are precisely the same in their touch, speed of 'hands-on' therapy and manual guidance. This is particularly relevant to those babies and young children who experience many unexpected spasms, uncontrolled reflexes and unreliable control of their posture and movements.

The therapists themselves are assisted and supported by other members of their team such as psychologists, social workers and paediatricians who work specifically with the families in 'family-centred care'. Family-centred care has broadened from being child-centred to include not only the child but also the practical and psycho-social needs of parents and families. As services have evolved for children with cerebral palsy, the concept of family-centred care has become central to service provision. A number of research studies on family-centred care by Rosenbaum *et al.* (1998), King *et al.* (1997, 1999), Larsson (2000) and Odman *et al.* (2007) give evidence of increased satisfaction with services with lower stress levels and better mental health.

It is reassuring that family-centred care continues to grow in physiotherapy. However, the collaborative learning approach differs from various models in that it emphasises that *learning processes* are involved not only in 'changing function of a disabled person's body but also in changing ideas, behaviour and attitudes' (Levitt & Goldschmied 1990). The person with disability and his or her family members and carers are changing as they embrace new ideas, new attitudes and behaviour as well as alternative ways of solving problems. Therapists also become learners as they deepen their understanding, gain new ideas, change any of their attitudes and give up old assumptions. A person's willingness to change is facilitated by desires to learn, achieve more and feel more satisfaction in daily life. It is the quality of rapport between a therapist and a disabled person and her or his family that is fundamental during mutual learning experiences in collaborative work.

This chapter focuses in a practical way on the role of therapists working with children, older people, their parents and families.

Family cultures

Family-centred care needs to be culturally competent in order to be sensitive to different cultural values of families. Therapists can be culturally aware but not culturally competent. Cultural differences are not right or wrong regarding the ways families adapt, cope and develop their own strengths in living with a child with a disability. Non-judgmental listening, avoidance of direct questions which may offend and a genuine interest in a child's family are needed even more than for families a therapist is familiar with in her or his own culture. There may also be a need for an English interpreter with positive attitudes to disability.

We are aware that families in our own culture do not all bring up their children in exactly the same way. In our multicultural societies, therapists are faced with more diverse cultural differences in their families. Diverse cultural backgrounds can provide challenges for the professional in terms of communication of functional techniques and appropriateness of the tasks given. For example, a therapist can learn from a Muslim family that a mother cannot be in a pool with her child during a swimming session unless the pool has a 'women only' time as this would be prohibitive for her. Special bath chairs and other equipment may not be appropriate for some parenting customs and a special chair may not be relevant to floor sitting used socially in a particular culture.

Normal motor developmental patterns differ in different cultures (Chapter 9). Lying on the floor or crawling may not be welcomed. Some consider floor work in the home as unhygienic. Some families do not expect play activities used for 'medical treatment' or child developmental guidance. Creative adaptations to familiar child rearing methods need to be made. In other situations, communication of unfamiliar methods does not need much verbalisation in parents' own language, as physical methods are demonstrated, pointing out immediate positive abilities revealed in a child or perhaps in another child similar to the child being treated. Parent–child groups are helpful as some mothers show willingness to try methods which inspire those more hesitant.

Therapists need to have a general practical knowledge of different cultural groups with whom they are involved. This can include likely health beliefs, religious practices and social customs. However, the collaborative learning approach offers therapists a direct working knowledge of the customs of individual parents and families (Levitt 1999). This approach for individuals avoids stereotyping a child, parent or family as being the same as all families in the cultural group. This stereotyping is less likely to happen when therapists are willing to learn from the individual older children, parents and family. A qualitative research study of physiotherapists' perceptions in cross-cultural interactions by Lee *et al.* (2006) found that some participants did not recognise that they stereotyped 'clients' perceptions of pain, the desire for passive treatments, dependency on family members and male dominance in specific cultures'. This small study shows implications for the quality of physiotherapy.

The collaborative learning approach

A child and his parents are offered:

- Opportunities to discover what they want to achieve.
- Opportunities to clarify what is needed for these achievements.
- Opportunities to recognise what they already know and can do.
- Opportunities to find out what they still need to learn and do.
- Participation in the selection and use of methods.
- Participation in the evaluation of progress.

Genuine participation in all these aspects by child and parents helps them feel more committed to the programme of work. It gives them some sense of control which decreases many of their anxieties and builds their confidence. They become more able and more willing to absorb ideas, information and practical suggestions from therapists.

Parents and an older child are accustomed to being asked 'What are your problems?' or 'What are your concerns?' This may well decrease their confidence as to them it emphasises the impairments, sadness and inadequacies. A positive, hopeful introduction about what could be learned and achieved is preferable. For example, a therapist might say 'Tell me what you would like to do better in your daily life'. More detail is given below.

The collaborative learning approach considers not only the views of parents and child but also the perspectives of therapists. There can be consensus and also different views between parents and therapists. Different views are managed by negotiation for an option both find acceptable. There can be a mutual understanding that there are different paths to the same common goal, which is carefully stated in the words of the parents. Early in the growing quality of the relationship, a professional can concede to follow the parents' choice until the relationship is strong (see also 'Participation in the selection and use of methods' below).

This style of work with parents coincidentally tunes in with the views of Bailey and Simeonsson (1988) in the field of developmental disabilities and that of Larsson (2000) among others. Bailey and Simeonsson found in their many studies that parents and families want the following:

■   Education and information.
■   Parental training in skills to help their child.
■   Emotional support.

This collaborative learning approach takes account of all these aspects. The studies of Sluijs *et al.* (1993) call for more education of patients by their physiotherapists and this approach offers a response to this as well by being more family-centred (Levitt 1991b). A pilot study by Ahl *et al.* (2005) found that parents' expectations were of a functional training approach in daily life settings. When such a programme was used, parents' perceptions of the rehabilitation process were enhanced. The collaborative learning approach focuses on parents' and child's choice of daily life functions (Levitt and Goldschmied 1990). Jahnsen *et al.* (2003) in their review of studies on parental experience with physiotherapy quote a number of studies which support many aspects of this approach and find positive responses in parents.

Opportunities to discover what parents and child want to achieve

Many parents are quick to say what their expectations from therapy are. Others want time to discuss this with their families. Some parents are unaccustomed to asserting what they want as they have anxieties and 'learned helplessness' (Greer & Wethered 1984; Seligman 1992). They may also not wish to upset their specialised therapist as they wrongly or rightly sense this might be so if they choose what therapy might focus on for *their* lives. Avoid using direct questions (which feature in some parent questionnaires) as this may feel like an uncomfortable confrontation with their many needs.

The therapist gains their trust by inviting them to talk about a typical day in their lives by saying which daily activities they would like to improve further and which daily activities are most stressful or time-consuming. These may be the same or different activities such as a child's feeding, washing, dressing, toileting, playing and a child going from place to place at home, school or in other environments. The therapist prompts parents and child to think about these activities as they are familiar to them. She explains that if she knows about their daily activities then she can plan a more relevant therapy programme with them. She also tells them that she can then clarify what she can offer from her profession for their wishes. If a child cannot communicate what he would like to achieve or do better, then he is observed to see what interests him. He may enjoy bath time, mealtime or special times for play with his parents. In a more specific situation, if possible in his familiar environment, a baby, child or a severely disabled individual at an early stage of development has facial expressions of pleasure and body language that can easily be observed, such as wanting to touch a person they like or a toy of interest. Their pathological symptoms may be used to show pleasure or displeasure, such as extensor thrusts or increasing involuntary motions.

It is essential to start with the priorities of child and parents rather than set aims or goals for them. Even if we set goals and then ask for their agreement, *we* are really setting the goals. This does not enable them to discover their own aims, formulate their own expectations and so improve their ability to share their ideas and feel more confident. Once parent or child states their wishes, the therapist repeats what they have said with a check such as 'Have I got that right?' This places parents and child in a more independent position. It is necessary to acknowledge when a child's wants differ from a parents' wants.

In their study on the values of activities of daily living in stroke patients with hemiplegia, Chiou and Burnett (1985) compared the choices of these patients with the choices made by their therapists. It was found that in 29 therapist–patient pairs, only one pair showed similar views regarding specific values placed on the daily activities. We need to recognise that professionals with clinical wisdom and experience do know what is needed for parents or patients, but do not really know what is needed for particular parents or patients at specific times. This leads to frustration on the part of both therapists and their recipients. Physiotherapists often say 'they [parents] do not really understand our aims' (Levitt 1986, 1991a). This is despite technical explanations clearly given by a therapist. It is the connection or marrying of a therapist's 'goals' with an individual's 'goals' that matters to facilitate mutual understanding.

Opportunities to clarify what is needed for these achievements, to recognise what they already know and can do and to find out what they still need to learn and do

These opportunities are given in the following ways:

(1) The parents themselves carry out the daily task on their own. This is the task they have selected, but they first need to learn what that task involves using their own experience of it. As a parent enacts the task, he or she is prompted to observe which *main* movements and postures are being used. They notice where they look, what they may hear and other sensations relevant to a task. Comments from a parent are encouraged so that a therapist learns something about their knowledge of, say, their own body movements and balance. She then only adds to their knowledge according to their stage of understanding and when this is relevant to their own child's function.

(2) The therapist herself may demonstrate their chosen daily task, drawing attention to the general aspects of balance, movement and some sensations. This is termed 'modelling' by some professionals. Some parents may prefer this before they carry out the task themselves.

In both points above, attention is drawn to the fact that observation is being made of able-bodied and adult actions. However, their child may then be observed to have achieved some of these, such as looking, listening, head control, hand-to-mouth movement, grasp or other components normally retained from infancy and the early years. Any 'normal' components already achieved by their child boost both the parents' and child's confidence. Parents begin to feel that their child is not 'all wrong'.

(3) A mother or father can then apply these educational experiences by actually doing the task together with their child. This can also be used to learn what is needed to achieve a task. However, it especially demonstrates what a child and parents can do already and what they still need to learn to do. The therapist first underlines what they can do before saying what is still needed for successful achievement of their task. In this way parents can feel they are managing some skills, which builds their confidence to learn more unfamiliar skills which develop a task or modify impairments.

(4) Direct questions about a child's functioning are also avoided so that parents do not receive an impression that their child should be doing something or is doing it abnormally. Rather say '*Tell me* more about what he can do' and 'How he likes to do it' and possibly 'When he does it really well'.

(5) The same procedure is used with a child who is invited to try and carry out his chosen activity as best he can. He experiences what he can do – which he often may not yet have recognised as perhaps adults have always manually (though lovingly) supported him or not given him time to try. The therapist emphasises what he can do, no matter how small, in simple words such as 'You can keep your head up' or 'You started to pull your sleeve down', according to the task. Even if not all words are understood, the parents appreciate what is being said as their child is reassured by the therapist's tone of voice and approving facial expression.

A therapist needs to continue her studies on task analyses in different types and degrees of severity in cerebral palsy so that she draws attention to the most successful components of functions (tasks) in each child. Parents are also learning from a therapist how to break down their chosen task into components needed for their own child. This is one of the ways that can be used to assist in solving a motor problem of a child. Each parent will have their own pace of learning this task analysis.

Although the therapist is also observing obvious impairments such as hypertonus, weakness, involuntary motion or deformities, these are not yet stated in these words. Her comments on such problems relate to 'what needs to be learned' such as a child 'still needs to stretch an elbow more' or 'still needs to learn how to sit more steadily' or 'how to stand up really tall'. This is a more motivating style.

Once child and parents show what they can do, the therapist validates their achievement and shares their pleasure. She might say something like 'That is good, and it could be even better if we try the following suggestions'. She can then demonstrate additional positioning, modification of the physical environment, appropriate manual support, handling or physical guidance to reveal more of their abilities and functions. As parents and child have had their capabilities acknowledged by a therapist, they are more willing to listen to what this therapist adds to the programme.

Task or functional analyses. The task analyses are also outlined in Chapter 6 about a child learning motor function. Analyses of components of a child's function are also given in Chapter 9, which outlines details of developmental functions, some of which are more detailed for therapists rather than for most parents. The motor learning models give more small achievable steps which are more clearly observed by parents and family members. This can show what has been achieved, no matter how minimal, for example, in a sequence of components, such as rising from a chair to standing. There are sequences of actions in activities such as feeding, washing and dressing which can be seen in small achievable steps, some of which may have already been achieved to show a baseline of abilities. This allows parents and child to experience initial success. This is a particularly encouraging way of looking at tasks to be learned and counters feelings in parents

or child of 'I'll never do this!' There is also a hopeful future that additional components and perhaps the full function will develop.

Once parents and child have stated their wants, these are analysed into steps. Steps or components towards parents' functional wishes are usually termed 'goals' because they are expected in a short time. Goals are clearly defined, apply to daily lives and once again checked that parents feel they know the goals and can achieve them at home. Goals are usually given by professionals (termed 'sub-skills' in the study by Ahl *et al*. 2005). However, this collaborative learning model enables parents to learn general task analyses so that short-term goals *are jointly created* with therapists. Facilitation interviews are used for parents who need extra support to create goals.

The therapist's specialised assessment. Once the motor and sensory components of a task have been observed by a therapist within a whole task, she decides how much more she needs to assess. She can then carry out more detailed assessments of components of the task and impairments of muscle work, joint ranges and tone, abnormal postures and other sensorimotor details. However, the advantage of first seeing all these separate aspects within a whole task reveals many ideas which challenge the accuracy of *only* using separate examinations of impairments or motor components (motor abilities, prerequisites) to plan physiotherapy home programmes.

The tasks or daily functions have been chosen by the parent or child and are thus being performed by motivated persons. Results of such an assessment tend to be more positive. There is interaction between all aspects of a task, so ability in one component activates any residual ability in another component. In my experience, tests of reflexes may be abnormal if carried out in isolation, but if observed within the context of parent–child interactions during daily activities, the assessment shows a more positive result. For example, a grasp reflex may become immediately modified as a baby places her hand on her mother's breast during feeding; an asymmetrical tonic neck response or a Moro reaction is modified or overcome as a child puts both her arms around her father's neck or holds her head up in eye-to-eye contact during social and specific daily activities (Levitt 1986).

Participation in the selection and use of methods

There is no sharp division between the assessments just described and methods. As mentioned above, a therapist's assessment methods of positioning, physical guidance and amount of manual support reveal more of a child's abilities and function. These methods then serve as treatment methods and are extended to include equipment, orthoses, furniture, footwear and playthings. It depends on the severity of the cerebral palsy together with the views of the parents, child or older person as to the content of the therapy programme.

As with a child, a parent is first observed practising his or her method of training his or her child and then guided physically or verbally by the therapist as they carry this out. This allows them to improve their method. Details are added according to what each parent can absorb and manage. Once their own style of parenting and handling is used, some parents welcome additional methods from therapists. Each parent also has their own pace of learning and some need many more repetitions of a method than others. Videos of methods with the child can be taken home for reviewing what parents have learned with their therapist and to show to their family. One parent may make notes or list exercises in their own words, whilst the other carries them out with the therapist.

As parents and child develop their confidence, they will share their own ideas with their therapist (Fig. 2.1). She always welcomes their ideas as they are showing an eagerness to take some responsibility in the programme and not become totally dependent on her. The therapist considers their suggestions, and if inappropriate, modifies them or shelves them for a later stage in a child's development. With any validation of the ideas of parents or child they become more able to cope with times when some of their ideas are incorrect. As parents have been learning and gaining information on their child's condition within a positive relationship, there can be negotiation on which methods are suitable. Clearly a therapist needs to become more flexible so she can be open to what parents and child offer. This means that she cannot stick rigidly to any system of therapy. The therapist also needs to learn what is realistic in the parents', carers' and child's daily

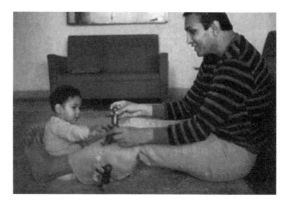

Figure 2.1   There is pleasurable interaction between this father and his child as the child's postural control with hand function is being developed. Father chose to use his feet to assist his child in symmetrical weight bearing on hips and weight shifting from side to side or forwards and backwards during play.

life. This includes cultural considerations, time constraints and a child's general health as well as the physical environment.

It is helpful to clarify who will carry out particular methods. If possible, the frequency and duration of a session for people using methods are recorded according to what can be realistically managed by a child himself, parents and others, including the therapist, who are involved in his development. This realistic record tends to be flexible or an approximate guide – unless it forms part of a clinical research project.

We avoid overwhelming a parent with a 'mountain of knowledge and tasks'. This may exhaust them and disrupt family life, creating additional feelings of inadequacy (Featherstone 1981; Hinojosa 1990; Ross & Thomson 1993). With the many demands on parents to provide for their child, family-centred care which expects them to take on the additional role of 'therapist' can be too much for some (MacKean *et al.* 2005). The collaborative learning approach, if appropriately carried out, enables parents to choose what is realistic for them, other family members and carers. In my experience, parents have phases in their lives when they can and cannot manage as much. During difficult periods for parents, a home programme can be largely replaced by the therapist giving a bout of more sessions with a child, encouraging another family member or friend to temporarily assist more if deterioration of his condition is expected. Deterioration is not always likely for short periods in all children.

Special physiotherapy techniques. Once a parent has some confidence in methods for the familiar, everyday tasks in childcare, they can add selected physiotherapy treatment techniques. Some parents are intimidated by unusual techniques whereas others overdo them. They believe or want to believe that these strange techniques are 'magical treatments' and overdo them at the expense of developing their natural parenting abilities and positive relationships with their child. It is these relationships which are fundamental to real progress. Exercises such as ranges of motion, stretching, specific balance training and strengthening exercises may be carried out in a didactic style which parents may have observed in a physiotherapist treating their child or perhaps treating some other person with another medical condition. A study by Kogan *et al.* (1974) found that mothers acting as therapists interacted negatively with their children. This was not the experience of von Wendt *et al.* (1984), who found positive interactions by well-supported parents. Jahnsen *et al.* (2003) reviewed 18 studies from 1981 to 1999 of parental experience with physical therapy which include positive parenting experiences and family satisfactions in many of the studies, all of which used specialised measures.

Physiotherapy within play activities. Any negative behaviour in parents or child need not happen if we first set the scene as described above and we find methods within play activities. For example, a child's postural mechanisms and movements are developed on his parent's lap, when being carried and handled during all daily activities and play (Figs 2.2–2.4). A child's spine and limbs can be stretched and moved within positioning for daily tasks as well as in water and during musical rhythms and action songs. When a mother also assists a child to enjoy his body parts which are being kissed, tickled and touched by her as well as moved to her song, she also develops a more positive view of her child's body. This pleasure in both mother and child contributes to their developing relationship in a creative way. It is important to develop parenting abilities at the same time as promoting a child's function, and methods can be found to do this (Figs 2.1–2.5). Parents usually bring their own playful ideas with a child once their confidence is cultivated. This also avoids an increased dependency and excessive demands on a therapist for 'magical treatments'.

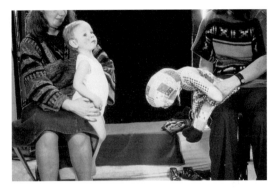

Figure 2.2   Therapist showing tilt reaction facilitation on a doll so that this mother can interact with her child on her lap playing a 'see-saw' game. The position of the adult's hands on the child's hips rather than on the trunk is important.

Parents need to recognise that their handling of their children is as important as special treatment sessions.

Other sources of 'best methods'. These may be from perhaps another parent or helpful family

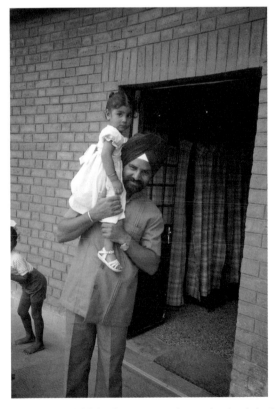

Figure 2.3   A child developing postural control on her father's shoulders in playful activity.

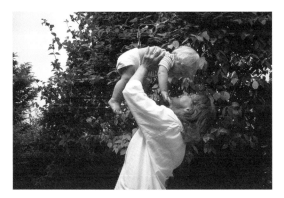

Figure 2.4 Stimulating head control in parent–child interaction.

member. Therapists can discuss whether this suits a child, as children do differ in developmental levels, severity, and likes and dislikes. Therapists using an eclectic functional approach can combine methods with other suggestions to suit a child. The internet has created easier access to written information; however, much of this is not peer-reviewed and can be confusing for the parents or child. This is confounded by the media's delight in promoting some types of therapies. The therapist's own clinical reasoning and experience will enable them to consider new approaches objectively, with emotional detachment, which is very hard for the parents of a

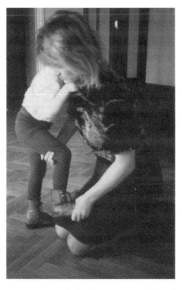

Figure 2.5 Learning early balance on one foot during dressing and undressing, washing or drying with body closeness between mother and child.

child with cerebral palsy. The role of the therapist in interpreting information for the child and parents is an important feature of clinical practice. There is further discussion about this in the section on 'Alternative and complementary treatments' below.

Participation in the evaluation of progress

Throughout the therapy sessions, it is reassuring for all to know how well they are progressing. Parents and child are asked to report on any new achievements based on the original assessments. They may have gained more of the steps in a sequence of actions in a daily activity or more postural control, more postural alignment or more hand use.

Improvements from a child's baseline abilities can be recorded on video, with graphs or in written records. Professionals use their own recording techniques discussed in Chapter 8. There are now a variety of outcome measures that can measure change over time. These special measures and clinical observations as well as results of consultants' special tests need to be explained to parents and, when understanding is available, to a child.

After joint discussions with parents, carers or any family member involved, there may be a need to modify therapy or new methods added for future progress. Equipment is checked together with parents to confirm correct size and function. The relevance of equipment to a child's home and lifestyle as well as acceptance of their aesthetic aspects is a continuing assessment with parents and child.

Behavioural progress

It is essential to comment on the progress of child and parents in their development of confidence, motivation, communication skills and personal relationships. It is after all not only functional gains that are important, but how much more viable life becomes for parents and child as a result. More qualitative research studies are being undertaken by psychologists and psychotherapists to evaluate these aspects (see discussions of qualitative research in Chapter 4 and section 'Review of a therapist's observations' in Chapter 8). Observations of videos made at home by both professionals and parents reveal progress to those experienced in parent–child interactions during feeding and other activities of daily life.

Parent satisfaction

Parent satisfaction with the service they are receiving, rather than specifically with therapy, is measured by the Measures of Processes of Care (MPOC) (King *et al.* 1997). Odman *et al.* (2007) used POCR and Ahl *et al.* (2005) used goal achievements, Gross Motor Function Measure, Paediatric Evaluation of Disability Inventory, MPOC and parent questionnaires in their research with parents and carers (see Chapter 8 on assessment for description of these measures). Parents' and carers' questionnaires are also used (Goldsmith 2000).

Parent–child interaction

When familiar daily activities are used in the programme, a therapist is able to see a parent and child functioning together. As Winnicott (1964) points out, 'There is no such thing as a baby, only a baby with someone else'. During these daily activities, there is normally mutual pleasure between mother or father and child. However, a child with disabilities gives unusual communications as clues for a parent to know how to parent such a child. If a child has a floppy head, a visual problem or hypertonus, this is not only a worry from a functional viewpoint but interferes with a child's response to a parent. Such a child cannot initiate communication with his head and eyes, hands or body to indicate his wants. Without head or trunk control, a child cannot turn away from his parents to show when he has had too much stimulation and may become irritable. Parents may find their child hypersensitive to touch, difficult to cuddle or exhibiting unexpected startles of distress. It is easy for parents already unsure of their parenting abilities to feel rejected and anxious. It can make the bonding and attachment difficult for some parents. The natural expertise of a therapist may make them feel more inadequate. There are, of

course, other parents who are especially responsive to their child and discover many subtle cues of communication from their child. They can clarify for a therapist what their child's body communications and sounds mean.

It is essential that during the joint assessments of feeding, dressing, bathing, playing and other tasks, the therapist points out that:

- A child's unusual body actions, hypersensitivity or increase in stiffness is due to the cerebral palsy and not to poor parenting.
- A child's fears, apathy, hyperactivity or poor concentration are due to the cerebral palsy and not to poor parenting.

Enabling a parent to position a child well, to handle him, cuddle and play with him not only modifies his neurological symptoms, improves motor function and daily care, and even prevents some deformities, but also enhances their communication and the quality of their relationship. It is not just correct handling but a positive reciprocal interaction between parents and child that is being promoted (Figs 2.1–2.7 for parent–child interaction, and also Figs 10.3 and 10.4).

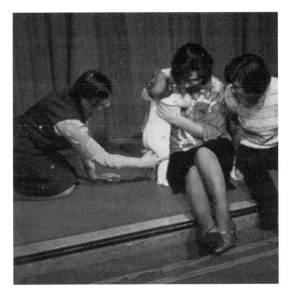

Figure 2.6 Physiotherapist enabling a mother and her key worker to learn how to activate early standing with close body contact as support.

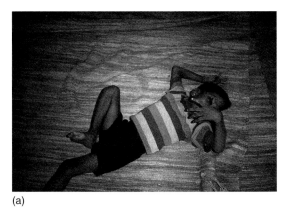
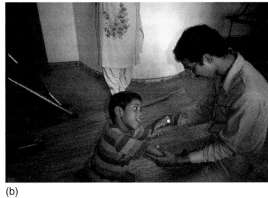

(a)   (b)

Figure 2.7 (a) Child with athetoid quadriplegia in supine. (b) Parent and child interact, enabling the child to master his symptoms.

Helping a child to learn motor control

This is discussed in Chapter 6. The therapist makes sure that a parent and carer are enabled to develop these behaviours to reinforce a child's learning. Points to note are:

- Give a child time to choose an activity or toy he likes and build in any desirable postures and actions.
- Wait for a child's initiation for a motor action and follow his lead.
- Wait for a child's response to the parent's initiation of an activity.
- Adjust a task so that a child can experience some success. Make it fun.
- Find ways to alert and maintain a child's concentration within his attention span.
- Show appreciation for a child's small and large achievements. Keep teaching a child even if gains are slow or minimal, eventually he learns and achieves at his own pace.
- Grade sensory input so that a child is not overstimulated. Avoid putting pressure on a child to perform.
- Make appropriate demands on a child so he needs to make some effort to achieve a task without excessive increase in hypertonus, athetoid motion, tremors or startles and spasms.
- Give time for the gradual development of parent–child relationships and be patient with oneself as a parent learning to interact with an unusual child. Many parents have *their own*

ways of managing which therapists must acknowledge, especially when cultural differences also exist.

- Learn from family members what their cultural and customary practices are in child rearing. They may have their own individual modifications and views (Levitt 1999).

Observation of parent and child interaction

There are psychologists and psychotherapists who are specialised in observing mother and baby interactions and the building of optimal relationships for a child's positive development (Stern 1985). There is increasing research effort on interactive styles of mothers with children with disabilities, some of which shows such mothers as being more directive as their children take fewer interactive turns with a parent (Hanzlik 1990). When a physiotherapist or occupational therapist assesses a child together with his parents, she can draw on the studies of psychologists or work closely with such a specialist on the team.

The therapist, therefore, observes not only the movements and postures which form the daily activities but also those that speak of the relationship between parents and child and between child and therapist. She informally notices the body language of how a mother and child look at each other, touch and move together. She notices how their bodies mould towards or away from each other. A child may initiate taking turns or need encouragement to do so in movement, eye contact or sounds and speech. The upright posture not only develops postural control but better communication and alertness. The way a parent supports and especially removes manual support demonstrates his or her anxiety and ability to trust a child to function alone. The parents' willingness to follow their child's lead and wait for their child's slow achievement can be very difficult for them. The therapist's support and confidence in the parents' developing skills in parenting are essential.

The therapist needs to include such interactions in the therapy methods and may have to avoid methods which decrease positive interplay between parents and child. The therapist herself also models how to play, feed, dress, enable a child to move and enjoy these and other activities. However, care is always taken to make parents feel as competent as possible at their stage of learning. Information is regularly given on the neurological symptoms, which can be modified to enhance non-verbal and verbal communication. Speech and language therapists can offer much in these areas. They also have the skill of enabling any adult interacting with a child to use an appropriate level of language (Winstock 2005; see also Chapter 10).

In this collaborative learning approach, a child is learning to make a choice by indicating his specific functional wishes at home and also his interests. Respect and serious consideration of these aspects by therapists and parents facilitate more positive parent–child interaction and avoid a number of difficulties with a child's lack of cooperation (see Chapter 6).

Emotional support

It is clear that therapy is not just 'a bag of tricks' to increase a child's motor function or independent daily skills. A therapist is not only showing practical ideas but needs to give time for listening to the worries of a parent. However, she is always balancing her time for the parents and for the child. Listening and observing a child's facial expressions and body language tells her about not only the appropriate pace of work with a child but his emotional needs in general. When listening to a parent's or child's anxieties, a therapist need not immediately

reassure them. It is a therapist's empathetic and attentive listening which serves them best. She needs to repeat back to each of them what she has heard them say and only later clarifies what she can do to help.

Therapists become aware of a variety of underlying anxieties in individual parents. A parent may be experiencing a complex mixture of emotions such as despair, anger, disappointment, frustration or guilt. This not only varies from parent to parent but in the same parent at different periods in their life with their child. Hall (1984), among others, perceives such emotions as part of the grieving process related to loss of the expected normal baby. There is hardly time for parents to work through this grief as they feel pressure to accept the very different child who is alive and may be making great demands on them physically and emotionally.

Therapists face a difficult situation in which their offer of help can make a parent feel more helpless and guilty. Some parents may then become more dependent on a therapist and burden her with excessive demands. Others resent their dependency, becoming angry that they should need professionals to show them how to handle their child. This anger can also be directed at the very professionals who are doing their best for such parents. Either way, the therapist needs to grow in maturity, and they become the 'patient ones' rather than the patients. To do this, therapists benefit from their own support groups and sensitive support from others in a team. This support is essential to maintain therapists' energy, understanding and motivation (Greer & Wethered 1984; Chapter 1 in Levitt 1984, 1991a; Price *et al.* 1991).

When a parent is particularly stressed, taking excessive time and energy from a physiotherapist or other professional, this needs to be discussed with the team or with a qualified psychotherapist, family therapist or specialised counsellor. The therapist will gain guidance on how best to manage such a parent and if *and* how to refer such parents for professional help from psychotherapy or counselling.

The collaborative approach described changes the situation of a professional being the helper and the parent the helpless one to that of more equal partnership. The therapist, therefore, is not placed in any position where her help is rejected which may understandably upset her, possibly inviting anger. The parent learns to ask for help instead of just receiving it. Parents who find it difficult to accept help may be able to do so in a more collaborative situation with therapists.

Social needs. Parents and family can have a variety of other worries, some of which are of greater priority than adherence to therapy. Unless these priorities are appreciated, attention to physiotherapy and occupational therapy may be difficult for parents to manage (Fox 1975; Tarran 1981). There are family strengths which support parents and child. Nevertheless, it is important that other team members provide information on schools, playgroups, parent support groups, special organisations, respite childcare, counselling and how to obtain housing and important financial advice for parents who want this. MacKean *et al.* (2005) found that many parents do not want the burden of making all the decisions themselves. Parents wanted to be working with a trusted and knowledgeable professional who could help them sort through the complexities of important decisions they have to make on these and other matters. Sometimes decision making is overwhelming for some parents. These worries, as well as coping with periods of crisis, need to be referred to psychologists, social workers, doctors or specialised nurses. Should social services not be available, therapists may need to have available a database of local organisations and agencies in the community.

Parents' health

Parents can become both physically and emotionally exhausted with caring for their child with cerebral palsy as well as caring for the rest of the family. Their child frequently has sleep problems, or may need special feeds or medication at night, all of which impinge on parents' health. They also have to cope with disturbance of sleep routines in the siblings due to the child with sleep problems. Besides the suggestions given above, physiotherapists are well trained to advise parents on where to learn relaxation methods and to care for their backs and for their general physical health. Improved physical health helps mental health. In Britain there are manual handling courses for therapists and nurses, which gives practical ideas that can be selected and taught to parents.

Teamwork with parents

The example of the collaborative learning approach can be carried out best with the therapist, sometimes together with another team member, as the key person or primary interventionist. This has the advantage of developing an ongoing relationship between therapist and child along with his parents and other members of the family. Parents find that visits from one professional are more desirable than from a stream of experts. They remain reassured that various experts are in support of their own primary interventionist. One person can coordinate the habilitation programme and avoid contradictory advice from different sources. This is particularly helpful in community work.

The key person, who may not be a therapist, will be designated by a team of professionals who will support her with their assessments and selection of ideas to suit the aims of parents and child. The key person will learn from the team when specialised assessments and advice are necessary and when any specialised 'hands-on' sessions are indicated. This applies to any other key worker designated by a team, who is also compatible with parents and child. He or she will judge the frequency of home visits so that dependency is not generated by them (McConachie 1986).

This type of teamwork is called the *transdisciplinary* model. There can also be an *interdisciplinary* model in which collaboration with parents can take place between each professional such as physiotherapist, occupational therapist, speech therapist and teacher. Each professional will integrate the ideas of the others into her sessions with child and parents. When professionals work as a multidisciplinary team, such integration is rarely attempted as each professional carries out her own assessments and therapy or teaching sessions in the area of his or her discipline.

There is such a wide variety of professionals who can offer their expertise. But first each professional needs to understand what parents' and family needs are, how well they are coping on their own and where the professional's expertise can truly be family-centred. A support team may consist of medical consultants in paediatrics, neurology, ophthalmology, orthopaedics, audiology and psychiatry for psychologists, physiotherapists, occupational therapists, speech and language therapists, teachers, nurses and social workers. Excellent progress has nevertheless been made by children with a much smaller and well-integrated community or centre's team including their parents and other family members, provided the whole child is considered. Liaison can be made with relevant specialists and agencies by a key worker or primary interventionist as well as by the team, depending on the needs of child and family.

The principle of teamwork varies from multidisciplinary, interdisciplinary and transdisciplinary approaches, and roles of different disciplines are discussed below and in Chapters 6, 10 and 12.

Effective teamwork does not consist of separate assessments and isolated specialised treatments of specific disabilities by each team member as if they equal the 'whole' child. Although specialised work is important, attention must be given to the interplay that exists between all functional areas of a child. Assets in one function may be used to develop another different and inadequate ability. For example, speech may reinforce movement, motor activities stimulate speech, and words and movement assist the training of perception and perceptual motor programmes, which in turn develop understanding and language. The work of Stroh *et al.* (2008) is an example of functional learning which integrates motor, perceptual and emotional needs in the development of understanding and language in children with developmental delay. Interplay between apparently different developmental aspects is outlined in a book on therapy for parents and carers of children with multiple disabilities (Levitt 1994).

An integrated approach

In both the transdisciplinary model and the interdisciplinary model, or combinations of both, professionals need to carefully learn the following in order to share this with an individual child and all those involved with his care. Therefore, this may be either through one or two key workers or directly by each professional as part of their own programme.

(1) Which postures and movements, including patterns of locomotion, to encourage so that a child develops them through practice in all environments?
(2) Which undesirable motor and other behaviours to discourage?

(3) Which positions make it easier for a child to see, hear, move and communicate?
(4) How to prevent and correct deformities?
(5) Which sensory, perceptual and cognitive experiences to encourage?
(6) Which aids, special furniture, equipment or orthoses to use to facilitate a child's function?
(7) How to lift and carry a child so that he participates and corrects his neuromotor problems, and how this is done to protect the backs of the adults?
(8) Which toys, playthings and recreational activities are specially recommended?
(9) Which augmentative or alternative methods of communication to use in those children who need them?

These aspects are managed in both anticipatory guidance and ongoing guidance based on a therapist's knowledge and experience.

All these areas of specialised information for the individual child are interwoven by a team of collaborative adults so that a whole programme is shared with a child. In Chapter 12, such collaboration is outlined when a child is in a peer group.

Teamwork is facilitated in many ways. For example:

■ Staff conferences in small or large meetings.
■ Staff meetings may or may not include parents, depending on the agenda and parents' availability.
■ Informal discussions with team members, including parents.
■ Visits to one another's workplace.
■ Combined sessions with different therapists, with teachers, with health visitors or with social workers.
■ Assessment by a number of professionals together with parents can be arranged using a one-way window so that the key person and child are alone together in a room. A parent may be in the room or watching with other professionals to learn about their child's actions and behaviour. Parents can then talk easily as they are not in front of their child and their comments add to everyone's insight. It is important to know whether a child's behaviour with professionals is typical or different from that at home (Newson 1976).

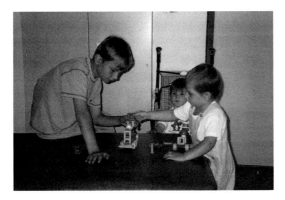

Figure 2.8 Therapeutic actions within play between siblings.

Siblings

Although a therapist is busy with a child, she needs to acknowledge the feelings of his siblings as well. Their normal rivalries are difficult to handle, especially when their brother or sister with disabilities receives so much extra attention. It is wise not to shoulder them with responsibilities for any treatment of their sibling. Although they may respond to their mother's need 'for an extra pair of hands', this should not be overdone. Brothers and sisters may respond to play activities which are therapeutic for the child with disabilities. They may invent their own games together (Levitt 1994) (see Fig. 2.8).

Simeonsson and McHale (1981) found many individual reactions in siblings which may be positive in many respects, especially if they are not over-burdened and given their own lives to lead as well. Craft *et al.* (1990) discuss an education programme for siblings of children with disabilities.

Records

These are discussed in more detail with current measures in Chapter 8.

Videos are useful for records of assessment, methods selected and evaluations.

Photographs or videos are given to parents as a record for the home programme.

Parents may be able to take videos of their child's performance at home, which can be different from the professionals' observations in their clinics. Parents do say 'my child can do this better at home'.

Child and parent reports are given under section 'Measures of daily activity and participation' in Chapter 8.

Records are made, in a collaborative style, of:

- The priorities of parents and of a child: *ultimate aims* such as mobility, a daily or community task.
- What parents and child can already do: *initial abilities (components)* and/or functional achievements.
- *Immediate goals or shorter term goals* or what parents and child still need to achieve. Future specific goals in the shorter term can be stated in their own words by more experienced parents and by a more communicative child/older person with a disability in joint decisions with therapists. Time for achievement is not always easy but estimates depend on a therapist's experience.
- Methods of therapy and management records. Also flexibly record frequency and length of sessions and the person who currently carries out specific methods.

Review of practical points for assessment, use of methods and evaluation

The arrangement of long-term and short-term plans is agreed between parents, child and therapist, and is also called a *contract* between them. The contract is made in the early sessions of the assessments during which there are clarifications of what the child and parents want to achieve and what the therapist offers them for their wishes, as well as what are the responsibilities of all in using methods for results in evaluations (Dale 1996). Individual 'goal setting' is discussed in Chapter 8.

As the collaborative learning approach may be new to some therapists or if a therapist feels it is not going well, reflection on some of the following points can be helpful. Check these points:

- Acknowledgment of parents' assets has been adequate. Quality of relationship is promoted.
- Clarify whether parents' wishes are the same or have changed.

- Clarify if other parental worries are more pressing than working on what they need to do for their desired achievements. Refer to other professionals or organisations skilled in handling parental concerns or crises.
- Check whether physiotherapy information or methods are currently overwhelming for parents, so needing repetition or modification with the therapist. Pace of learning differs in individual people.
- Make sure that emphasis has been on the therapeutic input contained in everyday familiar activities.
- Discuss with the team whether the programmes given by all the professionals make parents feel they have too much to do and assist any key worker with an integrated programme.
- Task analyses break down tasks into components (elements) manageable by individual parents and which are likely to be successful in a reasonable short term. For example, parents' apparently 'unrealistic goals' such as walking can be analysed into realistic components which build up towards a long-term goal of walking. More background knowledge for this approach is in Chapters 6, 8 and 9 dealing with tasks (developmental functions). Prognosis of long-term goals cannot be definite owing to many individual factors, as discussed in Chapter 1.

Alternative and complementary treatments

Parents may wish to mention an interest in or need to obtain alternative and complementary treatments, and the therapist needs to respect their needs and inform herself about what is to be carried out on the person for whom she is responsible. It is important to make clear that such treatments are no more able to cure cerebral palsy than traditional methods in Western medicine and therapies. However, parents of children with cerebral palsy and older people with cerebral palsy report improvements and a sense of well-being following such treatments. A therapist needs to continue to hear what is being done for those people for whom she is responsible. She should show understanding about the need of parents and other individuals to 'do all they can' to help their child. Her compassionate interest encourages parents and others to share what they need to explore so that discussion can take place. The theories underlying complementary medicine are very different from Western clinical medicine. There is always an extensive history and far-reaching information on the 'whole' person, including the individual's preferences for colours, odours, weather and seasons, as well as his fears and dislikes.

The physiotherapist or occupational therapist needs to observe any undesirable effects on an individual with cerebral palsy following alternative treatments and give an opinion on what she observes. She should draw on her knowledge and experience to say what she considers may be inadvisable for a child and his parents.

There are almost no research studies on the effects of alternative treatments in the field of cerebral palsy. Nevertheless, some positive effects due to relaxation associated with many treatments as well as a patient's strong beliefs do provide additional support for parents and some individuals with cerebral palsy. Some complementary therapies are briefly outlined for information (Hurvitz *et al.* 2003).

Acupuncture. This is conventionally used for pain, though other benefits are also claimed. The technique involves partial insertion of a fine needle into the skin or the use of pressure (acupressure) using fingertips.

Homeopathy. A minute dose of a well-diluted preparation (similar to that which causes the condition) is given to the patient. The patient's body is believed to heal itself by responding to this increase in the condition. The homeopath advises how long the healing process will take.

Herbalism. Medicinal properties of herbs are claimed and used, often being gentle in action. The dosage is dependent on the age of the patient. Like homeopathy, it aims to 'restore the healthy balance of the body and use its self-healing powers'. Herbal remedies are used for common health problems in all children such as cold, cough, catarrh or sore throat as well as sleeplessness.

Cranial osteopathy. A qualified practitioner gently massages or moves the bones and skin of a child's skull. It is believed that this affects the brain function and improves relaxation throughout the body, although this does not cure the cerebral palsy.

Reflexology. The soles of a person's feet are massaged, which is found to be relaxing and appears to increase circulation in relatively immobile children.

Pain and spasm are said to decrease in the limbs and body. It is claimed that areas of the sole relate to organs in the body so that reflexology improves their function. Therefore, constipation, congestion and dispersal of toxins in the body can also be treated.

Aromatherapy. Aromatic oils from plants and flowers and other substances are used and believed to have a variety of healing effects in conjunction with body and limb massage. Massage increases relaxation and improves circulation as well as helping to draw a child's attention to different body parts in a gentle and pleasant way.

Massage without aromatic oils is used in baby massage, which creates relaxation in both mother and child and helps mother–child bonding. The sensations of touch and smell are developed in a pleasant way for a young child.

Shiatsu massage does not use oils but massages certain 'meridians' beneath the surface of the skin, which is believed to contribute in the healing of a number of ailments.

Hyperbaric oxygen therapy. This treatment involves a child breathing pure oxygen in a special helmet whilst in a pressure chamber containing compressed air typically at a pressure of 1.75 atm. The treatment is for a period of one hour either daily or between 5 and 12 sessions a week. Many risks have been reported, particularly to hearing, vision and damage to lungs which cannot be dismissed. Although studies have been carried out, they have been inadequate and reports are anecdotal (Collet *et al*. 2001; Hardy *et al*. 2002).

Contraindications

Qualified practitioners must be used. A parent should not carry out any of the procedures from a lay person's guide. A therapist needs to have information from the practitioner as to what procedures will be used.

Any alternative treatment should not replace the drugs essential for controlling epilepsy. If this is attempted then there needs to be discussion with a child's medical consultant so that any drug is not suddenly stopped and parents are educated about the epilepsy.

Massage needs to be gentle and carried out by a qualified practitioner. A child may be hyperac-

tive if the soles of his feet are touched or the palms of his hands receive pressure. Hypertonic muscles, especially those with spasticity, may be hyperactive or hypersensitive to touch and pressure. Massage is preferably applied to the antagonists as mothers in various cultures feel they want to do this.

Parents and child may spend a great deal of energy and time as well as expense in visiting practitioners of alternative and complementary medicine. We understand that some treatment regimes create demanding schedules that dominate parents' lives. This can result in fatigue or exhaustion and can lead to neglect of the needs of siblings and perhaps a marriage and the wider family. As with any therapy programme, parents need to avoid overwhelming themselves with too much to do.

When some parents wish to explore alternative therapies outside their service, they are entitled to do what they feel is best for their child. This can cause conflict in professional responsibilities as to which treatment is being effective and who is responsible for injury or deterioration. Parents who explore other ideas are given a channel of communication should they wish to return.

Summary

A collaborative learning approach involves a therapist in a joint venture with a child and his parents, or directly with older individuals with cerebral palsy. It can be used with other family members, carers and with colleagues in a team. It is a radical departure from the traditional model in which a therapist takes full responsibility for assessments, treatment plans, use of methods and evaluation, or takes responsibility for a few of these aspects. Instead, all aspects are shared with parents and a child who can understand this. Their culture and values can also be directly learned from them.

This collaborative approach has similarities to family-centred approaches and thus welcomes the increase in family-centred teams. The difference, however, is that the approach discussed is a *learning approach* which includes learning not only to change a child or older person's motor function but also to change attitudes, feelings as well as behaviour by all involved in the process of therapy.

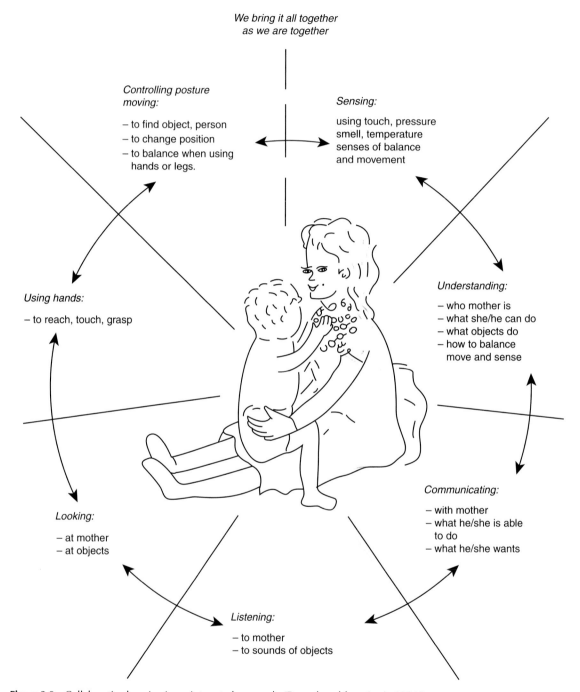

*We bring it all together
as we are together*

*Controlling posture
moving:*

– to find object, person
– to change position
– to balance when using
  hands or legs.

Sensing:

using touch, pressure
smell, temperature
senses of balance
and movement

Using hands:

– to reach, touch, grasp

Understanding:

– who mother is
– what she/he can do
– what objects do
– how to balance
  move and sense

Looking:

– at mother
– at objects

Communicating:

– with mother
– what he/she is able
  to do
– what he/she wants

Listening:

– to mother
– to sounds of objects

Figure 2.9   Collaborative learning in an integrated approach. (Reproduced from Levitt 1994.)

Emotional aspects are outlined in relation to parent–child interaction (Fig 2.9), as well as therapist–child and therapist–parent interactions. The education and other needs of parents and their priorities are given attention as well as care for their health. Therapists also deserve support in their own groups and teams. The collaborative learning model enables a therapist to develop both professionally and personally and to learn to knit together ideas from counselling, communication skills and the study of human relationships.

'Therapists and doctors often feel that they must advise parents and disabled people "to be realistic". This may not be necessary if the child and his parents are directly involved with their assessments and selection and use of therapy methods and equipment. In this process of rehabilitation they come to see for themselves the discrepancy between what their aims are and what their child is able to achieve. The therapist is there to support them and counter despair' (Levitt & Goldschmied 1990).

Parents who participate in physical therapy for their children with disabilities develop 'a more realistic view of their child's potential in terms of daily functioning' (Jansen *et al.* 2003).

Brazelton (1976) suggested that:

'the success of any intervention programme should be measured not only by the child's development but by increased family comfort, decrease in the divorce rate, lower incidence of behaviour problems in siblings . . . perhaps by pretty soft signs but they may be a lot more important as measures of effectiveness of intervention than is a rise in IQ or increased motor capacity on the part of the child'.

3

Outline of treatment approaches

There are many systems of treatment for cerebral palsy (Levitt 1962, 1976, 1987; Scrutton 1984; McKinlay 1989; Miller 2007). Various motor-learning approaches have added to the neurophysiological and orthopaedic systems (Shepherd 1995; Shumway-Cook and Woollacott 2001). Although all of these therapeutic approaches were devised for the cerebral palsies or applied from adult neurology for cerebral palsy, many of them are also used for treatment of children with other conditions of developmental delay and for traumatic brain injury and adult hemiplegia. It is not the purpose of this chapter to describe each system in full detail, and reference should be made to the literature and study observations of each system in practice. The author presents the essence of each system after many personal observations, discussions, practical work and reading of the work of the originators. In the next chapter, a review of research on various systems is included for evidence-based practice.

Muscle education and braces

W.M. Phelps, an orthopaedic surgeon in Baltimore, was one of the pioneers in the treatment of cerebral palsy who encouraged physiotherapists, occupational therapists and speech therapists to form themselves into cerebral palsy habilitation teams (Phelps 1949, 1952; Slominski 1984). The main points in his treatment approach were as follows:

Specific diagnostic classification of each child as a basis for specific treatment methods. He diagnosed five types of cerebral palsies and many subclassifications.

Fifteen modalities were described and specific combinations of these modalities were used for the specific type of cerebral palsy.

The modalities (methods) were:

(1) Massage for hypotonic muscles, but contraindicated in children with spasticity and athetoids.
(2) Passive motion through joint range for mobilising joints and demonstrating to the child the movement required. Speed of movement is slower for children with spasticity, increased for rigidity.
(3) Active assisted motion.
(4) Active motion.
(5) Resisted motion followed according to the child's capability.

The above modalities were used for obtaining modalities 6, 8, 10 and 12.

(6) Conditioned motion is recommended for babies, young children and mentally retarded children. This included a routine and the use

of the same song or jingle for the same movement modality (2–5).

(7) Confused motion or synergistic motion which involves resistance to a muscle group in order to contract an inactive muscle group in the same synergy. Mass movements such as the extensor thrust or the flexion withdrawal reflex were usually used. For example, using the hip–knee flexion dorsiflexion synergy, to stimulate inactive dorsiflexors by giving resistance to hip flexors. Confused motion is used by children when selective isolated movement is not possible.

(8) Combined motion is training motion of more than one joint, such as a shoulder and elbow flexion using modalities 2, 3, 4 and 5.

(9) Relaxation techniques used are those of conscious 'letting go' of the body and its parts (Levitt 1962), tensing and relaxing parts of the body. These methods are mainly used with athetoids. They attempt to lie still or relaxed or use contract–relax or active 'tense-up and let go' relaxation for grimacing and other involuntary motion.

(10) Movement from relaxation is conscious control of movements once relaxation has been achieved. It was mainly used for children to consciously control involuntary movements.

(11) Rest: Periods of rest are suggested for athetoids and children with spasticity.

(12) Reciprocation is training movement of one leg after the other in a bicycling pattern in lying, crawling, knee walking and stepping.

(13) Balance: Training of sitting balance and standing in braces.

(14) Reach and grasp and release used for training of hand function.

(15) Skills of daily living such as feeding, dressing, washing and toileting. Many aids were devised by the occupational therapists.

Braces or calipers. The appliances were designed and developed by Phelps. He prescribed special braces to correct deformity, to obtain the upright position and to control athetosis. The bracing is extensive and worn for many years. The children are taught to stand and step in long leg braces with pelvic bands and back supports or sometimes spinal brace. As they progress, the back supports are removed, then the pelvic band and finally they wear below-knee braces. The full-length brace has lock-ing joints at hip and knee, so control can be taught with them, locked or unlocked.

Muscle education. Children with spasticity are given muscle education based on an analysis of whether muscles are spastic, weak, normal or *zero cerebral – being unable to act*. Muscles antagonistic to spastic muscles are activated. This is to obtain muscle balance between spastic muscles and their weak antagonists. Athetoids were trained to control simple joint motion and do not have muscle education. Ataxics may be given strengthening exercises for weak muscle groups.

Others, including Rood (1962) and Tardieu *et al.* (1982), have also developed ideas on muscle education. Plum and Molhave (1956) advocated strengthening spastic muscles as well as their antagonists. However, Plum exercised the spastic muscles in their outer ranges as the muscles are usually shortened, whereas the antagonists are exercised in their middle and inner ranges. Tabary *et al.* (1981), in a 'factorial analysis', identified the specific problem in the muscles which gives rise to abnormalities and deformities. According to this careful analysis, treatment is given where indicated. Alcohol injections were used to diminish spasticity. Today, neurologists no longer recommend this due to side effects. Other drugs are used by them.

Tabary *et al.* (1972), Tardieu *et al.* (1982) and Dietz (1992) have shown specific changes in muscle length (*hypoextensibility*) of spastic muscles and also changes in the muscle structures which are quoted in current therapy literature. Studies by Tardieu *et al.* (1988) suggest prolonged passive stretch for 5–7 hours to obtain a change in length. This was carried out in braces by Phelps, but currently, better designed, lighter orthoses have been developed. The equipment suggested by the therapists in Phelps' centre continues to be used in occupational therapy and physiotherapy, with improvement of their designs as well as design of additional aids. For example, an upright standing frame was used but has also been improved in various currently used designs which are also adjustable in more ways. Weight bearing to prevent hip dislocation was advised by Phelps (1959). Current treatment to prevent hip subluxation stresses the use of modern standing frames for early weight-bearing and hip joint development (see Chapters 9 and 11).

Damiano (2007) refers to recommendations by Phelps to use resisted motion in cerebral palsy to develop strength. Researches by Damiano and others confirm the value of resisted exercises (Damiano *et al.* 1995a,b, 2002a). However, she recognises difficulties such as problems of poor isolation of muscle control (selective motor control) in some children with spasticity. Phelps called this 'confused motion', which therapists later generally discouraged by training selective motion of a particular muscle group as part of motor development.

Progressive pattern movements

Temple Fay, a neurosurgeon in Philadelphia, recommended that the cerebral palsied be taught motion according to its development in evolution. He regarded ontogenetic development (in humans) as a recapitulation of phylogenetic development (in the evolution of the species). In general, he suggested building up motion from reptilian squirming to amphibian creeping, through mammalian reciprocal motion 'on all fours' to the primate erect walking. As lower animals carried out these early movements of progression with a simple nervous system, they can similarly be carried out in the human in the absence of a normal cerebral cortex. The midbrain, pons and medulla could be involved in the stimulation of primitive patterns of movement and primitive reflexes which activate the handicapped parts of the body. Fay also described 'unlocking reflexes' which reduce hypertonus. Based on these ideas, he developed *progressive pattern movements* which consist of five stages (Fay 1954a,b).

Stage 1. Prone lying. Head and trunk rotation from side to side.

Stage 2. Homolateral stage. Prone lying, head turned to side. Arm on the face side in abduction–external–rotation, elbow semi-flexed, hand open, thumb out towards the mouth. Leg on face side in abduction, knee flexion opposite stomach, foot dorsiflexion. Arm on the occiput side is extended, internally rotated, hand open at the side of the child or on the lumbar area of his back. Leg on the occiput side is extended. Movement involves head turning from side to side with the face, arm and leg sweeping down to the extended position and the opposite occiput arm and leg flexing up to the position near the face as the head turns round.

Stage 3. Contralateral stage. Prone lying. Head turned to side, arm on the face side as in stage 2.

The leg on the face side is, however, extended. The other leg on the side of the occiput is flexed. As the head turns, this contralateral pattern changes from side to side.

Stage 4. On hands and knees. Reciprocal crawling and reciprocal stepping on hands and feet in the *bear walk* or *elephant walk*.

Stage 5. Walking pattern. This is a *sailor's walk* called by Fay 'reciprocal progression on lower extremities synchronized with the contralateral swing of the arms and trunk'. A wide base is used and the child flexes one hip and knee into external rotation and then places his foot on the ground, still in external rotation. As the foot is being placed on the ground, the opposite arm and shoulder are rotating towards it. As weight is taken on the straight leg, the other leg flexes up.

The Doman-Delacato system or the Institute for the Achievement of Human Potential (IAHP) (Doman *et al.* 1960), which follows the basic tenets postulated by Fay, also recommends periods of inhalations of CO_2 from a breathing sack, restriction of fluid intake and development of cerebral hemispheric dominance. Cerebral dominance is attempted by principal use of dominant eye, hand, foot and arm, and other methods. Children are also hung upside down and whirled around to stimulate the vestibular apparatus. They are also asked to hang and 'walk' their hands along a horizontal ladder as observed in apes.

The progressive pattern movements called 'patterning therapy' are first practised passively at least five times daily. One person turns the head, another person moves the arms and leg on one side, and another person moves the arm and leg on the other side. Locomotion beyond the stage of the child's patterning level is not permitted. A child who is not proficient in cross-pattern creeping is prevented from walking. There is a rigid and inaccurate view of development. 'Neurological organisation' is considered possible if each developmental level is established before going to the next level. This approach restricts itself to prone development and expects demanding daily regimes of treatment, amounting to 8–10 hours a day, 7 days a week in many cases.

Parents could not manage this without obtaining a number of volunteers. There was a high rate of inappropriate parental expectations with reports of excessive family stress as success or failure depended on the parents working intensively. Various medical organisations have made statements that there is no scientific evidence and that the theories are outdated and oversimplified. These organisations are American Academy of Paediatrics and American Academy of Neurology (1967), American Academy of Paediatrics (1999), American Academy of Physical Medicine and Rehabilitation (1968). Today, patterning therapy has almost disappeared in the United States (Miller 2007).

The British Institute for Brain Injured Children (BIBIC) and Brainwave originally acted in conjunction with the IAHP, but now function on their own. They use their developmental profile from Temple Fay (Fay 1954a,b). Play is notably absent and BIBIC's educational programme is superficial, according to a multidisciplinary appraisal and independent review (Morton *et al.* 1999). They found that the Doman-Delacato influences are strong, and emotional, financial and other demands on the family are considerable.

Synergistic movement patterns

Signe Brunnstrom, a physical therapist who worked with adult hemiplegia, assessed the stages of recovery and compared them with normal sequential neuromotor development in early childhood. Her studies consider flexion and extension limb synergies leading to isolated motion. She produced motion by stimulating primitive movement patterns or synergistic movement patterns which are observed in fetal life or immediately after pyramidal tract damage. The main features of her work are as follows (Brunnstrom 1970):

Reflex responses are used initially which a patient could 'capture' and use later in voluntary control of these synergies to move. Later, the flexor and extensor synergies were modified (broken up), and voluntary function with more variety that was possible was elicited and practised.

Control of head and trunk is attempted with stimulation of attitudinal reflexes such as tonic neck reflexes, tonic lumbar reflexes and tonic labyrinthine reflexes. This is followed by stimulation of righting reflexes and later balance training.

Associated reactions are used as well as *hand reactions*; for example, hyperextension of the thumb produces relaxation of the finger flexors. Resisted action was used on the unaffected side to activate

the affected side. The training of a patient's voluntary control is developed later in the therapy programme.

Sensory stimulation. Brunnstrom uses proprioceptive and other stimuli in her training, such as tapping or stroking for adult hemiplegia. We see some of these methods in the early Bobath approach and in other neurophysiological approaches which used hierarchical theories and sensory input.

Proprioceptive neuromuscular facilitations (PNF)

Herman Kabat, a neurophysiologist and psychiatrist in the United States, has discussed various neurophysiological mechanisms which could be used in therapeutic exercises. With Margaret Knott and Dorothy Voss, he developed a system of movement facilitation techniques and methods for the decrease of hypertonus, for strengthening, coordination and improving joint range (Kabat *et al.* 1959; Knott & Voss 1968; Voss 1972; Voss *et al.* 1985). The main features of these methods are the use of the following:

Movement patterns (called mass movement synergies) based on patterns observed within functional activities such as dressing, walking, playing tennis, golf or football. These patterns are spiral (rotational) and diagonal with a synergy or *chain* of muscle groups. Isolated muscle education was not used as a movement pattern could activate a muscle group within a chain of muscles. The movement patterns are therefore not the 'mass movements' seen after brain damage, but are functionally derived patterns. They consist of the following simultaneously activated components in hips, knees and feet or in shoulders, elbows, wrists and hands:

(1) Flexion or extension.
(2) Abduction or adduction.
(3) Internal or external rotation.

Sensory (afferent) stimuli are skilfully applied to facilitate movement. Stimuli used are touch and pressure, traction and compression, stretch or limb elongation and the proprioceptive effect of muscles contracting against resistance. Visual and verbal stimuli are included. All these stimuli provide clues for the direction of movement and are gradually reduced as the individual achieves the movement independently.

Resistance to motion is used to facilitate the action of the muscles which form the components of the movement patterns.

Special techniques

(1) *Irradiation* is the predictable overflow of action from one muscle group to another within a synergy or movement pattern or by *reinforcement* of action of one part of the body stimulating action in another part of the body.
(2) *Rhythmic* stabilizations which use stimuli alternating from the agonist to its antagonist in isometric muscle work.
(3) *Stimulation of reflexes* such as the mass flexion or extension which are now no longer used.
(4) *Repeated contractions* of one pattern using any joint as a pivot.
(5) *Reversals* from one pattern to its antagonist and other reversals based on the physiological principle of successive induction.
(6) *Relaxation* techniques such as contract–relax and hold–relax. Ice treatments are used for relaxation of hypertonus.
(7) *Timing* in using various techniques to train co-ordination or timing-for-emphasis to improve an element of movement synergy.

There are various combinations of techniques depending on the individual's physical condition and the therapist's goals. The use of stretch or traction and the optimal resistance needs careful use on unstable joints and level of muscle contraction.

Functional work or *mat work* involves the use of various methods mentioned above in training rolling, crawling, walking and various balance positions of sitting, kneeling and standing. As PNF is largely practised with adults, this was adapted for cerebral palsy using movement patterns within developmental motor functions (Levitt 1969, 1970b). PNF was also criticised for treating movement pattern in isolation from a whole function. Using them within developmental functions provided a better approach. Some examples of these are given in this book to use movements against resistance, which can simultaneously activate postural stability and counterpoising mechanisms in trunk, pelvic and shoulder girdles. Another example is the resistance to arm elevation which improves head control. In addition, the PNF patterns and resistance were used in combination with positioning other body parts

to minimise activation of spasticity. This combined PNF with ideas from the Bobath approach (Levitt 1969). However, the Bobaths disagreed as they were against the use of manual resistance. Today, resisted actions have been accepted for weakness.

Adler *et al.* (2008), using PNF with adults, have added principles of motor control and motor learning from the work of Mulder and Hochstenbach (2002). There are additional functional activities using PNF and additional techniques in different positions. As individuals achieve the movements and stability, there is 'hands-off' by the therapist, so that patients can then detect any of their mistakes in their motor patterns. These mistakes give 'feedback', allowing the individuals to learn and correct themselves as much as they are able to do. Ideas from Mulder are used in this book and quoted in Chapter 6.

Neuromotor development

Eirene Collis, a therapist and pioneer in cerebral palsy in Britain, stressed neuromotor development as a basis for assessment and treatment (Collis 1947; Collis *et al.* 1956). Her main points were as follows:

The mental capacity of the child would determine the results.

Early treatment was advocated before abnormal patterns could be established.

Management. The word 'treatment' was considered misleading in that besides the physiotherapy session there should be 'management' of the child throughout the day. The feeding, dressing, toileting and other activities of the day should be planned.

Strict developmental sequence. The child was not permitted to use motor skills beyond his level of development. If the child was, say, learning to roll, he was not allowed to crawl, or if crawling he was not allowed to walk. At all times the child was given a 'picture of normal movement' and, as posture and tone are interwoven, Collis placed the child in 'normal postures' in order to stimulate 'normal tone'. Once postural security was obtained, achievements were facilitated and developmental sequences were followed throughout this training.

The CP therapist. Collis disliked the separation of treatment into physiotherapy, occupational therapy and speech therapy. She established the idea of the *cerebral palsy therapist.*

The developmental sequences became much more sophisticated and less strict. The idea of a cerebral palsy therapist has some appeal in the concept of a developmental therapist or primary interventionist. The worries of mothers were assumed to be helped by the treatment and by her willingness to be able to help her child. One hopes there is deeper understanding of parents' predicaments and feelings today.

Neurodevelopmental treatment (Bobath approach)

Karl Bobath, a neuropsychiatrist, and Berta Bobath, a physiotherapist, based assessment and treatment on the premise that the fundamental difficulty in cerebral palsy is lack of inhibition of reflex patterns of posture and movement (Bobath 1965, 1971a,b, 1980; Bobath & Bobath 1972, 1975). The Bobaths associated these abnormal patterns with abnormal tone due to overaction of tonic reflex activity. These tonic reflexes, such as the tonic labyrinthine reflex, symmetrical tonic neck reflexes and asymmetrical tonic neck reflexes, have to be inhibited in order to counteract 'the abnormal patterns of released postural reflex activity, and at the same time facilitate normal reactions by special techniques of handling'. In time, the focus on reflexes was decreased (Bobath & Bobath 1984) but the Bobath system continues to focus on abnormal patterns and abnormal tone. The keystone of the approach still seems to be abnormal tone. There are many Bobath-trained physiotherapists who first spend time on reducing abnormal tone so that the child is 'prepared' for movement (Mayston 1992). Preparation involves stretching, handling and positioning by the therapist to improve quality of tone and therefore movement.

The practice of the Bobath approach or neurodevelopmental treatment (NDT) is different in different countries, in different parts of a country and in different centres. Physiotherapists have had to make modifications based on their clinical experiences and on the critical comments of others. As there is increasing scientific understanding of the brain and nervous system, the theories and concept of the Bobath system have been challenged by a number of therapists and other workers (Gordon 1987; Horak 1992; Shepherd 1995; Damiano 2004).

Howle (2002) suggests that contemporary theories developed by other approaches are now used for NDT. She quotes Mrs Bobath who maintained that the concept (or philosophy) had not changed through the years but the techniques have been developed and refined. A series of several photographs in Howle's book show a skilful Bobath treatment with handling not only with hands but also with the therapist's body and legs to position and treat a girl with cerebral palsy of a mild and moderate condition. These are familiar Bobath methods despite the 'new theories'.

Mayston, a former Director of the original Bobath Centre in London, states that 'little or no evidence is available to show that therapy offered by the "named approaches" is effective or that one approach is more beneficial than another' (Mayston 2004). Mayston has provided new thinking and self-questioning by physiotherapists wedded to this system. She also says that 'Bobath therapists' should and have become more eclectic (Mayston 2004, 2008). This is reassuring as the Bobaths (Bobath & Bobath 1984), referring to earlier editions of this book, firmly stated that 'Eclectic treatment, using a mixture of treatment techniques derived from various schools of thought which see the child's problems from different viewpoints, cannot result in a cohesive treatment programme'. Mayston (2004) also points out that conductive education (which is a learning approach) places more emphasis on the child's initiation, participation and practise 'which is different to the Bobath approach'. This is also different to any motor learning approach. The dramatic changes in theories underlying NDT make it no longer clear what this approach consists of in theory and practice and how different it is from other therapists who have never been dedicated to this approach.

Features of the approach which can be usually observed are as follows:

Preparation for movement patterns specifically selected to treat abnormal tone associated with abnormal movement patterns and abnormal posture. Key components such as extension, rotation and symmetry often form the basis for motor skills and receive treatment methods.

Developmental sequences were more strictly followed in the past, but are now modified (Mayston 1992, 2004).

Sensorimotor experience. The reversal or 'breakdown' of the movement abnormalities is said to give the child the sensation of more normal tone and movements. This sensory experience, now called 'feedback', is provided by the therapist's handling and is believed to gain more normal motion. 'Learning to move is entirely dependent on sensory experience' (Bobath & Bobath 1984).

Key points of control are used by many therapists to change the patterns of spasticity so that a child *is prepared for movement* and correct posture. The *key points* are usually head and neck, shoulder and pelvic girdles, as well as use of distal key points to aim to 'normalise' abnormal tone.

All-day management by parents supplements treatment sessions. Parents and others are advised on daily management and trained to treat the children. Nancie Finnie (1997) has written a book for parents on this all-day handling of the child in the home. This book is being updated.

Sensory stimulation for activation and inhibition

Margaret Rood, a physiotherapist and occupational therapist, based her approach on many neurophysiological theories and experiments (Rood 1962; Stockmeyer 1967, 1972). The main features of her approach are the following:

Afferent stimuli. Techniques of stimulation, such as stroking, brushing (tactile); icing, heating (temperature); pressure, bone pounding, slow and quick muscle stretch, joint retraction and approximation, muscle contractions (proprioception) are used to activate, facilitate or 'inhibit' motor response.

Muscles are classified according to various physiological data, including whether they are for 'light work muscle action' or 'heavy work muscle action'. The appropriate stimuli for their actions are suggested.

Reflexes other than the above are used in therapy, for example tonic labyrinthine reflexes, tonic neck, vestibular reflexes, withdrawal patterns.

Ontogenetic developmental sequence is outlined and strictly followed in the application of stimuli.

(1) Total flexion or withdrawal pattern (in supine).
(2) Roll over (flexion of arm and leg on the same side and roll over).

(3) Pivot prone (prone with hyperextension of head, trunk and legs).
(4) Co-contraction neck (prone head over edge for co-contraction of vertebral muscles).
(5) On elbows (prone and push backwards).
(6) All fours (static, weight shift and crawl).
(7) Standing upright (static, weight shifts).
(8) Walking (stance, push off, pick up, heel strike).

Vital functions. A developmental sequence of respiration, sucking, swallowing, phonation, chewing and speech is followed. Techniques of brushing, icing and pressure are used.

The sensory stimulation methods are sometimes used to draw attention to the part of a limb needing active motor control (Shumway-Cook and Woollacott 2001). Ice treatments are still used to reduce spastic hypertonus (de Souza 1997). The ontogenetic (developmental) sequence is a general outline of motor functions used as well as giving various types of muscle actions. Criticism of the approach is that stimulation may be overdone and care needs to be taken.

Reflex creeping and other reflex reactions

Vaclav Vojta, a neurologist working in Czechoslovakia and in Germany, developed his approach from the works of Temple Fay and Kabat (Vojta 1984, 1989; Von Aufschnaiter 1992). This approach is used in Europe. Reflex creeping and reflex rolling are present in newborns but persist in cerebral palsy. They can be used and adjusted by hands-on treatment for postural development and associated motion. The main features are as follows:

Reflex creeping. The creeping patterns involving head, trunk and limbs are facilitated at various *trigger* points or *reflex zones*. The creeping involves active muscle response to the appropriate triggering from the zones with sensory stimuli. The muscle work used in the normal creeping patterns or *creeping complex* have been carefully analysed. The therapist must be skilful in the facilitation of these normal patterns and not provoke pathological patterns. There are nine zones for triggering reflex locomotion.

Reflex rolling or reflex turning is also used with special methods of triggering.

Sensory stimulation. Touch, pressure, stretch and muscle action against resistance are used in many of the triggering mechanisms or in facilitation of creeping.

Resistance is recommended for action of muscles. Various specific techniques are used to apply the resistance so that either a tonic or a phasic muscle action is provoked. The phasic action (through range) may be provoked on, say, a movement of a limb creeping up or downwards. The tonic action, or stabilising action, is obtained if a phasic movement is prevented by full resistance given by the therapist. Therefore, the holding muscle action of stabilisation occurs if resistance is applied in such a way that it prevents any movement through range. *Rising reactions* are also provoked using resistance and all the methods above.

Vojta appeared to suggest that very early treatment could cure babies at-risk, but he did recognise that there are limits to the results with more severely impaired children. His methods were criticised for creating stress in children and their parents. The methods needed to be practised a number of times a day and parents found their child's crying during treatments disturbing. Nevertheless, a comparison between Bobath and Vojta methods found no significant difference in results on motor development (d'Avignon *et al.* 1981).

Katona (1989), like Vojta, suggests that in infancy, early patterns can be observed suggesting infants at-risk for cerebral palsy. Katona provokes early movement patterns different to Vojta. He considers these complex movements are precursors for later posture and movement. Treatment is six times a day for 30 minutes, carried out by parents. There is omission of sensory, perceptual and cognition with excessive focus on movements. Like Vojta, Katona claims this treatment 'cures' cerebral palsy in babies. However, we know that many babies spontaneously outgrow very early diagnosis of cerebral palsy.

Conductive education

Andras Petö in Budapest, Hungary, originated *conductive education*. After Professor Petö's death, the work was continued by Dr M. Hari until her death

(Cotton 1970, 1974, 1975, 1980, 1984; Hari and Tillemans 1984, Hari and Akos 1988; Beach 1988; Cottam & Sutton 1988; Tatlow 2005). The main feature is the integration of therapy and education by having the following:

A conductor acting as mother, nurse, teacher and therapist. She is specially trained in the habilitation of motor-disabled children in a 4-year course. She may have one or two assistants.

The group of children, about 15–20, work together. Groups are fundamental in this training system. There is also a mother–toddler group for early intervention (Seglow 1984).

An all-day programme. A fixed timetable is planned to include getting out of bed in the morning, dressing, feeding, toileting, movement training, speech, reading, writing and other schoolwork.

The movements. Sessions of movements take place mainly on and beside slatted plinths (table/beds) and with ladder-backed chairs. The movements are devised in such a way that they form the elements of a task or motor skill. The tasks are carefully analysed for each group of children. The tasks are the activities of daily living, motor skills including hand function, balance and locomotion. The purpose of each movement is explained to the children. The movements are repeated, not only in the movement sessions of, say, the *hand class* or *plinth work*, but also in various contexts throughout the day. The children are shown in practice how their 'exercises' contribute to daily activities.

Rhythmic intention. The technique used for training the elements or movements is rhythmic intention. The conductor and the children state the intended motion: 'I touch my mouth with my hands'. This motion is then attempted together with their slow, rhythmic counts of one to five. Motion is also carried out to an operative word, such as 'up, up, up' repeated in a rhythm slow enough for the children's active movement ability. Speech and active motion reinforce each other.

Individual sessions may be used for some children to help them to participate more adequately in the work of the group.

Learning principles are basic to the programme. Group dynamics with learning techniques are among the mechanisms of training discussed. *Cortical* (cognitive) or conscious participation is stressed, as opposed to involuntary and unconscious reflex therapy, or automatic reactions. They feel reactions to handling by a therapist cannot create active learning by a child. There is emphasis on a child's initiation, active participation and practice, and the promotion of self-worth.

There is also emphasis on their analysing of tasks in a 'task series' so that children will successfully achieve them. There is integration of cognitive, emotional, social, perceptual-motor and communication in the learning programmes.

Criticisms have been on quality of movements with the likelihood of deformities and contractures though the children gain motor functions. However, prevention and treating of deformities can be integrated with many practical methods selected from conductive education, as given in this book (see Chapters 9 and 11).

Sensory integration

The sensory integration (SI) approach was devised by Jean Ayres (1979) and developed by Fisher *et al.* (1991) to 'take in, interpret, integrate and use spatial-temporal aspects of sensory information from the body and the environment to plan and produce organised motor behaviour'. The approach relates sensory information to various types of learning behaviour, including motor, emotional and academic. Occupational therapists may use this approach for children with clumsy motor skills or developmental incoordination syndrome or perceptual-motor disorders. It has been used in other conditions as well as in cerebral palsy. Occupational therapists have focussed on perception difficulties in any physiotherapy approach for cerebral palsy as well as with the Rood or with the neurodevelopmental approaches (Blanche *et al.* 1995).

Children with cerebral may also have perceptual or sensory processing difficulties which need to be assessed and treated. Children with cerebral palsy very rarely have loss of sensation, but they do lack sensory experiences due to the paucity of motor repertoire. Sensory *information and its interpretation*, and not so much sensory input, need specific therapy. Stimulation of all the senses (touch, proprioceptive, vestibular visual and auditory) is provided in learning motor control with active motor function. Sensory integration has enjoyable motor activities, which can be selected and added to the physiotherapist's eclectic approach. Physiother-

apists and occupational therapists may overlap their work. However, specialised occupational therapy attends to specific difficulties of sensory integration or perception. Blanche *et al.* (1995) clearly separate the roles of NDT and SI so that there are separate sessions for the different neurological problems in a combined approach also seen in multidisciplinary teamwork in cerebral palsy.

Sensory integration expects an appropriate motor response or action in response to sensory input. Abnormal motor activity in cerebral palsy cannot easily be used in many children. The Southern California Sensory Integration Tests cannot therefore be used, as they are for other children with specific learning impairments.

Sensory input for children with low responses or with overresponses to stimuli is not the essential need from SI. Some children dislike sensory input or seek it out. I have observed that much 'hands-on' physiotherapy is not welcomed by a number of children with athetoid conditions (dyskinesia). Any overstimulation needs to be avoided, as this can be disturbing to those with cerebral palsy, causing sudden spasms or muscle tension. Others with poor sensory responses may well want such experiences. For example, children with severe visual impairment or intellectual impairments tend to seek out sensations and may rock, suck their hands, enjoy vibration and fans, music and familiar human voices.

Adjuncts to therapy

Targeted training

This option in physiotherapy for spastic cerebral palsy has been developed by Butler and Major (1992) using a biomechanical study for motor learning. In the training of sitting and standing balance, targeted training reduces the number of joints at which motor learning of control must occur. Specially designed equipment stabilises the joints below the targeted joint so that stability, weight shift and tilt are segmentally sequenced from the head downwards in the upright posture. This uses the cephalo-caudal development for head, trunk and pelvic control. The equipment replaces a therapist's manual support for training postural control in sitting and standing. The equipment is more precise for assessments and training of levels of spinal joint control and is, therefore, useful in detecting minimal and slow progress of postural control in severe cases. This would encourage parents and children who cannot see such progress due to the severity of the disability.

However, the equipment is expensive as is any equipment in research and in very precise evaluation of progress in postural control (Hadders-Algra and Carlberg 2008, Shumway-Cook *et al.* 2003). In Chapter 9, this book offers 'hands-on' training of postural control in the targeted biomechanical and developmental stages from head control (cervical spine) progressing downwards in a similar way to the research of Butler (1998) and Butler and Major (1992). In severely involved children, an interim stage of spinal joint control in these upright postures would be developmentally and biomechanically advisable and encourage parents and child to see progress, no matter how slow.

Targeted training selects children who are potentially able to gain control of relevant joints, and results have shown sitting achievement in a shorter time, even gaining sitting in a child for the first time at age 7 years. Intellectual ability is not necessary but epilepsy should not be present. Research continues in targeted training (Butler *et al.* 1992; Butler & Major 1992; Farmer *et al.* 1999).

Neuromuscular electrical stimulation or functional electrical stimulation

This is used for muscle re-education, strengthening, decreasing spasticity or as a biofeedback for training function such as gait pattern or wrist-with-hand function. The desirable action of a muscle within function is used to provide sensory feedback (Carmick 1993; Hazlewood *et al.* 1994; Comeaux *et al.* 1997). Shumway-Cook and Woollacott (2001) and others have used electrical stimulation biofeedback in adults, and its use with children is relatively uncommon. The evidence in children is still controversial and poor, especially for Carmick's studies (Siebes *et al.* 2002), but there is increasing interest in this therapy option, particularly for obtaining a local muscle contraction in children with poor selective muscle control in specific tasks (functional or neuromuscular electrical stimulation, FES or NMES). In cerebral palsy the child with multi-

ple disabilities and the young child with only motor disability can neither give reliable reports on discomfort nor comprehend the purpose, so motor learning can then be transferred to function without electrical stimulation. Improved strength of a muscle group does not necessarily lead to its use in function. In their study of hemiplegia with stimulation of tibialis anterior, Hazlewood *et al.* (1994) found increased range of active and passive motion and strength of this muscle but no change in gait pattern.

Kerr *et al.* (2004) published an annotation of 12 studies which met the criteria for inclusion. In all studies there was a variety of specific muscle groups in trunk, upper and mainly lower limbs stimulated with tibialis anterior being most common. They found three studies at best evidence Level I, three at evidence Levels III and IV, and six case studies with few subjects and other items of inadequate research evidence (Level V). Ages of children, in the best studies (Level I), were between 5 and 15 years with diagnoses of hemiplegia and diplegia, and one study with young children with diplegia from 8 to 16 months. Results of one of the Level I studies were no improvement with treatment, and two studies described improvements in strength and range of motion and one also in function in children between 8 and 16 months.

Like Kerr *et al.*, Durham *et al.* (2004), using functional electrical stimulation, point out the problems of various studies in parameters of stimulation, the appropriate muscle group to stimulate and duration of use. They faced limitations in their own pilot study and so more research was planned, though positive suggestions of results were indicated. Some children disliked the sensation of stimulation or were too young to cooperate and were not included, and compliance was a problem for some children in school settings.

Low-intensity electrical stimulation, 'threshold (therapeutic) electrical stimulation' which does not produce muscle contraction, has slight sensory effects and is tolerated during sleep (Steinbok *et al.* 1997b). The theory is that this electrical treatment promotes muscle growth associated with an increase in growth hormone assumed to be stimulated during sleep. This must be accompanied by functional physiotherapy treatments *over a year*. This electrical treatment is only used for children over 2 years of age. Kerr *et al.* (2004) found that three studies that were of evidence Level I, one at Level IV and two at Level V. Results found one support for threshold electrical stimulation (TES) and two found no effect of TES after a year of treatments. The one supporting TES (Steinbok *et al.* 1997b) recruited children who had previously had selective dorsal rhizotomy neurosurgery.

Kerr *et al.* (2006) carried out a randomised placebo-controlled study on NMES and TES with 60 children. No statistically significant difference was found for strength or function due to electrical stimulation of quadriceps in both legs in children with different types of cerebral palsies. They suggest further research for ambulatory children with diplegia.

Lycra suits and splinting

The UPsuit (Blair *et al.* 1995) cerebral palsy pressure suit and others on the market, as well as the compression Lycra bracing (Hylton & Allen 1997), are flexible supports used for stabilising trunk and proximal joints so that movements can be controlled by a child. Sensory input is provided by splinting a body part or the whole body and limbs, and whole body and shoulder and pelvic girdle. Each child needs to be assessed before appropriate splintage is planned. Nicholson *et al.* (2001) noted improvements, though not significant, in the reach and grasp scores in Paediatric Evaluation of Disability Inventory (PEDI) scores. Rennie *et al.* (2000) also used the PEDI and found functional change in ambulatory children, but this was not significant. Reliable evidence of results is not yet available, but parents and children as well as clinical therapists give anecdotal reports of more postural stability, allowing better hand function or better sitting, walking and gait, and also control of athetoid (dyskinetic) movements. The AACPDM report by Blackmore and three occupational therapists (Blackmore *et al.* 2006) of best evidence for soft splinting with Lycra or neoprene on upper limbs studied five acceptable articles and only found one randomised controlled trial (RCT) research paper which found no evidence for grip and abdominal strength in children who used or did not use the splint. There is no RCT trial to show evidence for differences in spasticity, range of motion quality of movement, postural control, proximal stability or sensory and proprioceptive awareness. Evidence remains weak for soft or

Lycra splinting and more careful research is needed. Disadvantages range from difficulties in putting on Lycra garments, discomfort when hot, and toileting problems among other practicalities affecting compliance. There is no adequate evidence of postural control without the Lycra splinting following its use at the moment and future studies may show this (see Fig. 9.211 of arm splint used in a child with hemiplegia).

Treadmill training

This is carried out with a body harness for body weight support or partial body weight support so a child is partially unweighted so that stepping is promoted without the need for balance. Some therapists guide the lower extremities for the best pattern of stepping. Gradually the partial body weight support is reduced. The work by Schindl *et al.* (2000) is often quoted by physiotherapists as support for treadmill training in children with cerebral palsy. Their study of 10 children, 6 non-ambulant and 4 slightly ambulant with help, had 3-month training, three times a week in 25-minute sessions, in addition to usual physiotherapy. Progress was positive on the Gross Motor Function Measure (GMFM) and on a Functional Categories Measure. Unfortunately, this study is not scientific enough for clinical use as the children were few, differed greatly in age (6–18 years, mainly older, mean age 11.4) and in diagnoses (spastic diplegia, tetraplegia, athetoid tetraplegia and ataxia) and were selected for cognitive and communication abilities and no contractures. There was no matching of pairs, so controls were absent and there were no follow-up measurements once treadmill training stopped (see Chapters 4 and 8). The quality of walking pattern was not assessed except in one 18-year-old person with athetosis.

Cherng *et al.* (2007) studied eight children divided into two groups of four each, matched according to the Gross Motor Function Classification System (GMFCS) (Levels I–III). There was 12-week treatment, two–three times a week of 20-minute sessions. A number of measures were used, including gait analysis. The results were improvement in some gait parameters (in stride length and double limb support) and some GMFM scores. But no significant change was observed in muscle tone or selective motor control. More research is recommended by these researchers.

Dodd & Foley (2007) studied seven children on the treadmill. There were matched pairs but no randomised controls and children were older. There was 6-week treatment, two times a week, up to 30 minutes a session. Children used gait assistive devices, special shoes and orthoses on ground before and after the study as they were in more severe GMFCS levels (two in Level III, five in Level IV). Results were that five children improved in walking distance, six improved in speed of walking. However, two became worse, one in distance and one in both distance and speed. The treadmill training added to usual physiotherapy. The controls who carried on with usual physiotherapy showed that three subjects improved in distance and two subjects improved with speed. Unfortunately, numbers are small and diagnoses were different with four athetoid quadriplegia, two spastic quadriplegia and one diplegia. The assessors were not blind to which child was a control and which on treadmill training. However, the results on speed and distance are very positive.

Mutlu *et al.* (2009) in a systematic review of seven studies found limited evidence for treadmill training despite positive reports in gross motor and functional walking and gait parameters. Numbers were too small and trials usually need further research to establish the benefits of treadmill training for clinical settings.

My own observations are that treadmill training is useful for keeping children fit and motivated to exercise, though the treadmill is an expensive item for parents to purchase. Treadmill walking practises walking without use of visual flow, spatial perception, change in direction, and needs supervision for safety. In clinical observations, once the child was not on the treadmill, there was no change in the abnormal gait patterns.

Horse riding

There are two types of therapy on a horse: therapeutic riding (horseback riding therapy) and hippotherapy. Therapeutic riding is in a small group carried out by a specially trained instructor and may be together with a physiotherapist. Hippotherapy is one-to-one carried out by a physiotherapist giving a child various exercises on the horse. A review of 11 quantitative studies by Sterba (2007) of horseback riding and hippotherapy suggests that both riding methods are individually efficacious. There is benefit for sensorimotor experience, rhythm, motor function (particularly in independent walkers). There is mobilisation of the pelvis, lumbar spine and hip abduction with improvement of sitting posture. However, the effect on impairments is inconclusive as sample sizes were very small, and 98% of children had spastic cerebral palsy and few follow-up measures. Further research is needed especially for the more severe children, who are able to carry out hippotherapy and able to sit with a rider behind them for riding a walking horse. Other more qualitative research would report on social and psychological benefits. Parents, children and therapists continue to give anecdotal reports of these benefits. Snider *et al.* (2007), in their review on horseback riding, feel that this activity is family-oriented in a natural environment and refers to conceptual frameworks. They also suggest favourable physical effects in a child, such as symmetry in trunk and hips.

Davis *et al.* (2009) studied therapeutic horse riding for 10 weeks with three Measures for Function, Health and for changes in Quality of Life with parents and child, and found that their randomised control trial showed no clinical significant impact. Family cohesion was encouraged (see Appendix 2 for address of the Riding for the Disabled Association).

Swimming and hydrotherapy

Exercises in water is hydrotherapy, which differs from swimming therapy. Both are recommended for health reasons, physical fitness and family participation. Both can be carried out in groups for social stimulation and peer encouragement. Both need to have a suitable and safe pool environment. Access to the pool such as hoists, chair lifts, ramps and hand rails are needed for a variety of disabilities. Many children need to be able to grasp the ledge of the pool. Other safety aspects and manual handling by therapists and assistants need to be checked with the organisations involved with hydrotherapy and swimming therapy (see Appendix 2 for addresses).

Hydrotherapy focuses on strengthening and passive range of motion and stretching. Movements in water eliminate problems of postural control and balance and reduce the risks of joint loading (Kelly & Darrah 2005). The buoyancy of water makes exercises in water more motivating to many children with significant movement limitations and is welcomed by any child post-operatively. Individual sessions are used for ensuring correct movements and adequate intensity of exercises.

There is currently no study to give evidence for hydrotherapy for cerebral palsy, but special swimming techniques such as the Halliwick Method (Martin 1981) continue to show achievement of swimming by children with cerebral palsy and a complete sense of independence of movement and enjoyment of games in the pool (see Appendix 2 for address of Halliwick Association).

Specialised medical treatments

Drugs to reduce spasticity, manage epilepsy and medical management of general health problems, particularly inadequate nutrition and chest infections, are important for individual children and adults. The therapist will obtain information from the medical consultants responsible and find out from them if there are any side effects. Drugs to reduce spasticity (Albright & Neville 2000) are usually baclofen (McKinlay *et al.* 1980; Lin 2004) as an oral medication or as intrathecal infusions into the spine (Albright & Neville 2000; Miller 2007). Localised injections of botulinum toxin A to reduce spasticity and allow muscle lengthening are also used (see Chapter 11). Treatment of spasticity with any drugs is planned together with therapists, parents and carers, as therapists' programmes are essential for best results.

Selective Dorsal Rhizotomies or Selective Posterior Rhizotomies to reduce spasticity are used mainly in the United States and Canada (Peacock & Staudt 1991; Oppenheim *et al.* 1992; Steinbok *et al.* 1997a; McLaughlin *et al.* 1998; Wright *et al.* 1998; McLaughlin 2000). Selective dorsal rootlets most responsible for spasticity at the spinal levels across L2–S2 are divided. Patient selection includes children with spasticity who have underlying voluntary power; who are ambulant, intelligent and motivated; and another non-ambulant group whose spasticity prevents bathing, perineal care and positioning for daily care and classroom activities. Intensive follow-up physiotherapy for 6–12 months is needed for the post-operative weakness and training

new motor patterns as well as stretching for range (Giuliani 1992).

Assessment of pain in children is important so that appropriate drugs and other management can be given in non-verbal as well as verbal children (Wong & Baker 1988; McGrath *et al.* 1998; Hicks *et al.* 2001; Hunt *et al.* 2004; see also http://pediatric-pain.ca). Performance during therapy cannot be at a child's optimum function unless they are pain-free and comfortable. Feeding problems, which cause poor nutrition and decrease in energy for therapy, are discussed more fully in Chapter 10.

Systems-based task-oriented approach

This approach is proposed by Shumway-Cook and Woollacott (2001) for the assessment and training of posture and movement in people with neurological disabilities and motor problems, mostly in the elderly population, and for stroke. Their theoretical studies in children are also given and evidence is available for training balance in children with cerebral palsy (Shumway-Cook *et al.* 2003; Woollacott *et al.* 2005). The main aspects of this approach are as follows:

(1) Constraints on a motor task are hypothesised as:
  - motor impairment and inefficient movement strategies;
  - cognitive impairment;
  - sensory impairment.
(2) The demands of a motor task include the person's interaction with relevant features of the environment in which the task is performed. For example, the task may demand motor, cognitive and visual abilities to manage locomotion on rough, slippery surfaces, the moment when terrain changes or whether the surface is moving, unstable or stationary. Movement solutions need to be adaptable and efficient for changes in direction and at different speeds.
(3) Motor learning strategies are used to train motor behaviour. The specific task or intended goal will have a number of possible 'goal-directed' movement strategies or a variety of potentially useful solutions. The same task performed in different environments demands different movement strategies. Therefore, motor

tasks need to be learned and practised in a variety of environments and situations.

(4) Augmented feedback is given to assist the achievement of the task.
(5) Treatment mitigates impairment or disabilities, or the environment is structured for achievement of the task despite the person's impairments and disabilities. For example, this involves adapting the home and providing appropriate equipment for function.

Therapists using task-oriented approaches are also influenced by dynamic systems theory on motor control proposed by Thelen (Thelen *et al.* 1989; Kamm *et al.* 1990; Thelen 1992) among others. For example, they state that 'Development of a particular motor pattern depends on a combination of mechanical, neurologic, cognitive and perceptual factors in addition to environmental contributions specific to both the task and the context of the infant's action'.

Shumway-Cook and Woollacott mention that methods for their approach are still developing and they include selected neurofacilitation methods for adults.

Shumway-Cook and Woollacott's motor control and motor learning approach has many similarities with the movement science-based model of Carr and Shepherd (1987), Gentile (1987), Horak (1992), as well as with elements in conductive education and in learning motor function in Chapter 6 of this book.

Mobility opportunities via education (MOVE)

This is a mobility programme using learning methods. The approach originated in California, composed by a teacher in special education and a physiotherapist (Bidabe & Lollar 1990). Thomson (2005) has given a review of theories supporting MOVE. A MOVE Europe (2001) has been published. The motor tasks are broken down into components well-known to cerebral palsy physiotherapists. It uses 'prompts' for guiding movement, which are decreased as the child achieves each component after repetition. Decreasing support and guidance not termed 'prompts' with the repetition of function are also traditional in physiotherapy but not as systematically structured as in this approach. What

physiotherapists may find useful are the systematic teaching methods used to develop motor control. The programme is best used for older children with severe and profound learning problems who have poor mobility. Results state that older children and adolescents have achieved sitting, standing and walking, although this was not expected and not enthusiastically pursued in the past. Teachers are expected to give an hour's practice daily and integrate motor control within the teaching day. Practice continues by the child on his own, if possible, or with a parent in the community.

Developmental stages are arbitrarily changed with many neurological omissions in the belief that there is no time for the child to follow developmental stages of motor functions other than sitting, standing and stepping. 'Treatment' is interpreted as being related to the impairments, so the MOVE programme is not called a therapy. MOVE relates only to gaining function. Supportive equipment is linked with the training programme, and is usually selected from the Rifton catalogue.

Recently, MOVE in some special schools in Scotland has been linked with visits from physiotherapists using NDT, presumably to treat the impairments which might cause deformities and contractures. This is presumably because MOVE has been criticised for not taking adequate account of the development of deformities.

Alternative and complementary therapies. These are discussed in Chapter 2. As Chapter 2 discusses, parents, family members and others involved with a child will usually value the views and comments of the therapists on procedures which claim to help their child. Therapists need to consider offering procedures which are rational, realistic and as effective as possible in the light of current knowledge and research.

Constraint-induced movement therapy is discussed in the section 'Development of hand function' in Chapter 9. It is a treatment system for hemiplegia based on motor learning.

Contemporary theories

The dynamical systems theory, or dynamical action theory, of motor development suggests that the acquisition of motor skills emerges from dynamic interaction of multiple subsystems. Multiple systems are spontaneously self-organising in the context of a task (Thelen *et al.* 1987, 1989; Kamm *et al.* 1990; Thelen 1992; Bartlett and Palisano 2000; Law *et al.* 2007). The number of subsystems to be considered varies with different authors.

Motor learning and motor control involve interaction between an individual, the task and the environment (Shumway-Cook & Woollacott 2001). These headings help to clarify the different systems involved.

Subsystems *within the individual child* are neurological, biomechanical, musculoskeletal, sensory, perceptual, cognitive and emotional. A child's own developmental levels of all these aspects influence whether he or she has the skills to do a task and is willing to attempt a task. For the latter, a child's temperament and motivation to do a task need to be included. Some add factors of a child's size and weight as well as cardiorespiratory and nutritional states, which relate to the energy that is required for motor tasks.

Subsystems *involved in the task* (what the child is trying to do) which affect motor behaviour, such as the position, shape, texture and weight of an object for reach and grasp, or the height of a chair or table that a child uses for sitting and pulling to stand.

The environment. Subsystems such as postural control and voluntary movement, and vision in a child and in the task are influenced by factors in the environment, such as surfaces on which motor function takes place, the effect of gravity, lighting, noise and obstacles in the child's path which include crowds of people. Dynamical systems theory points out that a particular system is rate-limiting if it has not yet developed. The other developed systems need to await the development of the limiting system before a function can develop.

Motor learning approaches are included in Chapter 6.

Neuroplasticity

This theory considers the nervous system in a dynamic way. The nervous system is adaptable and changing when there are demands from the environment, from new learning, developmental processes and from a variety of experiences. The following influence the changes in the structure and neurophysiology of a developing nervous system or damaged

nervous systems in children, adolescents and adults (Kidd *et al.* 1992):

■   Practice and repetition.
■   Task-related voluntary actions for learning.
■   Movements in the context or under conditions in which they are to be used.
■   Active and purposeful sensorimotor experiences which are part of a person's daily life.
■   Early treatment takes more advantage of neuroplasticity after brain damage in children, adolescents and adults.

There are responses in the nervous system if movements are regularly practised, but synapses are cut and neural pathways disconnected if motor activity is absent. Any repetition of abnormal motor patterns results in the nervous system adapting and establishing them. On the other hand, the nervous system can be influenced by the promotion of normal motor patterns with prevention of abnormal patterns.

The neuronal group selection theory

This theory suggests that the structure and function of the nervous system depend on repeated behavioural experience, motor actions and their sensory consequences. The nervous system is continually adapting to them (Sporns and Edelman 1993; Hadders-Algra 2000 (Annotation), 2001). Neuronal selection involves primary exploration of possible variations of movement, interactions and the selection of the most efficient patterns for a useful repertoire. Ultimately, a large variety of mature motor patterns, specific for tasks, are achieved.

Each neuronal group of strongly interconnected neurons is arranged in neuronal maps. There are reciprocal connections between groups to integrate activities. This theory seems to relate more than others to the experience of moving that activates sensory receptors.

A child uses active self-generated movement to develop coordination, accurate movement and functions which relate to a variety of tasks and environmental demands. Many functional synergies become available to accomplish a task in different environments, so no 'correct' synergy exists.

This theory suggests early intervention to provide a variety of postures and movements to increase sensorimotor experiences and active functions.

Implications for therapy in cerebral palsy

The main conclusions of dynamical systems seem to be that 'we should be aware that many factors are involved in the development of motor control'. This is an excellent notion. In fact, many thoughtful clinicians, particularly those working in interdisciplinary teams, have long been aware of this. Different expert professionals have shared ideas and methods with physiotherapists on many aspects such as vision, communication, perception, biomechanics, deformities and psychological aspects. In addition, attention to the human and physical environment of a child has been observed and managed by community therapists, often together with social workers and health visitors in Britain and elsewhere. There is recognition that the child's interactions in the human environment of family, friends, therapists and teachers influence motor learning, motor control and motor development.

Therefore, one welcomes these theories which appear to support familiar views that all aspects of the whole child, his or her family, teachers and others involved with him or her provide information for therapy and management.

Shumway-Cook and Woollacott (2001) review many more theories on motor control, motor development, motor learning and on learning processes. They also adapt ideas for their approach and find limitations in all the current theories.

What guidance do we receive for practical physiotherapy from all the theories outlined?

(1) All constraints to function should be assessed and eliminated or minimised. If one alters a constraint or trains a missing element, the whole function will improve. However, it is rare that only one constraint is present in cerebral palsy.

(2) Comprehensive assessments (motor, sensory, perceptual–motor, cognitive and social and emotional) continue to be essential but need to be integrated with motor function.

(3) The whole child is in the process of development and therapy is more effective if given at a child's levels of development. Therapy is particularly effective if given when a child is attempting a more advanced motor function, which is when an individual's motor behaviour is unstable. This is in the developmental transition phases.

(4) Provide experiences of a variety of movements and postures, and give many opportunities for exploration and discovery learning. Self-generated active motor patterns are more important than passive guided movement and overuse of 'hands-on' facilitation.

(5) If a subsystem is absent, such as postural control, give postural support to a child so the other subsystems can be activated. Adapt the furniture, toys and feeding and other utensils so the child can use what subsystems he has.

(6) Early treatment and postural management offer normal motor patterns so the brain, nervous system, and musculoskeletal system can adapt or learn and so grow and develop more normally.

(7) Modify environments so that a child can function in them. Functional motor patterns need to be practised not only in the clinic but also in a child's school, playground, home and other environments which may or may not have been modified.

(8) A child may not be developmentally able to function in all environments. Basic motor control and learning need development so that this can be possible in, say, moving surfaces and slippery, rough and other physically challenging environments.

(9) Functional activities should have meaning for a child and such functions motivate a child more than the treatment of specific constraints (specific muscle tightness, weakness, stiff joints and other impairments).

(10) Use appropriate equipment, walkers and, where indicated, give manual support or guidance so that a child can achieve function in any environment and there is a feeling of success.

(11) A child's emotional and social relationships in different environments need attention or need awareness, as this also greatly affects a child's motor development.

In the past, therapists have already attempted to give attention to all or most of these factors using information and practical ideas from other professionals to integrate into their work. These principles are stated in the eclectic approach in all editions of this book. As the writing on some of the theories can be obscure and lead to different interpretations, practical methods by therapists have understandably not yet developed and there are very few publications of the models tested in clinical practice. Selected hypotheses are taken by clinicians from current theories to support methods which are specific to particular systems favoured by them. These methods still differ from system to system, though boundaries are not as sharp as in the past. This is not surprising as there are limitations in the theories, and therapists select and interpret ideas which support their practice.

Examples of limitations are:

- A child with impairments cannot self-*organise* in a normal way. If left to do so, abnormal motor patterns in, say, gaits result, which may later cause pain and discomfort. Abnormal motor patterns are useful in some cases but others may be or become inefficient.
- A baby with poverty of movement has a limited repertoire with which to gain or receive sensory and other experiences. There are few, if any, primary movement systems for dynamic development of neuronal groups given in the neuronal group theories.
- Dynamical systems theory considers that all systems are equally important. There is no acceptance of a central motor programme but only interaction of systems. Yet, with damage to the central nervous system, there are devastating disturbances to many, if not all, systems such as motor, sensory, perceptual cognitive and emotional.
- Dynamical systems theory does not identify which of the constraints are most important and how they interact in different circumstances. Is it the stiff shortening muscles, connective tissues, joint and bone adaptations? Is it perception, adequate experiences, lack of learning abilities (cognition, attention, problem-solving, memory)? Researches by Thelen and others were carried out on a treadmill and not in a child's natural environment in their experiments to develop the theory.
- If self-generated active motion is very important in motor learning and motor control, then this challenges the long periods in different postural equipment and in orthoses. Perhaps very severe conditions with almost no movement may warrant so much equipment.

It is important to recognise that the contemporary theories above are largely from research on able-bodied infants or adults with or without brain damage or on subjects with normal cognition. Therefore, not all theories will apply to the heterogeneous population who have cerebral palsy. We use our interpretations of theories as hypotheses to plan therapy programmes. We still need to test these hypotheses in research on cerebral palsy.

Campbell (2006) states that 'we remain at the mercy of theoretical knowledge rather than hard evidence'. She points out that few publications have resulted to test the theoretical models presented in clinical practice.

Evidence-based practice

4

Research and clinical studies

Whenever available, research, clinical studies and experiences of expert therapists and that of other disciplines are quoted throughout this book. Good practice depends on all of these – none of them is adequate on its own. In evidence-based practice we need to 'integrate the best external evidence with individual clinical expertise and patients' choice, it cannot result in slavish, "cookbook" approaches to individual patient care' (Sackett *et al.* 1996).

After all, each physiotherapist or occupational therapist wants to know that her intervention or treatment produces benefit to a child and his family. Throughout the history of management of cerebral palsy, practitioners have kept records of their patients. Clinicians need to reflect on their own practice with careful observation and good records (APCP 2002). In this way, clinicians may be able to formulate questions for research or clinical studies to confirm their findings.

Research and academic therapists communicate current scientific studies by presentation and publication so that an up-to-date rationale for practice is developed. In a therapist's experience and knowledge, there are insights enabling them to be critical of published research. Ideally, there needs to be a dialogue between researchers and clinicians so that research is not isolated from practice. When there

is an absence of evidence of effectiveness, this is not evidence of ineffective treatment. Hence, further research is needed so that better evidence for effective practice can be gained.

Research on treatment approaches

All the various treatment systems claim good results. It is difficult to decide which system is superior, whether on theoretical grounds or on the basis of a scientific study. Clinical experience of many therapists, as well as my own, has not confirmed the superiority of any one approach.

As therapists 'want to know what is the best thing to do for children', there has been a focus on which therapy approach is superior. Perhaps this is not a worthy aim to pursue on theoretical grounds or research studies.

Theoretical grounds

Every therapist wishes to understand 'why we do what we do' and, unfortunately, may accept a therapy system because it offers a ready explanation. However, there is no all-encompassing theory which fully explains all the abnormal motor behaviour presented by people with the different cerebral palsies. In addition, theories may not adequately explain the effects of various treatment systems or, in some cases, of specific procedures. Theories also do not fully clarify mechanisms underlying motor behaviour from infancy to adulthood. Each therapy approach is based on scientific evidence available at the time, and the neurofacilitation systems are based on a number of controversial neurophysiological hypotheses. There are currently newer theories on motor learning and motor control. However, controversies exist, so current neuroscience and behavioural psychology do not favour a single model for motor behaviour. Therapists continue to work with an underlying theoretical framework with some scientific evidence but also with assumptions about motor control, motor development or motor learning. Increasing scientific understanding of brain function and motor behaviour will contribute to therapy and its knowledge base. Therapists will need to judge the relevance of such studies and advances and apply them to clinical work. It is still unwise to be dogmatic about a theoretical framework or about procedures which arise from that. Therapy techniques cannot fully rest on different and more current theories underlying motor control or motor learning. We still have to learn to live with these doubts.

Although the therapist should continue to ask herself why she is using a particular method, this enquiry should focus more on the careful observations of motor behaviour and any changes in behaviour after treatment procedures. Increasing clinical studies and research, together with clinical experience, will offer scientific evidence underpinning treatment procedures. Therapists need to draw on those studies which are relevant to their particular patients/clients.

Contemporary theories are discussed in Chapter 3.

Research studies

These are fraught with many problems and to date no study to compare the value of different treatment systems has convincingly dealt with all the problems. Firstly, the results of treatment are influenced by the methods dictated not only by the concept of an approach but by the severity of motor function and impairments, age and sex of an individual. Secondly, results are influenced by possible associated impairments and disabilities of vision, hearing, communication, perception, cognition as well as by the presence of epilepsy and poor health. A child's personality and 'drive' as well as his home background contribute to the results of therapy. One must also recognise that the therapist's enthusiasm, personality and her abilities to make positive professional relationships as well as her technical skill may have a strong effect on the results of treatment with any method.

There are other problems. The results of a scientific study would have to be obtained over a long period of time as progress is slow. At least a 6-month follow-up is now generally recommended. Crothers pointed out many years ago that one would really need a follow-up to adulthood to establish the ultimate effects of treatment methods in childhood (Crothers & Paine 1959; Levitt 1962; Paine 1962). However, this view needs to be reassessed with more current information on the deterioration related to specific physiological and psychological factors in older persons with cerebral palsy.

Reviews of research studies

The research studies that have been carried out on therapy interventions have been reviewed by Parette and Hourcade (1984) for the period 1952–1982, by Tirosh and Rabino (1989) for the period 1973–1988, by Siebes *et al.* (2002) from 1990 to 2001 and by Anttila *et al.* (2008) from 1990 to 2007. They all found in their reviews that the research designs were not rigorous enough and they discuss the problems facing researchers. Siebes *et al.* (2002) point out that although the methodology in research studies had clearly improved, this did not lead 'to a substantial improvement in the scientific foundation' of the motor interventions for children with or at risk for cerebral palsy.

Tirosh and Rabino (1989) suggest that a much larger number of subjects in a multicentre study should iron out many variables and that more reliable data might be obtained. They pointed out the importance of psychosocial influences. Bower and McLellan (1992) found pitfalls in eight major studies, most of which are included in Tirosh and Rabino's review. A review of studies specifically on the neurodevelopmental treatment (NDT/Bobath) approach by Butler and Darrah (2001), such as Siebes *et al.* (2002), classifies levels of evidence from I down to V. Both these reviews find that two-thirds of the studies are below Levels I and II. Furthermore, each of these reviews shows that the more scientific the study, the fewer the number of statistically significant results due to therapy.

Studies of specific treatment systems

Palmer et al. (1988) found NDT less effective than a global developmental programme. The NDT review by Butler and Darrah, approved by the American Academy for Cerebral Palsy and Developmental Medicine (AACPDM) Treatment Outcomes Committee Review Panel, has been mentioned above. They state that the 'preponderance of results did not confer any advantage to NDT over the alternatives to which it was compared'. Brown and Burns (2001) considered 147 articles of which only 17 studies met scientific criteria. These studies found insufficient evidence for NDT and the results were largely inconclusive. There are studies in the past which claim to support NDT, but their design is inadequate. For example, the study by Jonsdottir *et al.* (1997) did show that 'NDT seemed more effective than practice for improvement of postural alignment during reaching', but like other studies it only used a small number of subjects and for a short time of 5 days, without follow-up. In early treatment, Blauw-Hospers and Hadders-Algra (2005) found that specific or general developmental programmes had a positive effect whereas NDT was not beneficial. Of 17 papers, 12 were of high methodology (research levels I and II) in their study of early treatment.

The Doman-Delacato system was found unproven in results by Sparrow and Zigler (1978) and by Cummins (1988). Vojta's approach (see Vojta (1989) or von Aufschnaiter (1992) for recent account) received criticism by Jones (1975) and Forssberg and Hirschfeld (1992). Vojta's list of postural reflexes is not accepted by Norén and Franzén

(1982) as a reliable measure of diagnosis and results. The results of Vojta's very early therapy for babies at risk as well as any other early intervention such as that of Kong (1987) and Katona (1989) cannot show that it was the intervention that obtained results and not the fact that babies 'at risk' might have become normal anyway. Nelson and Ellenberg (1982) and Touwen (1987) point out how unreliable early diagnoses can be. Nelson and Ellenberg found in their large sample of infants suspected of cerebral palsy that there was a high rate of these infants becoming normal. However, neonatal studies by paediatric therapists continue and show positive value for intervention.

Carlsen (1975) showed improvement using methods from Rood (1962), sensory integration, proprioceptive neuromuscular facilitation and NDT compared to a functional occupational therapy approach. She had a small sample of 12 children.

Conductive education

Bairstow *et al.* (1991, 1993) carried out studies on conductive education (CE) compared with a neurophysiological and developmental approach in a selected group necessary for CE. No difference was found between these two groups. However, the assessors were aware which children were in the intervention group and which were in the non-intervention (control) group. Reddihough *et al.* (1998) carried out a comparative study of traditional therapy and CE which showed little difference in outcomes, provided equal intensity of therapy sessions were used. This is not always so with traditional therapy. Johanna Darrah with three physiotherapists (Darrah *et al.* 2004) carried out a thorough review of evidence for CE, approved by the AACPDM. Fifteen studies met the inclusion criteria. The studies included many aspects such as motor function, daily living activities, communication, various educational aspects, social skills and parent satisfaction. Only four studies are rated I and II, and there were many difficulties in obtaining information about the subjects' specific activities and the heterogeneity in various studies. The result is that there is no conclusive evidence in support or against CE as an intervention strategy. The focus of CE on daily life function and education may fit the needs of many families but cost, time, availability and effects on family dynamics need to be considered in view of current lack of strong evidence. Further research is recommended.

Odman and Oberg (2005) have carried out studies on Move&Walk, an intensive Swedish CE programme with conductors educated in Hungary, compared with an intensive rehabilitation programme with an eclectic approach called Lemo with two physiotherapists and a special educational needs teacher. Children were aged 3–16 years. Both programmes emphasised parents' and assistants' (carers') participation. No major difference in function was shown between the two training programmes. Odman *et al.* (2007) explored parents' perceptions in Move&Walk and Lemo, finding that high-level service quality and achieved expectations influenced parents more than their perceived functional improvements of their children. No difference was present in their perceived functional outcomes. Most parents perceived high-level service quality. The parents in the Lemo approach perceived better service quality than those in the Move&Walk and were more involved in discussions about expectations and knowledge exchange.

Research on specific procedures

Single-case studies to evaluate specific treatment procedures together with more sensitive and more specific measures for cerebral palsy are suggested in a review of research by Siebes *et al.* (2002). Single-case studies have increased and are useful for evaluation of procedures such as training methods for strength, for constraint-induced function in hemiplegia, methods for postural control with arm reach (balance), use of below-knee plaster casts (inhibitory casts), ankle-foot orthoses and similar procedures. For example, the research study of Damiano *et al.* (1995a) evaluated the effects of specific strengthening methods of quadriceps and showed that these procedures improved crouch gait.

Single-case studies, carefully designed, with an *appropriate* number of subjects offer useful results for research on therapy. Research designs are discussed below. Single-case study design is discussed by Kazdin (1982), Edwards *et al.* (1990) and Riddoch and Lennon (1991).

Other research

A series of research studies in cerebral palsy have been carried out by E. Bower and D.L. McLellan, investigating the effect of intensive physiotherapy with specific measurable goals. All the studies use the Gross Motor Function Measure (GMFM; Russell *et al.* 1989, 2002). The first pilot study (Bower & McLellan 1992) used a controlled series of single-case studies with only seven children. The trend was that increased intensity for 3 weeks with goal setting generally improved the rate of progress as compared to routine physiotherapy. The intensive treatment was carried out by the researcher.

In a subsequent randomized controlled study of 44 children (Bower *et al.* 1996), the subjects were assigned to four different groups of 11, with careful checks being made that each group was similar. Intensive physiotherapy was given for 2 weeks to two of the groups, one with general aims and the other with specific goals for physiotherapy. The other two groups received routine physiotherapy for 2 weeks, again one with general aims and the other with specific goals. The study showed that intensive therapy together with specific goals can accelerate the acquisition of motor function. There was no follow-up to see whether these gains were subsequently maintained.

A further study of 56 children (Bower *et al.* 2001) used four groups as before. However, the period of routine or intensive therapy lasted 6 months and, unlike the 1996 study, there was a period of 6-month routine therapy (about half an hour a week) with aims (baseline observation period) before the treatment period and a similar (follow-up) period afterwards. In the baseline period, there was some progress which accelerated with intensive therapy (average 3.5 hours a week). The mean total score on the GMFM improved by 5.9 percentage points on intensive therapy, whereas by only 3.1 percentage points on routine therapy. There was no difference as to whether aims or goals were used in the intensive or routine treatment period. The follow-up 6 months later showed that the average child did not maintain the lead gained during the intensive therapy. However, despite this obvious difference, Bower reports that the lead during the treatment period was not statistically significant.

Studies of rhizotomy by Steinbok *et al.* (1997a), McLaughlin *et al.* (1998) and Wright *et al.* (1998)

provide data on rates of progress on the GMFM during intensive physiotherapy alone. These show a range of average gains of 4.2–5.2 percentage points over a period of 9–12 months. This is less than the gain of 5.9 points from 6-month intensive therapy found by Bower *et al.* (2001).

Clinical experience with evidence-based practice

Today, what evidence of the evaluation of therapy is available to the clinician?

(1) *Professional experience*. We still use findings from long experience of our own and of acknowledged experts in the field. Careful observations, reflections and clinical reasoning from practical experience and from related existing studies remain important.

(2) *Measures of outcome*. Current practice continues to develop objective evaluations of outcomes (results) of motor training or treatment which are not biased by a school of thought or therapy system. There are still methods of assessment and reassessment which are often self-validating in terms of the theories of an approach. Because the theories or concepts are controversial, such evaluation measures of progress are not objective enough. However, objective measures themselves may not be sensitive or specific enough to pick up the outcomes. Therefore, measures need to be developed to be more specific and to reduce the risk of subjectivity of any measures. Measures for evaluation of clinical therapy outcomes are discussed in Chapter 8.

(3) *Research studies*. These are an increasingly valuable source of evidence for therapy. They offer quantitative or qualitative evidence for the value and effectiveness of physiotherapy and occupational therapy.

Quantitative research aims to measure the effects of a particular intervention and presents the results as numerical data. Such research uses experimental designs to test hypotheses, as discussed below.

Qualitative research aims to identify and describe the common experiences and relationships of all those involved in treatments, including the therapists (Patton 1980). It is exploratory by design and is often called 'client-centred' because it is concerned with the meaning that treatments and outcomes have for the patient (client). When the research involves a patient's family, the term 'family-centred' is more appropriate. Studies can show how therapy or specific therapy methods affect the individual's thoughts and feelings about their quality of life, their perception of their disability and of their ideas about changes in their bodies. The collection of data uses methods such as specialised focus groups, semi-structured interviews or open-ended questionnaires.

The different research styles of quantitative and qualitative studies provide different kinds of useful information and are complementary. They are each scientific in that their different methods are rigorous, systematic and disciplined (Stone 1991). Most of the research in cerebral palsy therapy has been quantitative, whereas qualitative research is relatively new in the whole field of rehabilitation. Some issues such as quality of life and empathy can be studied by quantitative methods using scales derived from counselling, psychology and psychotherapy. It is also possible to combine interviews of a sample of people and present some of the findings quantitatively (Bailey & Simeonsson 1988; Ross & Thomson 1993; Rosenbaum *et al.* 1998; Odman *et al.* 2007). There are also surveys on, say, attitudes which give numbers of the particular responses. This is not really qualitative research.

In order for the paediatric therapist to develop the skills of critical appraisal and so appreciate these studies and consider their clinical relevance, the following discussions can be helpful.

Systematic reviews

The best evidence comes from papers that systematically review all the research studies that have been published on a particular question. In a systematic review, the research design used in each study is assessed using a scale (or hierarchy) often called the 'Levels of evidence' (see below). Unfortunately, systematic reviews of research in cerebral palsy frequently conclude that there have been too few high-quality studies for reliable conclusions to be drawn – so 'further research is needed'.

Nevertheless, there are more and more reviews being published, particularly under the auspices of the AACPDM. The Physiotherapy Evidence Database (PEDro; www.pedro.fhs.usyd.edu.au) currently lists more than 35 systematic reviews related to cerebral palsy. It includes reviews from the Cochrane Library and AACPDM.

Another way of considering the results of a number of studies is a *meta-analysis*, in which data from a number of similar studies are combined and so the resulting larger sample size is more likely to give statistically significant results. In cerebral palsy at present, there are relatively few meta-analyses.

Levels of evidence

These are scales used to assess research designs derived from the original work of Sackett *et al.* (1996, 2001). Most of the scales have five levels, with Level I being the highest, although levels are sometimes further subdivided.

'In descending order, the designs are decreasingly able to demonstrate that the intervention – and not something else – was responsible for the observed outcome. Level I evidence is the most definitive for establishing causality, with greatest reduction in bias. Level IV can only hint at it; Level V only *suggests* the possibility' (AACPDM 2004).

For research into cerebral palsy, the most commonly used classification scheme is that adopted by the AACPDM (2004) in its 'Methodology to Develop Systematic Reviews of Treatment Interventions' (see the AACPDM website: www.aacpdm.org). An example of its use is in the botulinum toxin A systematic review (Lannin *et al.* 2006). Another scheme for levels of evidence was created by the Scottish Intercollegiate Guidelines Network (SIGN, www.sign.ac.uk), which has eight levels and is highly detailed. It is important to remember that the level of evidence is only one way to appraise a study for evidence-based clinical work. More details are needed for clinical evidence and these are discussed below under the section 'The appraisal of research studies for therapy'.

The AACPDM levels of evidence are as follows:

Level	Intervention (group) studies
I	Systematic reviews of randomised controlled trials (RCTs) Large RCTs (with narrow confidence intervals – high probability of certainty) (more than 100 subjects)
II	Smaller RCTs (with wider confidence intervals) (fewer than 100 subjects) Systematic reviews of cohort studies
III	Cohort studies (must have concurrent control group) Systematic reviews of case-control studies
IV	Case series Cohort study without concurrent control group (e.g. with historical control group) Case-control study
V	Expert opinion Case study or report Bench research Expert opinion based on theory or physiologic research Common sense/anecdotes

Definitions

Case-control study. A retrospective study which compares subjects who received the intervention (the 'cases') with subjects who did not receive the intervention but are otherwise similar (the 'controls').

Case series. A case series can be retrospective or prospective and usually involves a smaller number of patients than more powerful case-control studies or randomised controlled trials.

Cohort. A group of subjects with a common defining characteristic.

Confidence interval. The narrower the confidence interval, the greater the degree of certainty in the result.

Control group. A comparison group which does not receive the intervention but is as similar as possible to the group being studied.

Randomised controlled trial. Subjects are randomly assigned either to the treated group or to the control group.

The PEDro lists numerous *randomised controlled trials* and grades the quality of research design by using a checklist of 10 items, all of which should be present in the best design. The number of items present gives a mark out of 10. For cerebral palsy research, no study scores higher than 8/10 and many have much lower scores. Some studies which score high on this scale for significant treatment effects do not necessarily provide evidence that the treatment is clinically practical. This is where the therapist's own clinical experience and professional judgement are necessary to assess the relevance to their situation.

The appraisal of research studies for therapy

The clinical therapist needs to consider some fundamental issues when deciding whether a research study is relevant and worth applying for the child or children she is treating. Consultations with research workers as well as participation in journal clubs and discussion groups can facilitate critical appraisals of research.

The points below can be helpful in appraising a research study, which could be either quantitative or qualitative:

(1) *The questions asked.* A research study seeks information about specific questions. These need to be clearly stated, so that a practitioner can decide whether they are questions to which she too would welcome some answers or more information to improve her practice. Research questions may be on:
    (a) The impairment.
    (b) The motor function (task) or its components.
    (c) The participation in society as a result of therapy.
    (d) The organisation which affects therapy results.
    Questions which *assume* a particular theory or therapy system are controversial. This is especially true if the researcher is clearly wedded to that system.
(2) *The sample of children studied.* The characteristics of the children studied (subjects) must be stated, such as age, sex, severity, diagnosis and any associated disabilities that affect motor function. In some studies, culture, family and socio-economic background need stating,

as they are relevant. The clinician can then judge whether the sample of children in the study is similar to the individual(s) she is treating.

The sample size is very important. The larger the number of children in the sample, the higher the probability of obtaining statistically significant results. Furthermore, if there are only three or four subjects studied, then the results cannot be generalised to the population of interest to the clinician.

(3) *The intervention methods.* These methods or techniques need to be identified, as different therapists use different methods. For example, individual NDT (Bobath) trained physiotherapists frequently use different methods for the same aims of this approach. Eclectic physiotherapists may well use different methods for an eclectic approach.

There is increasing research into which specific method or strategy from a system or from an eclectic approach is responsible for results. This is important when a therapist uses a 'named' system which is a box of methods based on a concept. This is the question facing both researchers and clinicians which identifies which methods to use in an eclectic approach. We need the type of study that focuses on one well-defined treatment method aimed at a specific problem, such as plaster casts for a dynamically short spastic muscle group to evaluate a method.

The length of *time* of intervention needs to be reasonable. Some research shows that 'reasonable' in the eyes of a therapist may be a burden for a child or for his parent or anyone else who is involved in enabling the study to continue.

Some studies need to confirm ongoing cooperation in all the children and their parents. For example, Chappell and Williams (2002) have studied non-adherence to home physiotherapy in paediatrics. The reasons for lack of 'compliance' are a subject for both qualitative and quantitative research. Qualitative research may lead to quantitative research to complement understanding of an issue. On the other hand, as an example, quantitative research can lead to qualitative research (McBurney *et al.* 2003).

Cooperative children *practise* methods at home or elsewhere. We need to take account of this variable, as practice influences results. Other activities such as occupational therapy or therapeutic horse riding can also affect physiotherapy results.

Furthermore, *the length of a session* (an hour or half hour) and the *frequency of sessions* per week must be stated, as longer or more sessions may perhaps account for the results.

(4) The setting or environment may be relevant for a child or older person's competent performance (Tieman *et al.* 2004). Children may perform better at home during play, with their peer group, with a special friend or particular family member. For example, a study comparing motor function in a special adventure playground with function in a physiotherapy department found differences in motor performance (Levitt 1975). The setting of the research may need to be obvious or stated.

Specific points in quantitative research

(1) *Evaluation tools.* The measurement tools must be appropriate and measure what the research claims to evaluate. These measures of outcome have to be stated and be accepted as standardised and applicable to the clinician's interests. For example, measures used by doctors or psychologists do not necessarily have the details that interest physiotherapists (see Chapter 8).

One needs to consider whether the measures are suitable for particular questions. It may be more appropriate to use qualitative evaluation methods which are quite different from the 'numbers' used in quantitative research. These are outlined below.

(2) *Research designs.* The effect of a specific intervention or treatment should be evaluated by comparing it with the effect of routine intervention. The subjects receiving this routine intervention are called *the controls or control group.* Routine intervention can be either their usual therapy or only parent-handling at home. For example, Wright and Nicholson (1973) had a 'no-treatment' control group which received a parent-handling programme. But others compare physiotherapy or a specific intervention with passive range of movement as a control.

The comparison in a research design can be with the same subject in single-case studies where the subject is compared with himself so that he is his own control. A single-case study can compare the subject with a different group of subjects (the control group). A series of single-case studies can be used, provided the numbers of subjects are large enough to give statistically significant results.

(a) The simplest acceptable single-case design (the ABA design) starts with a baseline period (A) in which the subject receives everyday therapy or no therapy. This reveals the variations and the role of *maturation* in the behaviour (motor or other) of the individual child. This is followed by a period (B) in which the treatment to be evaluated is given and should be followed by another period of A. This second A period shows whether the progress, or lack of progress, measured in B, continues once the specific treatment is no longer given. The results of treatment may not be maintained once a specific therapy is stopped (Bower & McLellan 1992).

(b) The simplest control-group design consists of two groups: a treated group and a control group. If subjects are assigned at random to one of the groups, then it is an RCT. This randomisation aims to produce two groups that are as similar as possible but the researchers should demonstrate that chance differences are not biasing the results (see below).

If the study is an RCT, then it should be in the PEDro database (unless it is very recent) and should have been given a score as to its quality.

(3) *Sources of bias and error.* There are various reasons why the research may not be comparing what it is supposed to:

(a) The subjects in the control group may differ too much from those in the treated group. As well as random assignment, there may also be an attempt to match subjects in different groups. The research always needs to show that the groups are sufficiently similar. People with cerebral palsies are a very heterogeneous population and, consequently, matching subjects is difficult. The common characteristics which are considered are age, diagnosis, severity, intelligence and the presence of additional impairments. Moreover, the study should not be influenced by other variables such as social, emotional, cultural, economic and other unknowns. Variables such as occupational therapy and other activities should be similar in both groups in a physiotherapy study. An example of unmatched severity can be detected in the research of Kanda *et al.* (1984), who showed that early Vojta treatment under 6 months obtained better results than the same treatment after 9 months, but the younger group were less severe than the older group.

(b) The therapists carrying out the treatment should be independent of the research because therapists are expected to be highly motivated, to be helpful and see results of their work. It is wise to have a number of therapists carrying out a procedure to be tested, in case the research is really a test of one therapist's skill. All therapists should be of professionally acknowledged skill.

(c) The assessors measuring the effects should not know (be 'blind' to) which child has received which treatment; otherwise they may unwittingly bias their measurements.

(d) Ideally, the subjects (children and their parents/carers) and the treating therapists should be 'blind' to what treatment is taking place. In practice, it is pretty obvious that a different procedure is being used.

(4) *Analysis of results.* Graphs need to be clear when giving results to the clinician. They are useful for ABA research designs, as they can show trends during each of these three periods. For example, an upward trend in the first A period may be markedly increased in period B. The trend in the second A period shows whether any gains made during period B are *maintained*, once the bout of intervention has stopped.

Research studies differ from routine clinical measures and assessments in that statistical methods are used. Statistics are needed because people are variable and cerebral palsy is a heterogeneous condition. These statistics should be explained and not be so obscure that the clinician cannot decide on the value of the study.

Results are given as differences between the groups of children studied. These differences or changes in outcome may be positive, non-existent or even negative. However, the change may be a fluke or due to unknown factors which give a chance result, and the purpose of statis-

tical analysis is to show whether the change is genuinely due to the intervention. This is what the phrase 'statistically significant' means. This is stated as a *p*-value. A *p*-value less than 0.05 is taken to show that the results are statistically significant.

Remember, a statistically significant result is no guarantee that the research is worthwhile unless all the elements of the research are satisfactory. Clinicians and research workers are more knowledgeable about those elements than are statisticians. But even if the change is statistically significant, it could be quite small and may not be 'humanly significant'. Is it worth people making the effort in time, energy and money? Is it great enough to warrant a change to clinical practice? Changes in specific impairments or elements of function may only give minor gains in an activity (function). Quality of life can matter more than a large, statistically significant increase in, say, active ranges of movement.

Studies which use large numbers of children are more likely to give statistically significant results, as they can average out the variability. However, if a study is focused on one well-defined treatment procedure aimed at a specific impairment and if the effect is quite a marked change post-treatment, then a small number of children is acceptable. Even a control group is not absolutely necessary. Clinicians know the usual history of such cases in the short term.

Statistical significance cannot be calculated for only one or two cases. In addition, one cannot generalise from one or two cases to all children with the same condition. Certainly a marked improvement in a clinical case encourages the therapist to try out the treatment with other similar children. There are difficulties in recruiting enough children at a local level to participate in a statistically significant study, in which case a multicentred trial would be a good way forward.

Specific points in qualitative research

In considering the value of qualitative studies, Greenhalgh and Taylor (1997) have made some helpful suggestions. The paper by Greenhalgh and Taylor is 'How to read a paper: papers that go beyond numbers (qualitative research)', which may seem 'unscientific' to some workers accustomed to quantitative studies. As already mentioned above, there can be equal quality checks to ensure rigour and trustworthiness in this research approach.

In an appraisal of a qualitative research paper, one considers the following:

Was a qualitative research appropriate for the clearly formulated question?

Consideration of the methods used and that a number of methods needed to be included.

The results need to appear credible and also important.

The conclusions drawn have to be justified.

Consideration of whether the results can apply in other settings, that is generalised.

Examples of qualitative research methods (Greenhalgh & Taylor 1997)

Documents. Study of documentary accounts of events, such as meetings.

Passive observation. Systematic watching of behaviour and talk in natural occurring settings.

Participant observation. Observation in which the researcher also occupies a role or part in the setting, in addition to observing.

In-depth interviews. Face-to-face conversation with the purpose of exploring issues or topics in detail. Does not use preset questions, but is shaped by a defined set of topics.

Focus groups. Method of group interview which explicitly includes and uses the group interaction to generate data.

The additional aspects which need to be checked in a qualitative study are the following:

(1) Was confidentiality and anonymity assured in sensitive information?
(2) The subjects need to be able to communicate verbally. The children and parents need to be interviewed in some studies.
(3) The researcher needs to have checked with the subjects that their quoted statements in the transcripts of interviews about the issues are accurate.
(4) The quality control is also having the researcher's findings shown to other independent researchers to check any bias in the researcher's perspective.
(5) There are a growing number of assessments in qualitative research.

The use of qualitative research in health is devised or carried out by social scientists or medical sociologists.

The clinical practitioner needs to consult colleagues who are research therapists for further discussion.

The useful references on research methods are Kazdin (1982), Ottenbacher (1986), Hicks (2004), Whalley Hammell and Carpenter (2004) and Greenhalgh (2006).

Synthesis of treatment systems 5

The eclectic viewpoint in therapy

In Chapter 4, there is a discussion on the lack of scientific evidence for theories and methods of therapy approaches in cerebral palsy. Based on studies of many therapy systems, over many years, it has always been difficult to confine oneself to any particular system as each includes valuable contributions. Therefore, an eclectic approach has been and still is recommended (Levitt 1962, 1970a, 1974, 1976, and continuously developed, in the light of new ideas, in all editions of this book since 1977).

The eclectic viewpoint has become increasingly accepted. McLellan (1984), Griffiths and Clegg (1988), Dietz (1992) and Burns and MacDonald (1996) recognise elements of value in many different approaches and that selection of methods for an individual child is advisable. In the United States, Umphred (1984) and Farber (1982) suggested integrated approaches, quoting other colleagues who support this. Mayston (2004), a well-known proponent of the Bobath approach and former director of the Bobath Centre, London, states that 'little or no evidence is available to show that therapy offered by the "named approaches" is effective or that one approach is more beneficial than another'. She says that the Bobath approach is becoming eclectic (Mayston 2004).

Damiano (2004) discourages following any specific therapy system, pointing out that there are increasing numbers of research studies supporting specific treatment procedures which are not dependent on any system and its philosophy. Fortunately, research evidence is being accumulated for specific methods for an eclectic approach; yet there is still more research needed on methods found useful by observant and highly experienced physiotherapists. We still await research studies as to their value for specific children, at different ages, as to how often, how much and how early methods need to be used.

In Britain, studies by Bower et al. (1996, 2001) mention that most British physiotherapists use an eclectic approach, and also find that this best meets families' needs. Since 1990, the Association of Paediatric Chartered Physiotherapists in their guidelines for good practice (APCP 2002) have recommended that physiotherapists 'select appropriately from the various approaches for each individual child'. Their most recent guidelines (APCP 2007) continue to recommend this.

Different varieties of eclectic practice

It would be difficult to evaluate an 'eclectic approach' as there are different varieties of practice.

The diversity of the cerebral palsies, children's different ages and their variety of experience and different family backgrounds inevitably create individual eclectic programmes. Selection from different therapy approaches varies according to the knowledge, skill and experience of particular therapists, which is fortunately developing. Some therapists combine better teaching methods with neurodevelopmental techniques (Horn *et al*. 1995). Others select different neurofacilitation methods from either some or all the experts in neurofacilitation, such as Rood, Vojta, Bobath, Knott and Voss, but without understanding or use of any motor learning models. Others combine one complete system with another system, though one needs assessments for thoughtful selection from each. Combining two therapy approaches can even be largely contradictory in concept and methods for an individual child. Furthermore, two systems enthusiastically used for a child may well demand too many therapy sessions without regard for many other aspects of a quality of life for that child and family.

In developing my eclectic approach to create a synthesis, it has been necessary to try to understand the different rationales underlying the methods in various therapy systems. Contemporary research offers more rationales and should continue to do so.

At first, the systems appear different and even contradictory to one another. However, this is not really the case. Although there are differences, there are also areas of common ground. The following discoveries emerged in my comparative study of the theory and practice of various treatment approaches – neurophysiological, developmental, orthopaedic and motor learning:

(1) Different rationales are given by different systems for the same or similar methods. The common ground is the method, but the reasons offered differ.
(2) In some instances, the rationale and methods are not really different, but either the rationale or the methods are only couched in different terminologies. The common ground can be both the method and the reason for it.
(3) In other instances, the rationales are the same, only couched in different terminologies, but the methods suggested differ from system to system. The common ground is the rationale but methods differ. Currently, there are new theo-

ries (see Chapter 3), yet methods are not always quite different, and even old, habitual methods continue to be used and said to be directly related to these theories. This either supports or leads to questioning of the methods used.
(4) There are still differences in methods and rationale, which need understanding so that contradictory methods are avoided in an individual child at a specific level of development.
(5) Although methods may even differ, they are sometimes given the same name.

I have attempted to analyse and clarify this complicated field, over many years, in order to bring together isolated but valuable pockets of knowledge. During these studies, it has also been difficult to know which methods and ideas in any particular system are the ones which are responsible for the results achieved. In any system, there are methods and ideas which are superfluous. It is not correct that 'everything in a system depends on everything else'.

Methods and ideas have been selected rather more according to the functional problems of the children than according to the changing neurophysiological and different motor learning theories. In this way, a synthesis of treatment can be made. This continues to develop as research studies increase to show which methods improve specific problems, related directly to functions. Also, at which developmental stages are methods used and for which children.

Synthesis of treatment systems

A synthesis of therapy and management approaches is based on consideration of postural mechanisms, voluntary motion and perceptual-motor function intrinsic to function. It is particularly function that must draw on learning/teaching methods. Any synthesis for motor function development cannot be divorced from the emotional and social concerns of children, their parents and families. Synthesis also selects those methods which can enhance a child's functional experiences in his daily life in home, school, playground and community.

Despite different terminologies and methods, the following aspects of motor function are fundamental to various approaches of treatment and management of motor disorders in cerebral palsy:

(1) The postural mechanisms.
(2) Voluntary motion.
(3) Perceptual-motor function.

The postural mechanisms

The postural mechanisms are neurological mechanisms which maintain posture and equilibrium and are included in locomotion. Sensory information from visual, proprioceptive, vestibular and tactile input are involved with the postural mechanisms. The importance of particular sensory systems varies during typical postural development. Young children until about age 3 years find vision more important than proprioception for postural control, whereas adults depend more on the proprioceptive input for postural control (Lee & Aronson 1974). Fully developed postural mechanisms, other than tilt reactions, are exhibited by adults who are blindfolded. Tilt reactions need vestibular and visual perception.

Postural mechanisms have been described by various neurological workers (Martin 1965, 1967; Belenkii *et al.* 1967; Foley 1977, 1998; Marsden *et al.* 1981; Shumway-Cook & Woollacott 2001; Visser & Bloem 2005; Hadders-Algra & Carlberg 2008; among others). Paediatric physiotherapists first need to focus on postural mechanisms of stability and related postural adjustment, and add training of righting, saving and tilt reactions in both active as well as reactive methods to develop motor function.

Purdon Martin's presentation (Martin 1967; Foley 1998) has drawn on many neurological studies at the time and used their own observations or studies. Purdon Martin's clear functional scheme originally provided me with a practical observational framework for clarifying many terminologies and methods in different treatment approaches. In this book there have been slight modifications related to children with cerebral palsies and in view of new research.

Whatever the terminologies and different viewpoints, there are methods to stimulate or train postural mechanisms within most treatment approaches. However, particular systems have emphasised some, but not all, of these postural mechanisms. Some assessments for therapy such as Chailey Levels of Ability (Pountney *et al.* 2004) and Gross Motor Function Measure (Russell *et al.* 1989) omit examination of the tilt and the saving postural mechanisms as their therapy emphasises other aspects. Children with cerebral palsy with severe visual impairments, severe intellectual problems or with perceptual-motor difficulties are among those individuals who cannot function safely and fully independently without all the postural mechanisms (Levitt 1984, Chapters 9 and 14; Butler & Major 1992; Hirschfeld 1992; Butler 1998; Foley 1998; Shumway-Cook & Woollacott 2001; Hadders-Algra & Carlberg 2008).

It is important to draw on all treatment approaches which have methods for postural mechanisms to make sure that none of an individual's potential postural mechanisms are omitted. There need to be methods for a child's active initiation as well as for automatic or reactive aspects of postural control. Hadders-Algra *et al.* (1996) have shown that increased experience improves postural control in the developing nervous system of normal babies. Training postural control in cerebral palsy provides positive results in sitting (Hadders-Algra & Carlberg 2008, Chapter 4) as well as in standing (Shumway-Cook *et al.* 2003). Those therapy approaches that have given attention to all the problems of postural mechanisms have not necessarily suggested methods to cover the needs of all children and older people. Therefore, methods need to be selected from different approaches and from eclectic clinicians so that dormant motor controls of postural mechanisms can be activated in an individual as much as is possible. Whenever possible, postural mechanisms are activated in the context of a function desired by an individual with cerebral palsy. Suggestions are given in Chapters 9, 10 and 12.

The postural mechanisms are given mainly in the terminology of the functional scheme of Martin (1967) and illustrated in the practical chapters. Other terminologies are mentioned when known.

In outline they consist of the following:

The antigravity mechanism or the mechanism which helps to support the weight of the body against gravity. This provides a pillar of the limb for support against gravity. This firm pillar becomes more flexible with development of the postural mechanisms discussed above.

This is also known as the *supporting reaction* in infants, *leg straightening reflex* or *positive statzreaktion*, and similar to *infantile co-contraction*.

The postural stabilisation (automatic fixation) of parts of the body, including head on trunk, trunk on pelvis, stabilisation of the shoulder girdles and pelvic girdles and the muscular activity of lower jaw, tongue and pharynx. Postural stabilisation of the body as a whole takes place in a variety of positions. In upright sitting and standing, there is vertical alignment of body parts and symmetry of both sides of the body. In able-bodied people, stability is achieved in many other postures. Although quiet stability results, there are subtle adjustments called 'postural sway'.

Terminologies also used for this are *stability, heavy work* and *tonic activity*.

Counterpoising mechanisms are closely associated with postural stabilisation. They are postural adjustments of the trunk and other parts of the body so that a movement can be made whilst the person maintains posture or equilibrium. Movements are those of the limbs, head or trunk, which require these postural adjustments for equilibrium. Weight shift precedes limb movements and is minimal before any movement is started. Counterpoising or counterbalancing is an 'anticipatory' postural adjustment discussed below with voluntary motion. This is by proprioception and sometimes tactile as adults without labyrinthine function respond adequately.

Terminologies also used are *balance during motion, load shift, weight shifts,* and various *balance exercises* and *movement superimposed on co-contraction.*

Righting or rising reactions make it possible for the person to rise from lying to standing, or sitting to standing or for many other changes of position. It is not only rising into position but also returning to the original position. The rising involves a sequence of automatic 'righting reactions' or of intentional motor actions. The rising depends on turning over from supine to prone and later head and trunk raising which, in early development, include various head-on-body and body-on-body righting reactions. Intentional rising used by clinicians develops a child's ability to focus on different ways he might use to get up from one posture to another.

Terminologies used are *assumption of posture, moving into position* and *movement patterns*. The latter is confusing as there are also movement patterns which are voluntary movements and different from these automatic changes of posture. The rising or righting reactions above depend on tactile and proprioceptive input but other terminologies of 'righting reflexes' use vestibular or labyrinthine input. They are *righting* reflexes that have been studied in relation to being tilted down. When a baby is suspended and passively tipped downwards (forwards, backwards or sideways), this elicits *head adjustment to the upright and with further tilting the adjustments of the trunk.* In this book the terms of righting/rising are integrated responses which are functionally more important for rising to standing and changing positions (Martin 1967; Foley 1998). Others consider righting reactions to be part of 'equilibrium reactions' stimulated on stationary or tilting surfaces (Bobath 1980; Aubert 2008). The response differs according to the difference of the surfaces (see below).

Tilt reactions occur when a person is tilted well off the horizontal plane and adjusts his trunk so that he preserves his balance. This is seen on a therapy roll or on a tilting board. Tilt adjustments are anteroposterior, lateral or diagonal to each side with equal response.

Reactions to falling or saving from falling are various responses in the limbs which try to prevent the person from falling over, if the perturbation of a child is so great that tilt reactions cannot preserve balance. These reactions may be excessive if a child has no tilt responses. Normally, they do not, on their own, stop falling over completely. For example, the arms may be thrown out to save the person from falling forwards, sideways, backwards and in more complicated patterns. Once a person has fallen, the saving response may result in propping on arms or hands. Should the person be falling over from the standing position, he may stagger, hop or quickly place a foot out to stop the fall.

When a less vigorous push is given to the front of the body, threatening a fall, the person's reactions are ankle dorsiflexion or hip flexion. When a perturbation is particularly great, the person reacts with a forward leg placement to stop the fall (Shumway-Cook & Woollacott 2001). When the person is pushed from behind, he rises on toes. The arms may also be thrown out to stop falling. In sitting, kneeling and other positions, arms and legs also move in order to save a person from falling.

Terminology for these reactions is *protective responses*. Particular arm-saving reactions are also called *parachute reactions, protective extension, arm balance responses, precipitation reaction* or *head protective response.*

Equilibrium reactions or *balance reactions* are also terms used which mean a combination of tilt and the limb reactions. These terms are confusing as all the postural mechanisms above are involved with equilibrium or balance. Maintaining a stable posture alone or during movement is synonymous with maintaining balance even before equilibrium reactions develop. Also, limb-saving reactions need not be accompanied by tilt reaction, nor tilt reaction accompanied by limb-saving reactions. In children with cerebral palsy, either limb-saving or tilt reactions may only be present and then each is augmented, when on its own. This is seen particularly in athetoid and ataxic conditions. Perhaps the use of 'equilibrium' has led to the confusion that equilibrium reactions result in postural stabilisation and adjustment during limb and other intentional movements.

Besides the six main postural mechanisms above, there are also the following reactions:

Locomotive reactions, which serve to initiate, continue and stop stepping as well as enable turning in walking and running. They are also known as the mechanisms for propulsion or progression and control slow or faster locomotion. For stepping, locomotive mechanisms are initiated by slight forward lean, and for stopping by a slight backward lean. They operate with other postural control mechanisms in adaptation for human gait.

Visual postural reactions. Vision is of importance for babies and young children's development of postural control. Vision initiates and monitors both posture and movements. Vision compensates for poor postural mechanisms, especially the tilt, and is important during locomotion and when avoiding obstacles. Severe visual impairment delays the development of postural control, particularly tilt reactions (Sykanda and Levitt 1982).

Some physiotherapists stimulate each of the postural mechanisms separately, which does not necessarily lead to their use in daily functions. All these postural mechanisms need to be stimulated *within developmental functions* and in different environments. Postural control in different tasks and in different environments involves adaptation or orientation (Shumway-Cook & Woollacott 2001). This is learned through experience using higher level integrative processes for adaptive and anticipatory mechanisms for postural control. It is helpful to be guided by motor developmental levels, for as the child acquires functional motor control he is ac-

quiring these neurological mechanisms. However, the developmental sequences may vary in both able-bodied children and those with cerebral palsy. This is discussed below in the section on 'Developmental training'.

Voluntary motion

Voluntary motion which is purposeful, conscious, willed motion is sometimes confused with the active automatic movements which occur in the postural mechanisms such as rising or saving from falling. Although some of the automatic movement synergies are also seen in voluntary movement, stimulation of the automatic patterns only corrects some abnormal movement synergies (patterns) but does not contribute much to the training of voluntary motion. Physiotherapists contribute techniques to strengthen and stretch muscles and increase joint ranges to minimise muscular–skeletal problems, which interfere with voluntary arm and leg motion. These physiotherapy methods can be drawn from many systems of treatment and, as in the past, may still be treated separately from the functional training. In such case, these methods need to be immediately activated in functions. When a child is able to carry out functions at his own developmental level, it is preferable to include active stretching out and strengthening within function.

Voluntary motion of the arm and hand is important for many daily tasks. There is some difference of opinion about the use of atypical grasps, though there are specific atypical functional patterns that are acceptable. The section on 'Development of hand function' in Chapter 9 discusses fundamental fine motor development, including neurological anticipatory control in hands. Both musculoskeletal and neuromuscular methods for hand function are not enough for the development of voluntary motion which is involved with sensory experience, perception, praxis (motor planning) and understanding. Voluntary motion in able-bodied children develops many different coordinated upper limb patterns and there may be a great variety of patterns (synergies) in any one child for the same task. Therapy in cerebral palsy needs to offer a variety of motor patterns so a child can have a choice for a task and use what he can manage and also avoid those deformities which may hamper function.

In Chapters 9, various methods from different approaches are suggested in play and daily care with more details on daily life in Chapters 10 and 12. Additional information needs to be gained from other disciplines, such as occupational therapy, psychology and special education.

Voluntary motion and postural control

Voluntary motion is intertwined with the postural mechanisms. Postural mechanisms allow voluntary movement to take place and any voluntary motion itself further activates the relevant postural mechanisms. When a child makes a voluntary movement, he has to maintain his balance as he does so. If his postural stability and counterpoising are inadequate, the child may not be able to initiate or carry out the movement. Should he manage to carry out an active movement on a background of unstable posture, the movement can be imprecise, clumsy, uncoordinated. There are weak limb movements due to disuse as the unstable person is fearful of using them in case of falls. To stabilise himself, the arms and hands are used as supports rather than for voluntary motion. Clinicians understandably want to train voluntary movements giving external support to an unstable child. However, there is a need to avoid overemphasising training of voluntary movement of arms, hands and legs in isolation from the postural control. This can happen if a child is firmly supported, most of the day in, say, special chairs and standing frames. Postural adjustments cannot be activated in firmly supportive equipment. On the other hand, isolated training of postural mechanisms without a variety of intentional hand and limb motions is not sufficient.

Since Martin's work (1967), there have been many research studies to show that postural fixation (stabilisation) and counterpoising of limb movements are anticipatory postural responses (Marsden *et al.* 1981; Cordo & Nashner 1982). Nashner *et al.* (1983) found that in cerebral palsy, there is inability to activate postural muscles in anticipation of voluntary arm motion. Useful reviews by Mulder (1991), Hirschfeld (1992), Shumway-Cook and Woollacott (2001) and others quote many studies, including their own, showing that an anticipatory postural response takes place before an intended voluntary movement is begun. This is a 'feed-forward' mecha-

nism among others which are activated before voluntary initiation of movement. For example, von Hofsten (1992), in his many research studies of infants' visually directed reaching, had his infants fully supported as they did not have stability and anticipatory counterpoising under the age of 4 months. Amiel-Tison and Grenier (1986) manually stabilised an infant's head on his trunk to reveal pre-reaching arm movements which were not seen without postural control. von Hofsten's studies also showed that an infant's reaching became more successful as his postural control developed from 4 months of age. Anticipatory postural responses of their trunks were observed at the normal age of 9 months. There are also 'feedback' mechanisms to grade the size of the muscle responses of postural responses, which develop with experience.

Postural control of the head and trunk helps eye–hand coordination in voluntary movement. Oro-facial muscles function better with head control (Winstock 2005). Sugden (1992) and Van Vliet (1992) review vision, postural control and movement (see the section 'Motor development and the child with severe visual impairment' in Chapter 9).

Perceptual-motor function

The therapy systems explored in this book do not only mention the role of the physiotherapist but also emphasise the contributions of the occupational therapist and speech and language therapist to stimulation of all the senses, linking of sensations, sensory discrimination, developing body image, body scheme including identifying body parts, spatial relationships, and especially perceptual-motor abilities within self-care skills. Perceptual problems involve understanding concepts such as above, below, under and so on. There are also various dyspraxias which may be present with and without sensory integration problems. The psychologist, occupational therapist and teacher make specific structured contributions to these aspects. The neuromuscular techniques in the various therapy systems may be integrated with methods from one or more of the perceptual-motor approaches known to occupational therapists (Ayres 1979; Fisher *et al.* 1991) (see the section on 'Motor function and perception' in Chapter 10.)

Principles for a synthesis of therapy systems

The common ground between the different systems forms the basic principles of treatment. This is followed by my own additions from experience and from recent research studies. These common denominators will be discussed so that the therapist can understand where they exist and where differences are apparent or real.

General principles of management which are currently accepted by most practitioners:

(1) Team work (in various styles) (see Chapters 1, 2 and 11).
(2) Early treatment (see Chapters 1 and 3).
(3) Repetition or practice of a motor activity (see Chapters 2, 6, 9 and 10).
(4) Education, support and encouragement of child, parent or carer (see Chapters 1, 2, 4 and 6) and older person (see Chapter 7).
(5) Use of motor functions in home, school, playground or community (see Chapters 1, 8 and 10).

Specific principles of treatment. The common aims detected in the various systems of treatment with common factors and differences are as follows:

(1) Developmental training.
(2) Treatment of abnormal tone.
(3) Training of movement patterns.
(4) Use of afferent stimuli.
(5) Management of deformity.

Developmental training

Viewpoints differ as to whether to train a total motor function such as rolling, sitting crawling, standing and walking, as measured in various motor scales, or whether to break each function down into elements or components for treatment. Most therapists prefer to train elements or *bricks* which build up the motor function as well as train the total function (Rood 1962; Levitt 1974, 1986, 1991a; Bobath & Bobath 1975; Cotton 1980; Vojta 1989). However, views differ as to what these elements are. Some talk of different types of muscle tone, different reflexes, different muscle work and differ-

ent biomechanical ideas. In addition, various *basic motor patterns* are recommended as fundamental abilities which underlie many motor functions on the developmental scales. For example, Bobath and Bobath (1975) suggest head and trunk control, symmetry, extensor activity, rotation, arm support and equilibrium reactions; Rood (1962) suggests muscle work in main stages on an *ontogenetic developmental sequence*; Vojta (1989) suggests normal muscle work within the basic creeping complex and reflex rolling from which stabilisation and rising are facilitated. Fay (1954 a,b) and Doman *et al.* (1960) focused on mainly passive patterns of creeping, crawling and bear-walk; Cotton (1980) recommended symmetry, grasp, elbow extension, active hip flexion as fundamental in cerebral palsy. Green *et al.* (1995) emphasise load bearing on different body parts.

Motor learning approaches also use methods based on analyses of a motor function (task) into elements for learning. This is discussed in Chapter 6 and needs to be included in a synthesis of methods.

It is possible to contain all these viewpoints as one or a few may be relevant according to the individual assessment of a child. The assessment will of course not be bound by any one-therapy approach.

(1) Training postural mechanisms and locomotive reactions described above, as well as specific voluntary motion, includes attention to symmetry *and normal asymmetry*, grasp, head and trunk control, both flexion and extension, rotation, and other components (abilities) according to the assessment of individuals. It is important to look at the postural mechanism in each *part* of the body (i.e. head, shoulder girdles, trunk and pelvic girdles), which reveals weight-bearing patterns on all body parts. These neurological postural mechanisms are directly involved with aspects of biomechanics.
(2) Postural mechanisms of one part of the body may be more advanced than another part; for example, the head may be better than pelvis and vice versa; shoulder girdle may be better than pelvis and vice versa. One side of the body may be more advanced than the other. Methods are selected from any approach for these problems.
(3) Muscle work for activation and strengthening is included in training of postural control and voluntary movement within developmental motor functions and management of deformities.

Some therapists only carry out exercises for muscle strengthening separately, but there may not be an automatic transfer to developmental motor functions.

Development assumptions

The developmental training of the past trained first head control and only then rolling, next was sitting, then crawling and, only after all these, were standing and walking. This view of one developmental ladder may have arisen because these motor skills *appear* more or less in this sequence. However, in normal children, all these skills are developing simultaneously but are not fully achieved until different milestones (*motor ages*; development levels) are reached. At birth, the supported child is able to take weight on his feet and momentarily hold his head upright. These are the elements of standing, but it will take many months before the full achievement of standing alone. The same occurs for crawling, for rolling and for sitting. The therapist works on developmental sequences to build up motor elements for each motor function in, say, 'stages for crawl', 'stages for sitting' and 'stages for standing and walking' in the relevant developmental channels. It is now traditional to use prone, supine, sitting and standing as parallel motor developmental channels rather than one developmental ladder. This is more relevant to therapy (Levitt 1970a; Bobath & Bobath 1972, 1975). Parallel channels are also more task-specific biomechanically for muscle groups and joint ranges (see Chapter 9).

The use of parallel developmental channels by some therapists has also generated unproven assumptions. There are many examples such as: back extensors must first be trained in lying or use of the Landau reaction before upright standing; legs must first be strengthened in lying before walking; reciprocal leg movements must first be trained in reciprocal kicking, creeping or crawling before stepping in walking; rolling is necessary for the rotation component of sitting and reaching across or behind the body or for the gait pattern. There are assumptions such as that load bearing and load shift in lying will transfer to sitting and standing, and if sitting is not being achieved, then treatment 'goes back to lying' (Pountney *et al*. 2004). Yet, the influence of gravity, the muscle work and joint positions

are not the same in lying on a surface and being in upright positions. Body morphology changes and affects motor patterns. It is also of interest that Thelen (1992) mentions her research in which reciprocal kicking, though similar in pattern to stepping, continued after infantile stepping disappeared. Thelen also notes that an infant's legs can be strong but walking could not develop if other factors, including postural control, were absent. In this book, since 1977, the developmental sequence in standing position from manually supported infantile stepping, weight bearing to independent standing and walking is supported by research (Forssberg 1985) to show the effect of postural mechanisms and muscle actions on the development of walking.

The examples of the above developmental assumptions are usually clinical observations which appear to correlate motor components in different positions. But correlation is not causation. Therapists need more research to confirm the beliefs of what are the prerequisites of motor function. In individual cases, we also need to avoid confusion of sequence with consequence.

Therefore, postural mechanisms need to be activated in all the positions in which they underlie the sequence of specific developmental functions. Methods for strengthening, stretching short muscles, decreasing hypertonus/spasticity and mobilising joints in lying may show results, but will not necessarily transfer to functions in other channels of development against gravity. Methods for these aspects also need to be used in all parallel channels of development.

An accepted view by most therapists is that there needs to be recognition of other factors such as vision, sometimes hearing, as well as perception and motivation. The complexity is that these physical and psychological aspects may be at different levels of development to that of motor control. Comprehensive assessment by a team who are integrative assists individual therapy.

Biomechanics and development

Biomechanics involves the shape, size and weight of the body and includes the lengths and strengths of muscles and the degrees of joint ranges throughout the body. All this changes as a child develops. There are normal developmental stages against gravity which include biomechanics in a child whose size and weight is changing. For example, it is easier for the child to acquire postural stability of the head in a motor function at, say, 3-month normal developmental level than at, say, the more demanding functions at 6- and 9-month levels. Control of the head in supporting sitting (3 months) is easier than head and trunk control in unsupported sitting (7–9 months). Tilt reactions are easier in lying (6–9 months) than in sitting (9–12 months). Rising on to all fours (6–9 months) is easier than rising on to two feet (18 months).

These and other motor functions depend on the postural mechanisms, as well as on other aspects of biomechanics such as muscle lengths and strengths (forces). For example, at 9–12-month developmental level, the postural mechanism of rising from sitting to standing and return to sitting involves length and strength of muscles. In another example, at 4–6-month level, a baby in prone with postural stabilisation of the posture, propped up on the hands, strengthens and shortens hip and trunk extensors whilst stretching out hip and trunk flexors.

Aubert's 'progressions of development' (Aubert 2008) is based on a number of studies and her own observations of typical (normal) child development which draws attention to the biomechanics. The biomechanics also depend on the size and shape of a person and, consequently, are not always the same as in a baby, toddler or older child. Nevertheless, there are a number of similar biomechanical features in early normal motor behaviour which are characteristic of older children with cerebral palsy. Examples are as follows:

- Flexion of arms and especially of legs for weight bearing is present before extension. As stability develops, the centre of gravity is being raised with extension. Nevertheless, flexion returns at times of instability in both children and adults.
- Forward lean in sitting and standing with use of arm props before upright independent posture.
- Bases of support are first wider before smaller bases develop for stability.
- Younger children first hold onto supports in development of sitting, standing and walking, as well as when rising up against gravity from, say, kneeling or sitting to standing, before later independence without supports.
- Gait components in toddlers are similar to many used in older children with cerebral palsy

to balance during walking (see discussion on 'Typical toddler's gait' in section 'Development of standing and walking' in Chapter 9).

- Use of the long lever of a limb in movement improves when stability develops in trunk, shoulder girdle, or pelvic girdle, which then act as points of fixation.
- None of these patterns are due to hypertonus. Of course, hypertonus and especially weakness play a part in abnormal postures, but often the problems of motor control can be due to specific developmental motor delays. When hypertonus and weakness increase with age, there are changes in muscle lengths, creating secondary deformities, making biomechanics more complicated (see Chapter 11).

Individual variations

Individual assessment findings frequently suggest motor training at different developmental levels in each channel of development. A child can be ahead in one developmental channel rather than in another. In able-bodied babies, those who spend time predominantly in supine or in prone or in sitting position have motor abilities in a preferred position which are developmentally ahead of abilities in the other positions. This takes place as normal individual variations in Western cultures.

This is also observed in able-bodied babies in different cultures. Solomons and Solomons (1975) found that infants in Yucatan, Mexico, had a fine pincer grasp earlier than North American infants. The Mexican infants preferred different positions and sequences and were slower in walking than North American infants. In some cultures, parents rarely put a child down on the cold tiled floors or on rough unhygienic ground, so crawling and rolling were not used. Studies by Hopkins and Westra (1989) among others in cross-cultural studies show that mothers' expectations, parental training and especially opportunity create preferences which increase or 'delay' particular developmental functions in children in different environments. Physiotherapists, together with parents, in any environment, can also be an influence on developmental functions through training and practice as motor development is a learning experience and not only maturational. Even biological maturation is unique to each child. Therefore, in Chapter 9 on therapy procedures, there are also ranges of the developmental stages to take account of individual variations.

Variations within each channel also need to be recognised. The functional severity and age of each person determine how much of a repertoire of motor items can be achieved in each channel. It is unlikely that all items will be possible due to the abnormal nervous system or abnormal musculoskeletal system.

Developmental sequences

There are different views on developmental sequences with some therapists being meticulous in following sequences, though most therapists regard them as guidelines with a variety of views on modifications according to a child. The following summarises some ideas.

Some advantages and disadvantages of modifications of developmental sequences

(1) Fears or strong dislike by a child when placed in any posture leads to initial use of another posture and developmental channel. Prone can be disliked by children with breathing problems, gastrostomies, or severe visual impairment. Children, whether able-bodied or with disabilities, who become bottom shufflers dislike prone sequences. Children with severe upper limb involvement or hemiplegia often cannot use arm support and crawling in prone.

If head and shoulder control from 0- to 6-month levels cannot be activated in children who dislike prone, then train such control in a prone standing frame supporting the trunk, pelvis and feet. The child's head is forward with chin in and weight taken through forearms on a table. A child may also accept training of head and shoulder control in well-supported sitting, leaning well forward onto forearms or hands onto a table of relevant height. Training of head, arm and leg control may not be acceptable in four-point (crawl) position but might be practised in four-point standing on hands and feet with hands on a low box. If unstable, the individual is supported at trunk or pelvis (see Fig. 9.33b).

(2) Supine development normally has actions of head, arm and later leg, against gravity that a child finds difficult to do. Head, arm and hand functions and leg actions may be easier in side lying than in supine. The examples are bringing hands to midline, to touch body, grasp feet and play with toys. There are arm and hand functions which are easier with gravity assisting when in prone on a wedge or in crawl position with body supported.

(3) All techniques for arm and hand functions ideally need to be trained in many different positions. Supportive equipment is used when a child cannot maintain particular positions for hand function, perceptual-motor experiences and use of vision and hearing with and without hand function.

(4) Rising from either prone or supine may have to be a choice for some individuals so that they can manage the rising sequences. The disadvantage is that use of active rising in both prone and supine developmental channels offers more variety for increasing ranges of joints and muscles. A person also learns more strategies of turning in bed, getting out of bed or getting up from the floor.

(5) Development of standing and stepping seems to require training in the standing position. As in able-bodied babies at ages between 0 and 6 months, this can be activated early with appropriate trunk support. In cerebral palsy, well-designed fully supporting walkers are used, but the person is standing and stepping in these early patterns. This is a disadvantage if postural control is not being trained. The advantage is that a standing position provides the necessary visual, proprioceptive and spatial experiences. Vertical head stability may initially be stimulated in standing, but it is important to simultaneously emphasise development of head and trunk control in the upright sitting as well as in standing position. Sitting provides a wider and more stable base than standing for promoting independent head and trunk control.

Pre-walking skills of rolling, crawling and creeping have not been shown to need establishment before training standing and walking in adult neurology (Shumway-Cook & Woollacott 2001). This is similarly so in some children, provided these earlier skills continue to be established as far as possible.

A disadvantage of focusing on standing and walking or on sitting, standing and walking (MOVE programme – Thomson 2005) is that there may be omission or inadequate training of rising from lying to standing and managing bed mobility, components of which develop in the supine and prone developmental channels. This is likely to result in an individual remaining dependent on others to be 'stood up' for walking with and without walkers, and dependency in getting out of bed or for turning in bed. The advantage for a child, particularly one with severe visual impairment, is that mobility along the floor through rolling, creeping, crawling or bottom shuffling avoids deprivation of important spatial and other basic perceptual-motor experiences.

Summary

Parallel developmental sequences activate fundamental postural mechanisms and voluntary motion within developmental motor functions. They may be sequential or modified according to culture and individual conditions. Developmental assumptions and the biomechanics in development are discussed so that methods can be appropriately selected. In the practical chapters, ideas are selected from various approaches to train the motor activities according to each child.

Treatment of abnormal tone

Treatment of spasticity

The term spasticity or hypertonia is used in different ways by clinicians and researchers (Sanger *et al.* 2003; Lin 2004). It is a general term covering a number of motor problems which are not directly caused by spasticity. Katz and Rymer (1989) point out that spastic hypertonia is only one component and that other features may be more disabling. Weakness, fatigue and loss of dexterity are among the other problems. Therapy plans need to identify which problem is being treated (see Chapter 8). There is not only the velocity-dependent hyperactive stretch reflex but also abnormal postures, excessive co-contraction, muscle imbalance, atypical activation patterns and muscle sequencing. Spasticity also involves changes in the visco-elastic properties of muscle and other tissues which contribute to abnormal gait, increased resistance to passive stretch in limbs, limited joint ranges and deformities (Dietz & Berger 1983, 1995).

Spasticity is given particular prominence, for diagnosis, in orthopaedic approaches and for the use of botulinum toxin A injections. Physiotherapists may take their lead from such workers. However, spasticity is not of great significance for functional development (Levitt 1977). Too little attention is given to the absence of functional aspects.

If spasticity is reduced or even removed by, say, alcohol or phenol injections, the child will still be disabled (Nathan 1969; Pederson 1969; Sahrmann & Norton 1977; Dietz and Berger 1983; Carr & Shepherd 1987; Dietz 1992). Young and Wiegner (1987) state that 'spasticity may be partially responsible for joint contractures, it does not produce most of the functional disability…'; Giuliani (1992) in her many assessments of the results of dorsal rhizotomy to remove spasticity states that '… assumptions that spasticity is the underlying cause of disordered movement and that reducing or eliminating the spasticity will improve movement are unfounded. … Reducing spasticity may increase range of motion, but may unmask underlying weakness rather than underlying control'.

Dietz (1992) points out that various drugs can reduce stretch reflexes but this effect does not result in a significant improvement of function. McLellan (1977) reduced velocity-dependent stretch reflexes (spasticity) with oral baclofen, but co-contraction of quadriceps and hamstring muscles remained. Co-contraction can be used in function, as it compensates for lack of postural control, so the person can be propped up against gravity. Sometimes a moderate amount of co-contraction will assist transfers of individuals with severe conditions. Co-contraction is also used by able-bodied people coping with unstable or slippery surfaces. Recent research studies by Shortland *et al.* (2002), Gough *et al.* (2005) and Ross and Engsberg (2007) have shown that weakness is much more important than spasticity in causing functional disability.

There are situations when spasticity, now called 'spastic/hypertonus', is relevant to function. This is when spasticity together with weakness and visco-elastic muscle changes results in musculoskeletal problems. These problems are discussed in more detail in Chapter 11 on management of deformity.

Treatment of the spasticity varies from system to system. The neurophysiologists Hagbarth and Eklund (1969) stated that they supported my suggestion that therapists draw on different systems of treatment as there were various theories on spasticity. This eclectic view is also held by McLellan (1984) and Dietz (1992). Lin (2000, 2004) also points out that there are various mechanisms causing spasticity which affects medical decisions.

Methods from different therapy systems are now used to lengthen and strengthen short spastic muscles and shorten and strengthen overlengthened muscles, rather than a general aim to 'treat spasticity'.

(1) Lengthening short spastic muscles. There are methods using ice applications for 3–4 minutes, (Stockmeyer 1967; Voss 1972), manual stretches in warm water, prolonged stretching with inhibitory plaster casts for legs (Bertoti 1986; Cottalorda *et al.* 2000) and for arms and hands (Yasukawa 1990) and in equipment (Tremblay *et al.* 1990). There are different positions in which a decrease of spasticity allows muscle stretching (Bobath & Bobath 1984). There are many designs of orthoses, splints or equipment for daily or nightly stretching and positioning for limbs, head and trunk. Medical consultants also use antispasticity drugs, orthopaedic surgery and neurosurgery.

(2) Strengthening techniques. These are used to activate and strengthen muscles. There are strengthening methods in muscle education against resistance (Phelps 1952), with weights (Damiano *et al.* 1995b; Damiano & Abel 1998), quick icing, on muscles prior to their activation to increase action (Stockmeyer 1967), functional electrical stimulation (Durham *et al.* 2004) and proprioceptive neuromuscular movement patterns against resistance (Voss *et al.* 1985; Adler *et al.* 2008). The middle ranges need to be used more for muscle strengthening rather than inner ranges for short muscles and outer ranges for lengthened muscles. Functional strengthening can be carried out in circuit training groups (Blundell *et al.* 2003).

(3) If a child is being helped to move with a greater variety of motor patterns and as actively as far as is possible, then this will *include* minimising the stiffness as well as abnormal muscle

lengths of spasticity, whilst providing activation or strengthening of muscles.

Hypotonicity

Hypotonicity is also not necessarily correlated with strength of voluntary motion but seems more associated with the postural mechanisms (Foley 1998). Improvement of the postural control seems to coincide with improvement of the hypotonic muscles. 'Floppy babies' or Down's hypotonia improves as the postural mechanisms are activated. Tactile stimulation and other techniques aimed at increasing tone need to be accompanied by training of the postural mechanisms, or preferably replaced by this training. Proprioceptive neuromuscular techniques of joint compression through limbs while weight bearing with correct alignment assist postural control.

Fluctuating tone

Fluctuating tone or severe sudden spasms and involuntary motion seems to 'throw the child off balance', but may not prevent the development of the postural reactions. The association of these athetoid symptoms with postural reactions is not clear yet. Severe dyskinesia has disrupting spasms or tone fluctuations and severe disability in function. Nevertheless, in some children, voluntary motion can be trained, despite disturbance by the involuntary movements. Improvement of postural mechanisms seems to *decrease* the disrupting effect and sometimes the degree of involuntary motion. Excessive arm saving actions are due to poor postural stability, so they appear to decrease when postural stabilisation is improved.

Summary

The therapist should not collect techniques for abnormal tone *as such* but rather:

(1) Emphasise training the developmental motor functions which increases the variety of active motor patterns.

(2) Concentrate on threatening and established deformities to which abnormal tone may contribute, together with other factors (see Chapters 9 and 11).

Training of movement patterns

Movement patterns or synergies are made up of muscle groups or chains of muscles. Some therapy systems assess and treat individual muscle groups (Phelps 1952; Plum & Molhave 1956; Slominski 1984) and this muscle education is associated with orthopaedics (Samilson 1975; Horstmann & Bleck 2007). Others recommend only treating movement patterns in limbs (Bobath & Bobath 1984; Vojta 1984; Voss *et al.* 1985). Research by Damiano *et al.* (1995a) demonstrated an improvement in crouch posture (flexion of hip and knees) following strengthening of quadriceps. Although individual muscle groups may be treated *in isolation*, this is not possible with children who have more severe cerebral palsy. The children in this study were older and milder and were walking.

At early levels of development and in severe impairment, a child cannot easily carry out discrete or isolated movements. They lack 'selective motor control'. Such children and adults can only use mass movements or stereotyped synergies of muscle action or infantile reflex patterns. Tedroff *et al.* (2006) have found abnormal synergies and recruitment patterns in mild and moderate conditions in cerebral palsy. In some therapy systems, therapists have used reflex creeping complex, reflex rolling (Vojta 1984), withdrawal reactions (Phelps 1952) or 'immature stepping pattern' with trunk fully supported (MOVE Europe 2001). The activation of muscles within infantile patterns was used to avoid immobility and counteract deformities. Children themselves have used these early patterns when they have no other means of functioning.

More mature or different motor strategies need to be trained to achieve developmental functional stages. For example, a child uses stereotyped flexion of shoulder, elbow and hand. Treatment methods aim to vary these patterns by, say, training shoulder flexion with elbow and hand extension in reaching tasks. In the leg, the stereotyped movement of flexion at hip, knee with ankle dorsiflexion needs to be modified to carry out active dorsiflexion with knee and hip extension. This fractionation of stereotyped synergies is more mature.

Both specific muscle education and the fractionation of movement for selective motor control may not transfer to a motor function in some conditions. This is related to the variety of muscle actions in functions and the different muscle lengths involved.

Muscles are activated as prime movers, synergists or fixators when they contract during motion. Muscles have to shorten and contract (concentric work or isotonic), keep the same length and contract (isometric work) or lengthen and contract (eccentric work) in different motor functions.

For example, during dressing in supine, bridging hips is used. Bridging hips is concentric action of hip extensors whilst the 'hold' which follows is isometric muscle work. This also applies to head raise and then head holding in prone.

Summary

(1) Motor learning, discussed in Chapters 2 and 6, emphasises a person's use of movement patterns adapted to a task.
(2) However, separate movement patterns are devised for impairments such as muscle tightness, stiff joints, weakness and lack of selective movement control.
(3) When possible, take the lead from a child's initiation of motion to solve motor problems in his daily life and modify his motor patterns or train more mature patterns as far as possible. The severity of brain damage may not allow for a repertoire of normal motor patterns.

Use of afferent stimuli

There are differences between neurofacilitation methods and learning models such as conductive education and the approach of Carr and Shepherd (1987, 2003) and the Mobility Opportunities via Education (MOVE) programme. The neurofacilitation treatment systems use 'hands-on' afferent stimuli of touch, temperature (cutaneous) or pressure, stretch, resisted motion, joint compression or retraction (proprioceptive stimuli) as well as visual and auditory stimuli. 'Handling' obtains automatic active muscle activity. In learning methods, the adult's hands are used much less and then for guiding or minimally supporting a child. *Fixation* or manual holding of a part of the child's body is also used, but not in the same way as the methods from neurofacilitation systems. The handling methods help a child sense a movement or posture he cannot achieve himself. In time, this sensorimotor experience is said to help a child acquire the motion or posture on his own. Equipment for posture management in lying, sitting and standing and orthoses are believed to give a sensory experience which a child can achieve. However, this is passive correction and primarily aimed to correct abnormal postures or position of a body part. Passive posture and passive movements do not train function (Held 1965). A child develops movement and function through his active participation in association with afferent input, including the augmented proprioception given by manual resistance (Kabat 1961; Voss *et al.* 1985).

Motor learning takes more than sensorimotor experience and particularly emphasises active movement and postural control for achieving function. Although muscular activity is present in automatic neuromuscular techniques, what is not active is a child's own initiation of the function. His own actions enable learning and understanding as well as opportunity to use his own strategies for function.

It is important to recognise that movements and postures are automatic *after* they have been learned. In the process of training motor function as, say, in learning to drive a car, play tennis or ice skate, there is a person's concentration on the active movement and control of equilibrium. Children should concentrate on, say, movements for rising from the floor, on maintaining balance, on putting their hands out to save themselves from falling. For example, children with severe visual impairments have been taught to save themselves with verbal instructions to 'put out your arms'. Later this becomes automatic. Automatic postural reactions may be possible in some procedures and should also be actively learned as well as reactive to a therapist's handling.

During training, there are times when a child should have his attention on the afferent stimuli used by the therapist, as they are often cues to direction or to parts of his body and convey what movement is required. In addition, afferent stimuli need not be used when a child can learn to respond actively to 'pull', 'push', 'stretch up', 'try to sit alone' and so on. Some children, especially when younger, respond better to concentration on an incentive for a particular motion, 'touch this', 'catch this', and on the motivation of toys and play.

The Petö approach (conductive education) is particularly careful to use the child's concentration on control of motion (Cotton 1970, 1974, 1975). However, this approach does not carry out every aspect of motion with concentration. The active efforts may focus on, say, voluntary arm motion whilst automatic head and trunk postural stability and postural adjustment are simultaneously activated. Voluntary movements that are selected do not aggravate spasticity as these active motor activities are not too far ahead of the child, so that he is *pushed* to make abnormal efforts to achieve a movement.

Taub (1980), Rothwell *et al.* (1982), Gordon (1987) and others have drawn attention to research that shows that movements can be achieved without afferent input. However, Rosblad and von Hofsten (1992) demonstrated that sensory input is essential for fine coordination (see also von Hofsten & Rosblad 1988). There is a central motor programme in a child's central nervous system which can be used without afferent stimuli. Afferent stimuli are, however, needed to modify the child's actions and achieve accuracy of motor control. 'Hands on' sensory stimuli are therefore not always necessary. Vision and cognition with language may assist a child's acquisition of motor function.

Summary

(1) It is advisable to show the child how and where to move by the therapist's afferent stimuli for movements and postures. However, as soon as possible and even in the same therapy session, check whether the child can carry out the motor activity on his own, even though it will be partial or unreliable.

(2) A child may be able to concentrate and practise the motor function without being handled or touched by the therapist. The motor activity selected should be just beyond his level of development so that he can achieve something on his own. Depending on the severity of the condition, appropriate support by equipment or furniture may initially be needed.

(3) When the child is so severely impaired that there is little activity possible on his own, manual support and afferent stimuli or handling may be the only way to begin motor activity.

Interaction between body parts

There are methods which different clinicians use which activate one part of the body to facilitate action in another part of the body; for example, arm elevation simultaneously activates head elevation and back extension, creeping techniques triggered at the legs facilitate activity in the whole child. Stimulation of one part of a synergic movement pattern activates the other muscle groups within the same synergy. These facilitation techniques involve normal *overflow* of activity from one area of the body to another. Feldenkrais (1980) has made an intensive study of such interactions in the normal body acting as a whole.

In a person with cerebral palsy, it is, however, possible to activate undesirable actions in other parts of the body; for example, grasping may increase flexion in the elbows and shoulders in a child already round-shouldered and flexed, use of the arms may increase abnormal postures in the legs and grasping with one hand may be associated with clenching of the other hand. Physiotherapy techniques, which use resisted motion, must be used in such a way that the rest of the body does not become abnormal (Levitt 1966, 1969, 1970b). This is a combination of positioning (Bobath & Bobath 1984) and proprioceptive neuromuscular facilitation (Voss *et al.* 1985). Active movement against resistance is facilitated in one part of the body while the rest of the body must be *positioned* so that abnormal overflow

does not occur. Vojta's techniques use resistance to a creeping complex but, as the whole body is moving in a corrective pattern, positioning is unnecessary. Also, much rotation within motor patterns in people with spastic hypertonus prevents associated abnormal motor activity in other parts of the body.

There are interactions between body parts in all the postural mechanisms. A scoliosis can correct during tilt reactions, an inactive hemiplegic arm is activated in a saving reaction and the 'constraint-induced methods' include activation of an inactive body part when the more able body parts are constrained (Taub *et al.* 2004).

Summary

(1) Any action in one part of the body should be accompanied by careful observation of the whole child and not only of the part being activated. Physiotherapists can learn more about normal interactions of body parts in their own experience in 'Feldenkrais classes' (Feldenkrais 1980).
(2) There are a number of different methods which use or constrain one body part in order to activate another less able body part.

Management of deformity

Every system aims to prevent, minimise or correct deformities and contractures. There are many methods to counteract deformity as well as various viewpoints as to the genesis of deformity. Chapter 11 is devoted to this aspect.

6 Learning motor function

Physiotherapists have been treating motor control separately, drawing on one or more neurological and orthopaedic approaches. Studies and clinical experience have shown that activation of muscles or motor patterns on their own can show an improvement, but this is a performance in a therapy session and is not necessarily learned. The improved motor performance does not transfer into the actions of daily life (Goldkamp 1984; Gordon 1987; Mulder & Hulstijn 1988; Mulder & Hochstenbach 2002). The therapist needs to recognise that:

■ A child does not move by neurophysiology alone. The ability to move is also dependent on learning processes.
■ Learning depends on active movement initiated by a child as much as possible.
■ Strengthening of muscles and decreasing stiffness of muscles, soft tissues and joints improve the motor apparatus but not necessarily the everyday motor functions.
■ Achievement of motor control in a clinic (or research laboratory) does not necessarily carry over into daily life, which includes self-care, school activities, play, hobbies and household chores.
■ When a child learns to use motor function in the context of his life, this motivates and also activates his motor control and promotes the motor learning.

■ Special clinical therapy sessions are important but need to be used simultaneously with therapy sessions within other contexts of a child's life.
■ Carry over from the treatment sessions to a child's everyday life depends on motor learning.

In which therapy aims for a child do learning principles apply?

■ A child with brain damage *learns* motor functions such as sitting, standing, changing postures, using hands and the various forms of locomotion.
■ A child *learns how* to use equipment such as walking aids, wheelchairs and playthings.
■ A child *learns to* use his motor functions to achieve activities such as self-care, play and interaction with people and objects in most daily tasks.

In Chapter 2, my priority was to start with motor patterns and functions in the context of the daily lives of children with their parents, originally based on the need to translate my technical knowledge into what has meaning for them in our culture (Levitt 1991b, 1994) and in other cultures (Levitt 1991a, 1999). This is followed by specific therapy for motor patterns which are observed to be useful for what parents and child state they want to achieve in their daily lives. This includes specific activation of motor actions which are dormant but necessary for any daily life activity. On the other hand, therapy minimises those motor patterns which are inefficient or block motor function relevant to daily tasks. In Chapter 2, a collaborative learning model shows how therapy programmes relevant to daily lives of parents and people with cerebral palsy can be jointly created involving therapist, child and parents in a learning process (Levitt & Goldschmied 1990).

Learning methods

Many experienced paediatric physiotherapists and occupational therapists do intuitively select training methods which suit an individual's learning style. This art and common sense of therapists can be supported by some of the knowledge and research presented by experts in the behavioural sciences. It is nevertheless of much value to learn from such experts so that a therapist comes to understand more deeply and analytically what she is already doing so that she can be more precise in the way she works. This also allows the therapist to further develop her way of working. These studies are quoted by therapists and psychologists who also offer theories for our work, and new ideas are being developed (Carr & Shepherd 1987, 2003; Forssberg & Hirschfeld 1992; Russell and Cotton 1994; Shumway-Cook & Woollacott 2001; Mulder & Hochstenbach 2002; among others).

Learning methods are also developed through interaction of paediatric physiotherapists with occupational therapists, teachers and other professionals. Child psychologists experienced in child development and disabilities give therapists many ideas about learning. These ideas need to be adapted for learning motor control. Community therapists interested in motor learning in different environments have found home, playgroup and school visits enlightening.

A behaviour

This is a term used by psychologists and teachers to convey any action of a child that can be observed. When behaviours are troublesome for therapists and parents – in that a child refuses to cooperate, dislikes handling or having splints applied, these are discussed with team members. A clear description of what a child does, when he does it and people's response to his behaviour is discussed so that a constructive approach can be worked out.

The behaviours which are more directly the concern of physiotherapists are motor acts. A description of what a child does with the criteria for success of a motor act is called a *behavioural objective* for therapy or training (Presland 1982; Steel 1993). For example, 'Sitting on a potty for one minute independently without extending backward or falling to the right' (Bower & McLellan 1992). This gives the motor act, how it is done and for how long. This is also called 'setting a goal' with a child and his carer. We need to go further than setting a goal and clarify a carer's or a therapist's response to a child's efforts and his motor achievement as is done with other behaviours. This will affect a child's learning of any motor function.

'Feedback' by a therapist on 'goal-directed' trials made by a child and on his end results either assists learning or may cause feelings of pressure, of fears of failure and of disappointing people whom he likes and are helping him.

Emotions and learning

There may be feelings of discomfort or distress in a child when a change in that child's familiar motor behaviour is expected by a therapist. The responses of children when confronted by new tasks may be fear, frustration and anxiety. These emotions in such situations have been interpreted as fear of the unfamiliar and self-protection against failure or from past experiences of failure. This is understandable caution and hesitation about change. On the other hand, many therapists know that using specific play activities, most children may be motivated to try new motor skills and derive pleasure in positive achievement. However, there are children who even find a new toy or novel play activity too unfamiliar and hesitate to act. This is especially so when a child prefers not to use a part of their body for play which previously resulted in failure and frustration. Children have also experienced medical language focused on their abnormalities during the making of a diagnosis, when using a measure of impairment and during treatments which aim to correct abnormalities. Statements and words such as 'he or she can't do this', 'no', 'that's wrong', 'you're not trying', 'stop that movement' are some examples.

There are children who may not understand what is expected of them or how to use a toy. Children who have no or minimal speech, especially any words to express feelings, when asked to carry out a task, will cry or scream, show anger or withdraw. Children use their extensor spasms, involuntary movements and total flexor posturing to show that they are upset. These strong feelings of unease are also shown for all the situations above.

The significant tasks for adults to manage when they are involved with a child are as follows:

(1) Their own protective impulses. They need to balance their wish to challenge a child to develop with a desire to protect that child against possible failure and fears.

(2) Their own examination about failure. A child learns from the mistakes he makes so that he can improve his function. So-called failure can be a spur to better function. Failure may also not be true failure if the task is too far beyond a child's developmental stage or too easy so he is not interested.

(3) Their body language and words so that adults learn to reframe their language in a more positive way.

There are various options that therapists already use to achieve this, and the following need special emphasis:

■ Therapists first need to examine what a child can do and which activity is familiar and then build on that. Offer variations or add manual resistance to actions all within an individual child's competence.

■ When training a new function, gradually give less manual support, less guidance and less supervision. Use equipment for one part of the body so that another can function, and decrease use when a child's abilities develop. A task is broken down into smaller and smaller components so success is possible.

■ Therapists understand and feel that mistakes are learning tools so they do not show disapproval or disappointment when a child does not manage a task. They wait calmly, when those children want to 'try again and again' and find their own way of achieving a task.

■ Therapists offer information for achievement of tasks or for improving them, but while doing so avoid conveying assumptions of inadequacy of a child or disapproval of a child's own abnormal efforts. Otherwise a child can be discouraged and feel a failure. This can increase what might be a 'normal' anxiety about an unfamiliar task.

■ The therapist gives information for initial or better performance through 'hands on' procedures, or other methods given in this chapter and Chapter 9. There are methods to manage fears of falling in procedures given in Chapter 9.

■ Therapists share a child's success and pleasure of achievement with smiles, looking approvingly at his actions, commenting on what was specifically achieved. However, overenthusiasm on children's achievement may well make many children feel that only success pleases adults and earns approval. Children's mental and emotional energy is then wasted on fear of failing to please adults helping them. We therapists need to reflect on how our responses to the 'failure' or achievement by a child will be sensitive to a child's needs to be accepted and valued as a person.

■ Therapists assess whether tasks are developmentally appropriate for individual children. This is likely to ensure success. The task includes developmental levels of understanding, perception and motor function. An individual child is offered tasks which he can just manage to achieve (the 'just right challenge').

■ These tasks need to be interesting and enjoyable for a child as well as challenging at his level.

All these suggestions facilitate and depend on the positive relationship of a therapist with a child. In the security of this relationship, there is trust which assists a child to cope with the unfamiliar tasks he needs to achieve. The trust is by a therapist for a child's developmental potential and trust by a child for a therapist's emotional support and for discovery of what and how he can achieve.

The development of a child's attention and learning

The cerebral palsies may create apathy, hyperactivity and fleeting attention in children. Besides the brain damage which causes these difficult behaviours, they may be due to some drugs, fatigue and emotional stress of a child. Parents find their child's demand for non-stop attention with play activities and his restlessness very difficult. Their child cannot maintain concentration and play on his own. Parents are enabled to understand that therapy tasks need concentration for learning and therapy is not necessarily only a set of procedures during which a child 'receives treatment'. Therapy with learning tasks of interest to a child will, therefore, improve not only the motor tasks but also a child's attention span. The child's general behaviour improves with successful experience of achievement through active learning of tasks.

Practical ideas to promote attention and learning

(1) The suggestions for a child's choice of an activity (see Chapter 2) and those above in the subsection 'Emotions and learning' all promote attention and learning.

(2) Use small steps within each stage or modify a task so that achievement is possible. Successful achievement maintains attention (see section 'Cues for learning').

(3) Impairments are known, so the influences of other disabilities are appreciated.

(4) Difficult and new motor tasks need to be interspersed with easier ones. Rest periods may need to be interspersed.

(5) Ensure that the therapy session does not have too many activities and that priorities are chosen.

(6) The time of day must be considered. A child may be better in the morning or some time after a meal or rest. Clearly, concentration of a child is not enhanced if he is taken away for therapy from his favourite lesson in school or from a special hobby or play activity.

(7) The length of a therapy session must relate to the child's attention span and pace of learning.

(8) Avoid distractions of too many people moving around, too much noise or non-stop television or radio during sessions. Later, *following achievement*, train the motor function in the presence of distractions by grading the degree of distractions in his natural environment.

(9) Keep a child looking at what he is doing with an object, toy or walking aid, and not at the therapist. He learns to attend to what he is doing and when trying to manage his problems for himself.

(10) A child's attention is best appreciated in terms of his stage in the usual sequence of development of attention, so that too much is not expected of him. Infants normally attend to more of their internal activities and to stimulation very close to them. Around the age of 6 to 12 months, their attention can be focused on stimuli of sight and sound further away from them. Fleeting attention in infants becomes longer in duration until they focus rigidly on one thing at a time. Later they will allow an adult to shift their attention and become more flexible in use of their attention (Cooper *et al.* 1978).

(11) Swings, movement on wheels, on rocking apparatus and actions with musical rhythms as well as activities devised by any therapist are challenging for learning motor control. Enjoyable activities also focus a child's attention on pleasurable body movement.

(12) Activities such as swimming, horse riding, sledging and abseiling with appropriate assistance teach balance and movement in social contexts and give pleasure. The associated development of fitness and health provides positive feelings.

Learning a motor function

When a child focuses his attention on a motor task, he is more likely to learn it. The therapist clarifies for him where he needs to concentrate. In the first stage, a child focuses his attention on the purpose for moving. This is his *intention* to move or the *action goal*. This may be a child's daily living activity of, say, eating, washing, dressing or interacting with his mother or another family member. It may be exploring an object or getting to a place where he wants to be.

Once focused on the goal, the child uses what are called *goal-directed movements* together with postural mechanisms. His attention is kept on the task as he learns which motor actions are used to achieve this goal. Therapists need to avoid *goal confusion* by their emphasis on the *best motor pattern* rather than maintaining a child's attention on the goal (Gentile 1987). Once some understanding of what to do is shown by a child, his attention shifts more to how to do it. The action of movement and posture is therefore not separated from the purpose of that action. Van der Weel *et al.* (1991) in a cerebral palsy study showed how using pronation and supination in order to bang a drum obtained better action than pronation and supination as an exercise.

Goal-directed movements should not be isolated from postural control as both are interwoven and need to be learned together. This presents a challenge to those who use much equipment to control and correct posture during hand function.

A child's own goals and strategies

A learning model often involves an adult explaining in reassuring ways what a child is going to do, showing him how to do it and keeping his attention on these aspects. However, if one precedes this approach with discoveries of what a child himself wants to achieve, he may not need to have explanations of what he is going to do. If a therapist also observes how he goes about trying to achieve his own goal, *she* learns about his motivation and what he can already do using his choice of postural controls and movement patterns (see Fig. 6.1a,b). These may be the following:

- ■ An approximation of the whole task.
- ■ An initiation of the task without completion.
- ■ An unusual way of doing the task.

The therapist can then show that child how to develop or modify the task if his approximation of a task is at a *lower developmental stage* of performance, *uses symptoms* of his type of cerebral palsy,

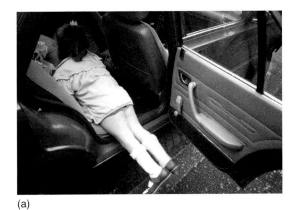
(a)

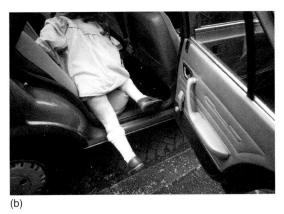
(b)

Figure 6.1   (a, b) Child finding her own strategy of getting into a car; Part (b) is more desirable as she herself corrects spastic adduction of her legs.

increases deformity or shows *disuse* of any part of his body or muscle groups. Once a task is initiated by a child, the therapist assists him to complete it. When unusual ways of performing a task are seen, careful consideration is needed as these patterns do not always cause deformities or disuse and may be a variation of performance, much like normal variations of motor function are acceptable in able-bodied people. When a child uses immature, pathological or biomechanically compensatory patterns which do cause deformity, block further development or demand excessive energy, they are corrected and alternative patterns encouraged. However, the 'undesirable' motor patterns may be the only ones possible for a child to achieve independence in a particular skill. It is then important to plan other motor activities in his day which use motor patterns to counteract the choice of his abnormal patterns for independence. Additional splinting and treatments are also added to counter undesirable motor patterns. Accepting abnormal motor patterns for independence in a skill depends on the age of a child as younger children have more potential for correction and variety. The severity of the physical condition, the degree of intellectual impairment and the degree of visual disability lead to some compromise on the use of abnormal motor patterns for selected motor tasks.

Task analysis

In order to assess which movements and postures to improve, develop or discourage for a function, a task analysis is done. The child's actions are compared with those in his age group and with those at an earlier stage of normal development. Task analyses include the following:

- A sequence of actions such as getting up from the floor through various postures. There is a sequence of actions for eating, drinking, washing and other daily tasks. There is a sequence of actions in using walking aids, wheelchairs and transfers or play equipment.
- The postural mechanisms at a particular developmental stage together with patterns of voluntary movements (synergies).
- The motor action and its related sensory, perceptual and cognitive areas. This involves analysing where a child looks and what he hears, smells, tastes and touches during the motor action. At the same time, he senses what he is doing in both movement and postural control (vestibular input and proprioception). Finally, what he understands as the purpose of his action and all the senses which inform him of the motor plan and of its achievement.

When analysing a motor function for an individual, consider the ways a therapist can augment the residual or established abilities of sensations, perceptions and level of a child's cognition and motivation. Suggestions also need to be gained from psychologists, teachers and others in the team.

The physiotherapist also contributes to the motor components of a task by considering how the following affect the quality of motor function:

- Ranges of joint motion.
- Muscle lengths and strength.
- Postural alignments including asymmetries.
- Deformities, both fixed and unfixed.
- Involuntary movements, spasms or reflex reactions which interfere with motor function.

These aspects are discussed in Chapters 8, 9 and 11, which cover assessment and methods.

There are different viewpoints on the analyses of tasks, not only among physiotherapists but also between professionals. It is therefore necessary for members of a team to share their views on a child they all know. Common ground between physiotherapists has been discussed in Chapter 5. Research on motor analyses progresses, and therapists need to continue their studies so that better task analyses are developed in the future. Interdisciplinary studies and experience also add to better task analyses involving sensory, perceptual, cognitive, emotional and motor interactions. Tasks in different environments need adaptations which influence task analyses.

Cues for learning

Cues for learning need to be clearly given in therapy. Each child will respond to different cues according to his stages of development and the presence of specific impairments. Cues are given for the starting position, during the action and for the final result of the action. A child needs to detect or be informed of any errors in his performance as well as his success (Winstein & Schmidt 1989; Winstein *et al.* 1989).

Therapists may use sensory input, verbal guidance with positive language to help a child learn motor control. Experts in motor learning call cues about the child's function as *feedback*; they not only are given by a therapist but are intrinsic to the child's own experience in actively achieving any task. Feedback by a therapist needs to be skilfully given. Winstein and Schmidt's research (1990) shows that too frequent feedback makes a learner too dependent on an instructor and dependency can be demotivating.

In some situations and according to a child's ability and motivation, a child can initiate or *feed forward* a specific function.

An example of an approach which may be adapted for different individuals is as follows:

(1) *Set the scene such that a child can actively manage* what he can on his own. This means modifying the environment by having non-slip mats, place mats, appropriate toys, sturdy furniture and equipment according to the child's size and providing adequate light and colour to encourage achievement. Placing toys or objects in different areas activates and provides success in the training of movements. In this way, a child's own action gives him feedback for learning. He senses errors so that he can correct them through his motivation and understanding of the task and how to move. The use of motor patterns *he* discovers is best for learning, provided they do not seriously increase his symptoms.

(2) *A therapist's hands can physically guide* a child through a whole task to demonstrate what is to be done and how to do it. She must then immediately remove her hands at any time that a child takes over this action from her. This may be at the beginning, middle or in finishing the task.

(3) *A therapist gives minimal support* to a child's body, shoulders or hips so that a task can be actively attempted and practised by a child. She may use equipment to support a child, allowing active movement of the body or limbs that he can begin to control (see Fig. 6.2).

(4) *Appropriate manual assistance or resistance* to a child's movements or stabilisation of his head, body, hips and shoulders allows him to sense what to do and how to do it. Joint compression also alerts his sensory understanding of postural stabilisation (fixation). Once correct postural alignment is manually given by a therapist, the child is encouraged to actively hold the posture. Starting positions are first assisted so that a child's action on his own is more effective for his purpose. The therapist's appropriate manual resistance also conveys to a child which body part to move and in which direction to move it. Other neuromuscular facilitation methods offer this as well.

(5) *The problem presented by too much neuromuscular handling* is that sensory input is provided by a therapist handling the positioning and movements of a child while the child is concentrated on a goal which he wants to achieve.

It is perhaps not always clear in every case that such excessive sensory input can be processed, and then understood and motor planning created by that child so that motor function or skill emerges and is learned. This is an important consideration for assessment.

Motor learning also involves a child's concentration on the goal-directed movements and postures underlying what he wants to achieve. This may not be given enough attention when too much 'handling' is given. Although when children have severe conditions or multiple impairments, specific handling by therapists receives more emphasis to prevent and minimise deformities. However, there are careful observations of any active actions by a child, which may emerge. These need practice with active learning methods.

(6) *Visual feedback* can inform a child of what he is to do and how he is doing it. Encourage him to look at his own body and at what he is doing. Mirrors may help, though the reversed image may sometimes cause difficulties. His own observation of another child with cerebral palsy similar to him is most helpful. He may observe the therapist or his parents carrying out a task which he needs to learn. Observing others directly or on video can only be used for children who are able to imitate others. Thus, severe visual impairment or severe learning impairments may make this impossible. Videos of themselves may be used by some children if they are not upset by seeing their inadequate performances. A child's best performance or desired behaviour should rather be videoed for feedback. A child's achievements need emphasis and what can still be achieved presented with positive expectation by a therapist, if this is likely.

(7) *Feedback with sounds, visual displays or vibration* can inform a child on the results of his actions. These biofeedback techniques may also be arranged to augment the most desirable motor patterns of posture and movement. However, like therapy 'exercises', they do not transfer to daily living if feedback on isolated actions is given (Mulder 1985). Babies and severely intellectually impaired children who cannot understand *cause and effect* are not able to use feedback. They have to be enabled to learn that their movement created a sound or switched on a light.

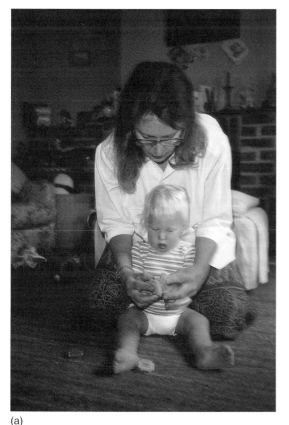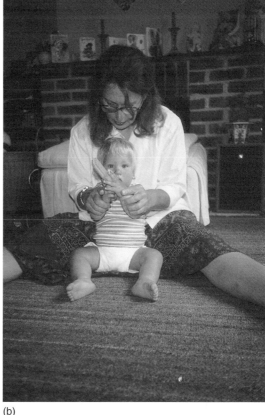

(a)   (b)

Figure 6.2 (a, b) Physical guidance for learning arm and hand functions.

Verbal guidance

This is only possible when a child understands words. It includes all or some of the following verbal instructions:

(1) Informing a child, in a reassuring style, what is going to happen or the purpose of the motor patterns; for example, 'You are going to ...'.
(2) Suggesting the starting position, the movement or balance and, once carried out with appropriate assistance, commenting on the positive results of these motor patterns. This may be done together with physical guidance. For example, when showing a child how to stand up from a chair, verbalise the skill by saying, 'Keep your feet flat, go forward over your feet and stand up'; and if active participation of the child happens, share his pleasure with 'you stood up well!'

However, it is usually best if minimal verbal guidance is used with young children. Sometimes an operative word like 'step, step, step' or 'push, push, push' can be helpful. For many children, especially those who are multiply disabled, it is advisable to set the scene and physically guide or use clear gestures for communicating what is expected in a task. Also, use specialised (adaptive) equipment and toys. It is then best to be quiet and attentive as a child learns from his own experience. Quiet encouraging looks at the task and glances towards a child avoid distractions from the task to what a therapist is saying. Such an approach encourages better focusing of that child's attention on the task.

Comments on the results of a child's efforts may not always be necessary if he clearly understands that he has achieved what he has set out to do. Motivation can be maintained by phrases such as 'you sat nice and straight' or 'you stretched your elbows well'. This provides the feedback of information and praise so that the task can be learned. Praise for the achievement of a component ability within a task is as important as the completion of the whole task. However, a child needs to learn the component within the whole task and not on its own. Unless well understood 'in context' of a task, components can be less motivating.

Remember: Care needs to be taken that physical guidance and words do not themselves distract a child. A child with visual impairment or multiple disabilities may become attracted to a therapist's touch or speech rather than keep his attention on the task to be learned. One needs to avoid a child becoming passive and dependent on your physical guidance or *facilitation method*. It is wise to remove your hands as soon as possible.

Rewards

Children can gain intrinsic reward in their own achievement of a task. This is especially satisfying if children have chosen the particular task themselves. However, there are those who have such profound impairments that hamper their making a choice or if enabled to show what they want to do, cannot physically carry this out. Despite such difficulties, if a child does achieve something, then he warrants additional rewards which are extrinsic. Many teachers recommend giving a child with profound intellectual impairment a reward *immediately after* he has completed a task or even *the intention* to try to do it. Smiles, words of approval and of information may not be understood. Very basic rewards, which do not depend on language or social development, are suggested. There are many possibilities and each child is observed to discover what he prizes most as satisfaction. This may be food, juice, music or lights. A variety of tactile stimuli such as stroking, patting, cuddling, blowing on his face and vibration may please him particularly. The goals for a child must be tangible so that he can be rewarded, rather than fail to achieve goals well out of his range of abilities. It is important to observe when a child has had too much of the same reward and become bored with it. This applies to all children who enjoy the incentives of a variety of toys and play during daily tasks. We continually use our imagination to find satisfying rewards for children.

Apparent rewards of 'good boy', a hug and other social praise should not be used indiscriminately as, for example, when a child is not doing anything constructive, such as he is slumped in a chair or carrying out undesirable movements or mannerisms. This does not help learning and confuses a child as to what adults expect from him. Of course, hugs and showing pleasure in knowing a child as a person are worthwhile.

Natural rewards of enthusiasm and delight, together with clear information on what a child has struggled to achieve or tried to initiate, are recommended. When basic rewards need to be used, these are decreased as a child with profound learning disabilities learns and retains the achievement of a motor task (Levitt 1982; Presland 1982).

Older children and young children who can appreciate it may be given a progress chart with ticks for abilities gained, or collect stars or tokens for achievement. They are also rewarded when their friends, classmates and their family members approve their hard work and specific achievements.

Practice and experience

In Chapter 2, the collaborative learning outlines ways of sharing the practice of a motor task with others assisting a child's development. Practice of a motor task incorporated into activities used by teachers, playgroup workers and family members is planned with them. A motor function is also practised on its own. The stages of learning are as follows:

(1) A consistent way in which postural control, postural alignment and movements are first practised so that some ability can be initiated and developed.
(2) In the therapy session, a child may have tried out various different motor patterns to accomplish his goal and improved on them with a therapist's suggestions. When his own strategies were unsuccessful, he will have been shown alternative patterns by his therapist. The successful patterns are those that will be practised so that they are consolidated. Whenever possible, the motor patterns discovered as successful for a child's purpose by that child are used. They

may be unusual but not deforming nor increasing symptoms of motor dysfunction.

(3) Once consistency of practice has led to abilities, these are immediately used in a variety of situations. A child is encouraged to use his motor function to explore inside and outside his home and school. He rolls, crawls or walks on different surfaces indoors and outdoors. Surfaces may be stationary at first, but moving for later motor control. This may happen when a child is taken on visits to shops, the zoo, the countryside and other places for his education as well as for his motor experiences. During these visits, time and patience need to be given so that he can use his movements and balance as he acquires sensory, perceptual and cognitive experiences. Various play experiences with sand, water, snow and many other materials are at first presented so that he uses his motor abilities or emerging abilities in play. Control of posture, movements and the use of his hands develop further during his own spontaneous exploration.

(4) It is best to develop and practise a task in a child's familiar environment. This offers him well-known clues for learning motor function. When home visits or school visits are difficult, a clinic or centre needs to create situations similar to those known by a child so that transfer of motor function learning can be achieved.

(5) The training of the motor components of posture and movement needs to happen at home either following or preceding their use in the whole motor function or daily living activity. In this way, training motor components is not reserved for a clinical session in one venue and use of these components in their meaningful context in another venue. Training and practice of components are only necessary if these need to be separated due to the complexity of particular tasks. To help learning, a child needs to understand the relevance of components to the whole task, as outlined in Chapter 2.

A word of caution: A child should not be made to feel that unless he is achieving a motor skill he will not be loved. He needs to feel loved and appreciated for the person he is, whether he is working hard or not and whether he is successfully achieving or not. There are many ways of building this attitude into relationships with a child.

Summary

Learning motor function needs to be integrated with the purpose or meaning of such motor function to a child. Consideration needs to be given to the emotional aspects of learning a motor function, as well as the ways of helping a child learn the function either on its own or within a daily activity. Consider the following:

(1) Developing a child's attention.
(2) Discovering a child's own goals and strategies and following this lead.
(3) Analysing the task for learning for each child.
(4) Giving cues for learning performance for what a child wants to do, is going to do, how he performs and the results of what he does.
(5) A child's own actions and results of them provide him with sensory information for learning a task.
(6) Sensorimotor experiences need to be understood by a child using active attention for learning. The clear links with an individual's choice of task need to be clearly given in therapy.
(7) Verbal instructions are usually minimal but are useful in working with children who understand them.
(8) There is intrinsic reward in achieving the task itself. However, external rewards may also be incentives for individuals with severe multiple disabilities.
(9) Practice is necessary to develop motor function. It needs first to be consistent and then within a variety of situations. A variety of movement experiences helps to stimulate as well as reinforce motor learning.

7 The older person with cerebral palsy

The aims of therapy stated in Chapter 1 remain as lifelong aims. These are as follows:

(1) Communication, either verbal or non-verbal.
(2) Independence in activities of daily living.
(3) Recreational activities.
(4) Independent mobility and/or some form of locomotion.

The priorities of these aims depend on the individual's choices and, for the older person, are even more focused in the context of social, educational and employment situations. It is particularly recommended that the collaborative learning model outlined in Chapter 2 is used directly with an adolescent or adult with cerebral palsy.

The collaborative learning model provides for fundamental emotional needs during the changes of puberty and for the autonomy of individual adolescents and adults. For example:

A sense of control, opportunities for individual choice and opportunity to use more of an individual's problem-solving skills. Collaboration makes new strategies and an individual's innovation possible, especially as educational progress increases an adolescent's understanding. Authoritarian behaviour in professionals and parents provokes rebelliousness and non-cooperation. Avoidance by therapists of negative patronising comments is associated with their calm, firm manner and sense of humour. Therapists overcome any sense of intimidation by adolescents through negotiation, concessions and offering constructive professional knowledge without threats.

Sensitive listening to individuals and demonstrating action on what adolescents and adults discuss is essential in the collaborative approach. This respect and personal value are very much needed by an adolescent facing the consequences of long-term disability and experiencing biological changes at the same time.

Adolescent distancing from parents and preparation for adulthood are particularly difficult when physical independence is not fully achieved due to disabilities. The collaboration with individuals gives them support and respect so that independent views can be expressed and responsibility developed as far as possible. Parents and siblings also need support and encouragement so that their many years of help can be gradually withdrawn. Such anticipated withdrawal needs to be discussed in late childhood, around the age of 10–11 years, to prepare the individual and his family for future changes.

The older individual can choose which activities he will practise and which motor skills need improving for daily life, and can be given responsibility for carrying them out. Plans and methods are jointly discussed as to when, how often and where activities can be carried out. The older person is expected to say when time can be found to practise a motor activity or exercise. Being collaborative and specific about therapy programmes avoids feelings of doubt that time for physiotherapy is unrealistic and also irrelevant in an older person's daily life.

The therapist focuses and negotiates short-term goals and methods which will demonstrate success. The adolescent's responsibility and related success are helpful to parents so that they can feel able to withdraw their help. At the same time, successful independent achievements by any adolescent promote confidence and self-esteem. If possible, differing views of parents and siblings are not given priority over that of the adolescent, but much tact will be needed.

More severely affected individuals, who cannot make decisions, can show their distancing from parents by carrying out enjoyable activities in peer groups. An adult facilitator of peer group exercises, discussions, games or other educational activities is often particularly useful. The therapist either works with groups or suggests functional positioning so that communication and social interactions are assisted. Self-help groups, especially for adolescents and adults, are appreciated and also foster independent decision making, which some have not experienced for many years.

Confidentiality. When physiotherapists carry out slow stretches or ranges of motion to counteract deformities, there are opportunities for an adolescent or adult to have conversations about their anxieties, concerns or problems. What emerges needs to be kept in confidence so that trust is maintained with an individual. The therapist may sometimes be an advocate for an individual. Counselling sessions with a qualified professional are recommended if desired by an individual.

Role of the physiotherapist and occupational therapist

The role of a physiotherapist is valuable as maintained or any increased motor control may contribute to an individual's participation in social, educational and work activities. Environmental restrictions need to be discussed and problem-solving carried out with the individual and others involved.

Occupational therapists work together with physiotherapists in assessment and supply of equipment for different environments in which the individual finds himself. Specific aims of physiotherapy and occupational therapy are:

(1) To maintain motor abilities decreased by disuse.
(2) To prevent and decrease deformities wherever possible.
(3) To learn a healthy lifestyle, including physical fitness.
(4) To develop appropriate community mobility.
(5) To continue the training of self-care skills.
(6) To teach the individual all he or she needs to know about the condition.

These aims are discussed below together with health and other concerns of individuals. Ongoing research studies related to prognoses of function are firstly outlined for older people.

Studies of function

A number of studies of health and function have found a deterioration in adolescents and adults with cerebral palsy (Thomas *et al.* 1989; Wilner 1996; Bottos *et al.* 2001; Bottos & Gericke 2003). However, many recent studies are more optimistic.

McCormick *et al.* (2007), using the Gross Motor Function Classification System (GMFCS; Palisano *et al.* 1997), found that 91% of 33 children who were walking without aids (GMFCS Levels I and II) at around age 12 years were still walking without aids at about age 22. They also found that 96% of 48 children who were using a wheelchair as their primary or only mode of mobility (GMFCS Levels IV and V) at the age 12 years were still wheelchair users at about age 22.

Day *et al.* (2007) made a retrospective study of walking in 7550 adolescents and 5721 young adults. Their graphs show that children with cerebral palsy with mean age 10 years, who walked well alone (GMFCS Levels I and II), had a high likelihood (77–89%) of still doing so over the next 15 years. They also found that 54% of children who walked well but needed some assistance in climbing stairs (GMFCS Level II) stayed the same until age 25. Those who changed were equally likely (23%) either to decline in walking or to improve in stair climbing. Children who walked only with support or unsteadily (GMFCS Level III) but did not use a wheelchair had only a small chance (11%) of losing walking (ambulation), whereas those who used a wheelchair were more likely (34%) to lose walking.

In adults with mean age 25 years, the graphs of Day *et al.* (2007) also show that 71–84% of those who walked well alone (GMFCS Levels I and II) were still doing so over the next 15 years. The graphs also show that of adults in GMFCS Level III who did not use a wheelchair, 15% achieved stair climbing by age 40 whereas 11% lost walking by that age.

Strauss *et al.* (2004), in a study of 904 adults aged 60 years, found that 60% were still walking alone or with support. By age 75, 40–50% of those survivors who had walked well alone at age 60 could still walk but with a decline in skill. They also frequently lost the ability to dress themselves completely. Nevertheless, other skills of speech, self-feeding and ordering meals in public were well preserved. These research workers note that their subjects were more severely disabled than people with cerebral palsy as whole.

Andersson and Mattsson (2001) found 79% of 77 adults with spastic diplegia had achieved walking ability with or without aids, but of these, 51% claimed that their walking ability had decreased in recent years and 9% said that they had stopped walking. The reasons reported by these adults for deterioration of walking included decrease in muscle strength, in balance and in their condition. Experience with adults is that either therapy services are focused on children or they are tired of physiotherapy. They found that a specific strengthening programme showed positive results. MacPhail and Kramer (1995) also demonstrated improvement in function and walking following strength training.

Butler and Darrah (2001) pointed out that neurodevelopmental physiotherapy showed no general agreement on the long-term efficacy of focusing on achieving walking.

All these studies generally give a mostly encouraging picture, compared to past views. Prognoses for walking in older people have improved where services and physiotherapy methods together with psychological and social factors have developed for adolescents and adults. Walking may become more difficult for those who develop contractures, joint problems and a decrease in strength, as well as in the presence of fatigue. Prognosis for walking in children is discussed in the section on 'Development of standing and walking' in Chapter 9.

Issues of concern in the older person

Pain. This can be due to many factors. There are abnormal biomechanics causing joint and muscle pain. Excessive range of athetoid motion and muscular dystonia can cause spondylosis of the neck or arthritic changes in joints. There may be overuse syndromes in efforts to keep dealing with daily life (Pimm 1992). Inability to change postures increases joint and muscle pains and skin pressure points. Hodgkinson *et al.* (2001) found hip pain the main concern of non-walking adults with cerebral palsy. Abnormal shoulder girdle postures, especially if pulling in a downward direction, may cause nerve traction. New health problems related to ageing, such as urinary and bowel problems, can cause severe discomfort.

Pain may not receive adequate medical attention or may not be reported by the individual owing to inexperience or due to communication difficulties of cerebral palsy. This also applies to many other health problems in cerebral palsy.

Fatigue. Many are functioning and moving at their peak of performance with little rest. Locomotion is at a high physiological cost for both health and neuromotor problems. The older person is unaccustomed to working out strategies to conserve their energy. For example, the effort to speak need not accompany movement which makes greater energy demands. Distances may be better managed with wheelchairs rather than walking so that energy is conserved for any social or other activity desired by the person. Adults significantly reported more physical but not more mental fatigue than the general population in Norway. They suggest that it is the challenges of work and daily life rather than motor impairment that create fatigue (Jahnsen *et al.* 2003). Early loss of walking can be attributed to the fatigue and high energy cost of having to make efforts to walk (Bottos & Gericke 2003).

Early and minor deterioration. This is often not detected by the person and increasing compensatory motor patterns are therefore used to 'keep going'. These motor patterns can cause increased deformities, stiffness and pain, which add to the person's fatigue. Speech and swallowing problems also increase in some and they may need regular monitoring by a speech and language therapist and medical practitioner. *Swallowing* problems (dysphagia) are reported mainly in people with athetosis (dyskinesia/dystonia).

Urinary problems appear in older persons because either their locomotion has deteriorated and they cannot reach toilet facilities in time or there are bladder problems needing medical attention. Retention of urine is known to occur if adductor tightness has increased, and so initiation of urination is prevented.

Increased musculoskeletal deformities due to biomechanical changes, increased spasticity, weakness and disuse may occur as more time is being spent in sedentary academic or social activities. There is an increase in weight and height, which makes more demand on the neuromotor and musculoskeletal systems, leading to compensatory biomechanical response which can result in deformities, pain and fatigue.

New environments of schools, homes and in the community offer new problems not easily overcome using familiar strategies. More help is needed due to a person's increased size. The older person needs to be educated in how he can let people know what assistance is appropriate for him or her. Therapists' communication skills need to be fine-tuned so they can let teachers, instructors, youth leaders and others know what the physical needs of older persons might be. Unless others are informed of what assistance is necessary, a person with cerebral palsy remains at home and cannot join in community activities, as ageing parents are unlikely to have the capacity to help him do so.

Discrimination in society. Teachers and social workers and disabled people themselves do assist in dealing with discrimination against people with disabilities in society. Therapists are involved in pressing for access, environmental adjustments and attention to other physical needs of the person with disability with whom they are working.

Services for older people. These have been poor and a link-person is really helpful in knowing what is needed and how to obtain health, educational and leisure opportunities and adapted physical activities. This is particularly needed during a child's transition to adolescent and adult services. The need for therapy services is discussed below. Management is particularly important; though therapy needs may not be ongoing, management must be appropriate. This consists of postural management, especially in chairs and wheelchairs, standing frames, positions in bed and appropriate shoes with or without orthoses. Scolioses and other spinal postures need monitoring to avoid deterioration, pain and respiratory problems as well as additional difficulties for carers. Adult teams for adolescents and adults with cerebral palsy are being strongly recommended by many professionals, families and the individuals themselves (Thomas *et al.* 1989; Murphy *et al.* 1995; Bax 2001).

There are many older people who continue to be independent and do not wish to have therapy. They do, however, need monitoring if there are abnormal postures, pain and health problems to enable them to maintain their best level of function. Adults with cerebral palsy are living longer than in the past (Strauss *et al.* 2008).

Motor abilities and self-care activities

Recent research on the growth and development of brain structures and neural pathways (Paus *et al.* 1999; Sowell *et al.* 2002) suggests that potential for learning continues to mature. Although Bottos and Gericke (2003) and others have considered that walking would deteriorate or not be expected in older people as it was not essential for a person's lifelong rehabilitation, the Europe programme with teachers and therapists (MOVE Europe 2001) reported successful teaching of sitting, standing and walking in adolescents.

As many paediatric physiotherapists have focused on children, and plateaus of motor achievement have been reached by adolescence, further potentials have not always been adequately explored. In addition, social and educational needs have correctly received emphasis and time for specialised treatments discouraged (Goldkamp 1984; Cantrell 1997). However, when more up-to-date motor learning approaches are used, functions can be maintained or activated with particular emphasis on daily life activities (see Chapter 2).

The main motor functions needed in school, social situations and in the community are sitting, rising to standing, standing and walking, as well as hand function. This book offers many practical suggestions for learning these functions independently, with assistance or with equipment such as special chairs, wheelchairs, walkers and walking aids.

Although 'a child' is given in the text, this can often be an older person with modifications for body size and weight.

Some individuals may still want to re-learn or learn to walk with or without appropriate walkers. Designs of walkers and equipment have developed since the person with cerebral palsy was much younger. This re-learning or learning may well be possible in the home and in some other environments. An individual may feel more independent, participate more in transfers and manage to exercise with a walker rather than remain seated most of the time. Individuals with severe motor disabilities may actively participate in their care by 'bridging' hips for dressing, rolling over, using minimal arm and hand actions or grasping a support. Participation by an individual with disabilities, no matter how minimal, avoids passivity and a feeling of helplessness.

Carers may also find an individual's participation useful, especially if abilities in sitting, standing and stepping are maintained or trained. Carers may well be able to make less effort and save time. If an individual's active participation is adequate, then this can minimise the demands on carers. The use of two carers may then not always be necessary. A manual handling assessment together with therapist and individuals is necessary to confirm this. There are electric lifters into standers and other hoists and equipment which need to be selected. However, they may not always be manageable in all environments. It is always important to explore the views of both carer and the individual with disability to assess what is realistic in different situations and to assess what potential for assisted or independent function is present in an older person.

If an individual is interested in having specific training sessions, and if these sessions draw on motor learning models, then they need to be supplied by neurological therapists together with teachers, carers or others involved with the individual (Umphred 2000).

Motor developmental assumptions

Some professionals consider that in older children, adolescents and adults, only training in sitting, standing and stepping functions is worthwhile be-

cause the individual no longer needs the child developmental sequences observed in prone or supine lying. Depending on the energy of an individual, this may be appropriate. However, the analysis of tasks needed by the older person involves the selected functional abilities observed in early child development, but they should nevertheless be age-appropriate and relevant to the task desired by individuals and carers.

All people need to turn in bed, get out of and into bed, and get up to sitting or standing from lying. All assisted or independent transfers involve selected elements of head control, reach and grasp, support on arms, half-roll or full roll-over, push up from lying to sitting with legs over the edge of the bed, lying change to supported upright kneeling and up to supported standing. It is especially valuable to have the ability to use early postures in a transitional phase in any sequences of rising from lying to sitting or standing. An older person can draw on the early childhood series of rising observed in prone or supine developmental stages in this book. Such early childhood patterns are the easier motor patterns and therefore may be more useful for an adolescent or adult with disabilities. Naturally there will be adaptations of postural stability, counterpoising and changing of positions so that the developmental sequences are modified according to an individual's condition in specific environments. Generally, creeping, crawling, knee stepping and use of arms and hands in lying and floor sitting with and without equipment are not age-appropriate. Use of hands in lying in bed is naturally useful if an individual can pull up his blankets or use hand grasps to get into and out of bed or to switch off an alarm clock.

Deformities

These are discussed in Chapter 11. The physiotherapist plays an important role in preventing secondary musculoskeletal problems and correcting as many as possible of those that are inevitable. Plaster casts are also used for the older person (Bertoti 1986; Mosely 1997). The tightness of spastic muscles appears to increase with age, especially as muscles become bulkier and do not grow as fast as bones. Botulinum toxin, baclofen and other muscle relaxants are used and need to be associated with a physiotherapy programme (see Chapter 11 on botulinum toxin injections).

Scolioses, pelvic obliquities and hip dislocations are more common in older people than in children (Strauss *et al.* 2004). Orthopaedic surgery is often indicated and surgeons have different approaches and post-operative physiotherapy regimes. Bony operations are often delayed until after growth spurts have ceased in adolescents.

Cervical problems may occur in athetoid (dyskinesia and dystonic) people due to excessive cervical lordosis in compensation for flexed spines or due to persisting involuntary movements of the head and neck (Levine *et al.* 1970). Botulinum toxin A injections have been used for neck dystonia and surgeons may suggest other procedures, though there are many difficulties.

Physiotherapy methods continue to be important, and prolonged stretching, positioning equipment, orthoses, range of motion exercises and position change are particularly recommended in the older age group. Active exercises, strengthening and actions within daily life activities need special attention. Rhythmic stabilisation and other methods from proprioceptive neuromuscular facilitation appeal to teenagers and adults as part of their strengthening and balance training. Damiano *et al.* (1995a,b), Dodd *et al.* (2003) and Damiano (2007) in their scientific studies firmly recommend strengthening. Andersson *et al.* (2003) used progressive strength training or heavy resistance with good results for people who were walking with or without aids. MacPhail and Kramer (1995) found strengthening improved function and walking. McBurney *et al.* (2003) carried out a qualitative study of the value of strength training from the perception of young people and their parents.

Stretching with manual methods for trunk and hips used in the Bobath Centre, London, are followed by the individual's active maintenance of the new alignment in sitting and standing as well as by specific facilitated walking patterns (Christine Barber, personal communication, 2001). Conductive education groups for adults focus more on function than on deformities, though there are corrective movement synergies (Kinsman *et al.* 1988).

Young people who can understand are motivated by measurements of increased range, strength and number of times they can carry out an activity.

They enjoy biofeedback training on force plates with video feedback of symmetrical weight bearing and weight shift, and other records of specific achievements (Winstein *et al.* 1989; Hartveld & Hegarty 1996).

Explanations are given to educate an individual about why motor activities are necessary to minimise the effect of growth spurts, disuse, increasing weight with immobility. Deterioration of motor functions may decrease confidence in physiotherapy. Young people need explanations such as that shorter spastic muscles are bulkier and tighter in older people, that growth spurts lead to bone growing faster than muscles and cause deformities, and that deterioration is not due to poor physiotherapy or primarily to their lack of practice. Unwitting habits of prolonged sitting in one posture or repetition of movements in only a few patterns may lead to deformities.

Physiotherapy treatment for aches and pains need to be offered and responsibilities for attending treatment appointments are given to those who need them.

If possible, adolescents should be shown how to apply orthoses and given responsibility for doing so (Fig. 7.1). If hand function or balance does not allow independence, then the individual instructs someone in such applications. If speech is poor, then handout sheets can be prepared by the therapist with an individual. Computers enable many individuals to communicate care needs and exercises to carers. These are examples of developing autonomy in growing adolescents and adults.

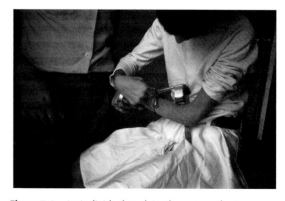

Figure 7.1 An individual applying her own orthosis.

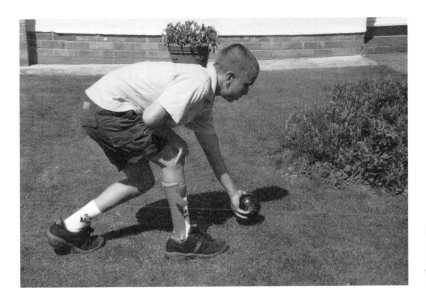

Figure 7.2 Keeping fit with bowling and other motor activities. A hinged ankle–foot orthosis is worn on his right leg, allowing ankle motion.

Healthy lifestyle

The quality of life for an older and especially ageing person with cerebral palsy is improved if the following are available:

(1) An understanding general practitioner who makes community resources available when an individual has pain, ordinary health problems or depressions. Blaming the cerebral palsy condition is not addressing the quality-of-life needs of a person.

(2) Communication problems due to speech and language disabilities result in a person not conveying their needs well enough and thus not receiving health care as any other citizen would. As a person with cerebral palsy may be using special communication aids and methods, then the advocate for that person with cerebral palsy needs to educate his hospital nurses and anyone involved with that person about his special communication aids and methods.

(3) Adolescents and adults with disabilities need to have had education since late childhood about healthy lifestyles. However, this is even more important in adolescence and adulthood. Care with regard to nutrition, weight control, keeping fit and positive mental attitudes or stress management improves quality of life. The strength training studies with references above

contribute much to these aspects of physical and mental health. Counselling or peer group discussions as well as health education in groups are valuable for different individuals. Others may prefer health workers or therapists in one-to-one sessions. This preference may be relevant when sexual and bodily functions are to be discussed.

Exercising on stationary bicycles, rowing machines or treadmills as well as sports are useful for keeping fit (Fig. 7.2). The person with disabilities needs supervision by a therapist in case deformities are threatened by the movement patterns and efforts of the person. However, this is weighed up against the quality of life of each person. Darrah *et al.* (1999) positively evaluated a community fitness programme for adolescents. Fatigue needs to be avoided when such activities are overdone by enthusiastic people. Pimm (1992) has drawn attention to physiological burnout in adults who try to maintain their motor levels in the presence of deterioration of strength and energy.

Respiratory problems may arise in later years due to immobility, scolioses and lack of ordinary health care. General exercises, aerobics and respiratory physiotherapy may well be needed. Swimming as well as exercise are recommended by most therapists for aerobic capacity and fitness, which may prevent fatigue (Vogtle *et al.* 1998).

Develop appropriate community mobility

In order to access social clubs, meet friends or participate in education and work, it is essential that appropriate wheelchairs and transport are considered. Electric wheelchairs and correct seating have improved considerably through seating clinics and technological advances. Occupational therapists often provide assessments and, together with a physiotherapist, an individual is enabled to learn the correct use of a wheelchair. In severe conditions, the therapist assesses which part of the body an individual can reliably control or learn to control for using joysticks or switches to manage electric wheelchairs.

Using a wheelchair does not automatically deter a person with cerebral palsy from learning to walk with a walker, with the help of friends, carer or independently. The energy and motivation of an individual are crucial and realistically he may often wish to walk only within the home or in school rather than in the community. The distance, roughness or smoothness of the ground and weather determine the decision to walk outdoors. Once again, discussions with the individual and comments by his family and friends contribute to planning. The physiotherapist considers the individual's weight-bearing abilities, stepping and adequate hand function for walkers (see Chapter 8 on assessment for equipment and Chapter 9, section on 'Development of standing and walking').

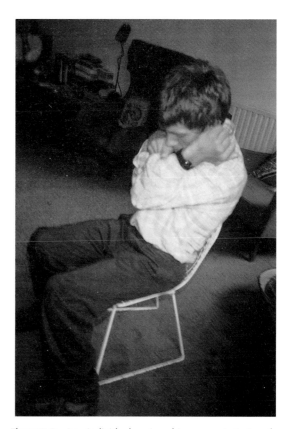

Figure 7.3 An individual using his own strategies for independence in fastening sleeve buttons. No resultant deformities.

Training of self-care and cosmetic appearance

This is discussed in Chapter 10 on motor function in daily care. The speech therapists, occupational therapists and physiotherapists, all contribute to training of eating, dressing, washing, bathing, toileting and hygiene abilities. Therapists also need to respect an individual person's own strategies, especially when deformities are unlikely to result from such strategies (see Fig. 7.3).

Age-appropriate activities such as hair setting, hair cuts, use of cosmetics, clothes and the interests of any normal adolescent are important parts of the programme. An interest in one's appearance has motivated some adolescents to practise good posture and keep-fit exercises. Sadness about appearance due to cerebral palsy is not uncommon. Counselling and emphasis of all assets of a person need consideration. Skills with a hobby such as bird watching, photography, or social assets give confidence to people and all need to find out what these assets are.

Knowledge about the condition

Teach individuals all they need to know about their specific condition. This is implicit in the collaborative learning model. If parents have already received this information over the years, they also convey this to their adolescent son or daughter. However, this needs additional education from a professional who explains aspects in a different style. In addition, adolescents who are feeling anxious or depressed may not have absorbed medical information. They are more 'grown-up' and need direct education for themselves and answers to their own questions.

Sex education is important and there are organisations and groups that offer information in this area.

Therapeutic motor activities

There are an increasing number of activities for people with all levels of disabilities. They not only keep an individual fit but also maintain motor abilities and opportunities for treating deformities. Swimming is particularly enjoyable and useful for maintaining ranges of motion as it includes stretches. There are a number of clubs promoting horse riding for people with disabilities, which helps individuals in maintaining balance, abduction and use of hand grasp (see the section on 'Adjuncts to therapy' in Chapter 3). Sailing, angling, skiing and abseiling are some of the many activities which are beneficial. In Britain, there are adventure holidays and imaginative activities designed for people with disabilities. Social skills and friendships develop in the clubs which often have both the able-bodied and people with disabilities.

Measures

Reports by the individuals themselves are important. Jahnsen *et al.* (2006) found that self-reports by adults with cerebral palsy agreed with the professionals in using the GMFCS (Palisano *et al.* 2008). Older individuals report well on the decrease in falls, increase in any daily function, distance walked, wheelchair control and bed mobility and transfers.

There are a number of tests of balance, arm reach with postural control, spasticity and weakness that are used in adults with neurological conditions. These can also be adapted or used in cerebral palsy (Bower & Ashburn 1998; Umphred 2000; Shumway-Cook & Woollacott 2001).

Assessment for therapy and daily function

Approach to assessment

The framework for all assessments is outlined to synthesise various approaches. This avoids use of assessment methods focused on any one therapy system.

The framework consists of the following assessments:

(1) The task(s) individuals want to achieve. Their choice may be a daily activity in self-care, play, social interaction or during recreation.
(2) The motor functions for the individual's chosen task, for example sitting, standing, using a form of locomotion and using hands. The individual's developmental level of motor functions is identified.
(3) The component abilities of each motor function needed for the chosen task. This includes specific postural mechanisms, relevant voluntary movements and perceptual motor abilities which may be present but abnormal or are absent.
(4) The impairments which may be preventing achievement or causing abnormal performance such as limited range of motion, weakness, abnormal reflex reactions, abnormal movement patterns, postural malalignments or limited

repertoire of movements for the task. The impairments are primary and secondary. These impairments include any medical conditions such as pain, fatigue, poor nutrition, respiratory problems and general health in individuals.
(5) The constraints on motor functions and their components by other impairments and disabilities of vision, hearing, perception, understanding and communication.
(6) The abilities or residual abilities of these components of vision, hearing, perception, cognition and communication and general motivation which can reinforce the learning of motor functions.

This process of assessment is discussed in Chapters 2 and 6 to show how specific assessments of posture, movements and use of sensations are observed in the context of whole daily functions or tasks which individuals want to achieve and the family background which enables achievement. This chapter addresses the specific assessments and objective measures by a physiotherapist and occupational therapist, which grow out of the collaborative learning models in Chapters 2, 6 and 7.

Assessments of motor functions, their specific components and impairments, often take place in physiotherapy rooms in hospital units and special centres. Whenever possible, these daily functions are best observed in individuals' natural environments most relevant to the tasks chosen by them and the specific people involved with individuals. Therefore, depending on a therapist's workplace, appropriate organisation is made to include the important observations of individuals in their own environments. The therapist is then enabled to complement the clinical examinations and to have assessments of the following:

- Which tasks, functions and component abilities are actually used and which are not being activated.
- Which physical obstacles in the environment prevent use of a task, functions and component abilities or block further development. Assessment, both indoors and outdoors, shows, for example, whether access is available, ground is uneven or slippery, furniture is inappropriate or there are no stable objects or bars to grasp. Recommended special equipment needs to be assessed as useful in different environments.
- Which attitudes and behaviours of people in the individual's environments may influence a child's motor or whole daily functions and the use of components or whole of a task.
- Whether a child's motivation and behaviour vary in different environments.

Occupational therapists in different places have expertise in environmental assessments and share their information with centre-based physiotherapists. Simultaneous visits of physiotherapists with occupational therapists to an individual's environment are desirable whenever possible. Community paediatric physiotherapists and occupational therapists are well placed to obtain the broad perspective of a child's function in home, school and community.

Purpose of assessment and outcomes

(1) *To respond to the reason for referral*, which may be for additional medical information, for educational placements, for parental needs or for social or legal considerations. Some adolescents or adults with cerebral palsy refer themselves and state their reasons. People paying for therapy will want assessments indicating the need for physiotherapy and reassessments of outcomes.

Therefore, the type of assessment varies according to the referral. Physiotherapy assessments need to relate to what information is wanted and how it will be used.

(2) *To add to medical and other diagnostic* information as specific assessments before *and* during therapy involve long periods of time and close contact with a child and his family. Information may be revealed to a therapist when not obvious in shorter consultations with different medical consultants. A therapist will also detect any unusual deterioration which needs referral to a neurologist in case a progressive neurological condition rather than cerebral palsy is becoming obvious. Deterioration in function due to neuromuscular, deformity, health or behavioural problems may be detected so that referral can be made to other professionals.

(3) *To participate in screening and follow-up* of children 'at risk' of developing cerebral palsy and to decide whether specialised physiotherapy or monitoring is indicated.

(4) *To plan a specific physiotherapy and occupational therapy programme based on the child and parents' needs*. There are programmes of selected treatment methods focused on function and the component abilities and for impairments constraining function. Therapy includes a management programme with information and practical ideas for all involved with a child or older person.

(5) *To evaluate progress (outcomes)* in reassessments which may lead to continuation, modification, changes or periodical stopping of specific therapy methods and sometimes of specific therapy sessions. The evaluation also changes practical suggestions for others involved with an individual.

(6) *To share assessments and evaluations* with child, parents and families, and others involved with a child and to receive their reports and views.

(7) *To contribute to research into the effectiveness of therapy* by using standardised measures within a research study. Clinical assessments and measures discussed in this chapter also detect questions for research (see section 'Research and clinical studies' in Chapter 4).

Review of a therapist's observations

Observations are made during joint assessments with a child and parents or with an older person. There will also be other joint assessments with another professional and with carers. They are continued during specialised 'hands-on' assessment and evaluation as well as during ongoing therapy and management. Observations need to be as unobtrusive as possible and must precede 'hands-on' examinations and measurements to gain rapport with child, parents and any family members present at assessments.

(1) *Behaviour.* Observe whether a child is alert, apathetic, irritable or fearful in a session or during particular activities. A child or older person may become fatigued easily, make undue effort, or show discomfort or fear during an activity. Find out what motivates any actions. Is it a particular situation, a person, special plaything or hobby? There may be fear of falling, of augmenting musculoskeletal pain or due to space perception problems. Behaviours are detailed in Chapters 2, 6, 7, 10 and 12.

(2) *Communication.* Observe how the child and parents interact (see Chapter 2). Find out whether a child initiates or responds with gestures, sounds, hand or finger pointing, eye pointing or uses words and speech.

(3) *Attention span.* What catches a child's attention? How does a parent assist him to maintain attention and what distracts him? Distractibility is due to brain damage and/or environmental overstimulation.

(4) *Understanding.* Observe if a child follows suggestions to move or promptings to act. What does he appear to understand? (See section 'Development of communication – brief summary' in Chapter 10.)

(5) *Position.* Notice which position he chooses to be in and if he get into that position on his own or with help. Observe if a parent can place him in a position and if he participates in any way. His limbs and head may move more easily in some positions than in others. Involuntary movements may be decreased in some positions.

(6) *Postural control and alignment.* Observe how much parental support is given and check a child's own ability in postural stabilisation and counterpoising (postural adjustment) in all postures. Parental support may be excessive or reasonable. Check whether a child bears more weight on one side of his body, or on one hand or foot. A child may collapse to one side, twist to one side, or tilt and turn his head to one side. Observe any fears of falling in a child due to poor balance experience. Parental anxiety about falling may increase a child's fears.

(7) *Use of limbs and hands.* Observe limb patterns in changing or going into a position as well as using them in a position. There may be excessive flexion, extension or rotation in one part of the range. Observe whether one or both hands are used, type of grasp and release. Inaccuracy of reach and hand actions also indicates a possible visual problem. Observe any involuntary movements, tremors or spasms which interfere with actions.

(8) *Sensory aspects.* Observe a child's use of vision, hearing, touch, smell and temperature in relevant tasks. Does he enjoy particular sensations? Notice whether he enjoys being moved or having his position changed. He may show an increase in tension and apprehension on being touched and handled. Are his hands persistently fisted so sensation cannot be experienced?

(9) *Form of locomotion.* On entering the room, observe how a child is carried, if he uses a wheelchair or walking aids. During the session, create interest which motivates him to roll, creep, crawl, bottom shuffle or walk to where a daily activity is to be carried out. A child may have unusual ways of getting about, such as dragging himself along his stomach, along his back, *bunny hopping* on both knees, *running headlong* and a variety of abnormal gaits.

(10) *Deformities.* Observe any recurring positions of the whole child as well as of parts of his body in all postures and in the movements he uses in motor functions and daily living activities.

Impairment and function

The observations above are predominantly functional. The observation of impairments which constrain function will vary with age and any changes in diagnostic classifications (see Chapter 1).

There is a functional view of the impairments as subtypes of cerebral palsy. For example, hemiplegia tends to be less disabling in motor function than diplegia, and diplegia less than tetraplegia. Dyskinesia tends to be more severe than spastic hemiplegia, diplegia and ataxia (Ostensjo *et al.* 2004). However, other research studies with a large number of participants have a few subtypes of spastic tetraplegia and of dyskinesia present in milder levels of functional disability, and a few of spastic hemiplegia in more severe levels. Spastic diplegia can be present at any functional level (Beckung *et al.* 2007; Voorman *et al.* 2007).

Chapter 9 gives details of impairments linked with functional aspects so that they can be immediately related to simultaneous functional therapy with minimising of impairments which are constraining the specific function. The suggested therapy and management methods do not separate impairment from function but integrate them so that a quality of function may be gained as far as possible. However, in the very severe conditions, more attention is given to minimising deformities whilst activating whatever minimal function can be achieved.

Teamwork and the influence of other disabilities

The therapist will need a comprehensive assessment from a team (see Chapter 1; Thylefors *et al.* 2000). She will learn from the different professionals what modifications to make for specific visual, hearing and sensory impairments. She will adjust her communication with a child in relation to any speech and language difficulties and find out what communication systems are being used, for example Paget, Makaton, Bliss or electronic communication aids. If a child has perceptual problems (sensory processing difficulties) relating to body scheme, space, distance and timing, then adaptations will be recommended by specialists in the team.

Medical consultants inform therapists about a child's or older person's health, nutrition problems, fatigue, possible pain and other medical impairments which affect energy, motivation and attention span. The health problems of parents are also relevant to therapists' home programmes for their child.

General points for assessments

- Assessments need to be playful, interesting and non-threatening.
- Assess a young child, as much as possible, on a parent's lap.
- Observe a child among the familiar toys as well as with selected toys to activate interest as well as reveal dormant abilities.
- Keep sessions within the bounds of a child's concentration.
- Have an unhurried atmosphere.
- Have easy, successful actions of a child interspersed with difficult tasks.
- Avoid undressing a child, especially an adolescent, until he is happy about this.
- Time is needed for a child who is unhappy about a new environment, new professional or new experience of being assessed in a different style.
- An individual needs time to attempt new abilities in the assessment.
- Consider a child's state of health and energy.

Assessments can take from one to four sessions, depending on each child's severity, mood, level of energy and cooperation. It is usual to create a final plan of therapy and management after a number of assessments, especially if a therapist meticulously checks her assessment findings with the variations in daily behaviour of a child. It is surprising that daily variations are rarely checked by some therapists as it is well known that a child has good and bad days in function. Assessments need to relate directly to therapy methods and evaluations so that parents appreciate the relevance of specific professional assessments. It is wise to select some home therapy on the first visit, so parents feel 'something is given' for them to do which will help their child.

Assessment and measurements

Clinical assessment includes both careful observations and measurements. There is a growing importance of measurements for evidence-based practice. However, in cerebral palsy there are still observations of unique abilities and difficulties discovered in careful clinical assessments of an individual. These are significant for therapy and for a child's own strategies. The observations for clinical assessment cannot always be easily measured using current measurement tools (measures).

It is also recommended that a therapist's assessments are not limited to existing measures. Although measures are important, they should not reduce her own innovative observations. In addition, current measures are based on values which may change in the light of research. For example, measures were focused on spasticity for many years and functional measures thought to be dependent on them (Bobath & Bobath 1984; Haas and Crow 1995; among others). In some references in Haas and Crow's review (1995), in Levitt (1977, Physical Ability Chart) and in Shepherd (1995), spasticity was not given great significance and functional assessments and measures were valued much more.

As in previous editions, Chapter 9 continues to present clinical assessments of function in prone, supine, sitting and standing positions and use of hands so that treatment and management suggestions (sometimes called 'tactics or strategies') are immediately related. A developmental framework is used to show how the components of motor functions are normally developed and how an abnormal performance may be normal at an earlier age. For example, asymmetry is normal in a number of early actions and postures, and so weight bearing on one side of the body in lying is expected at the 0–3-month developmental stage. A person's stepping in a walker giving full trunk support is similar to the manually supported stepping of an able-bodied baby at the developmental level of around 6 months. The normal gait of a toddler uses components such as co-contractions, wide base, flat foot contact and more double leg support, which are also seen in older children with cerebral palsy. A developmental framework also shows a therapist the degree of motor delay which has an effect on other areas of child development.

The examination of the individual in channels of prone development, supine development, sitting, standing and walking development, and hand function also shows any influence of impairments in the functions. Impairments which create deformities are treated within these developmental functions and

also discussed in an additional Chapter 11 on specific problems of deformity in cerebral palsy.

Clinical progress is assessed when supports by equipment, walkers and orthoses are decreased or eliminated. Walkers can change from wheel-walkers to elbow crutches, quadripods or sticks.

Current measures used in cerebral palsy

The traditional therapy measures in physiotherapy and occupational therapy are for impairments and motor functions and participation in self-care skills such as eating, washing, toileting and dressing. These measures can be linked with the International Classification of Functioning, Disability and Health (ICF), World Health Organization (WHO 2001) aspects of body structure and function (impairments), with activity (daily functions and self-care skills) and with some aspects of participation. Participation and quality of life have received consideration in occupational therapy, social work and psychology. The teamwork with other professionals, families and others involved in the life of the young or older person with cerebral palsy adds information to the therapist's assessments of environmental and personal factors which are stated in the ICF. There are parent or child questionnaires which are being increasingly used by therapists. There are also measures for environmental factors used by professions other than physiotherapists and are given below.

Measurements of impairments

When assessments of impairments are made, a therapist assumes which of the impairments appear to primarily constrain function. This assumption is studied by Ostensjo *et al.* (2003, 2004) and discussed in relation to the International Classification of Functioning, Disability and Health (WHO 2001). This study found that the measure of abnormal selective motor control links more with overall motor function than spasticity and range of motion. 'Motor function is strongly related to accomplishment of essential tasks in daily life' (Ostensjo *et al.* 2004). Voorman *et al.* (2007) support the view that selective motor control and strength are most important for gross motor function. However, in a study by Bartlett and Palisano (2002), spasticity, topographical distribution and range of motion (ROM) were listed by paediatric physiotherapists as the most important impairments which contributed to change in motor function. Selective motor control was not listed and weakness was not given emphasis.

There was no correlation of true spasticity with function at Gross Motor Function Classification System (GMFCS) Levels I to III (Palisano *et al.* 1997) in researches by Ross and Engsberg (2002, 2007). They used KinCom, an instrumented dynamometer, to measure spasticity and strength in the same subjects, and showed no relationship between strength and spasticity, nor between spasticity, motor function and gait. They pointed out that their research did not include children in more severe classifications.

A number of research studies now find that *weakness rather than spasticity* is particularly significant for functional disability in cerebral palsy (Damiano & Abel 1998; Damiano *et al.* 2002a,b; Ross & Engsberg 2002, 2007; Shortland *et al.* 2002; McNee *et al.* 2004).

Weakness

Strength is the ability to generate force to either move a body part or stabilise a body part and resist movement. These two aspects need assessment for physiotherapy exercises and functional activities. Strength may be measured isometrically (no change in muscle length), isotonically (shortening of muscle length) or isokinetically (concentric and eccentric work during a specific velocity of movement). Endurance is measured by the number of repetitions of a motor function. Cardiovascular measures of fitness relate to energy consumption and endurance. A child can be 'weak' when not fit (Miller 2007). Parker *et al.* (1993) found that aerobic power and anaerobic power of the legs, but not of the arms, were correlated with the total score and the scores for the standing and walking, and running and jumping subsections of the Gross Motor Function Measure (GMFM).

The isotonic (concentric) and isometric (eccentric) muscle actions are measured clinically and the isokinetic measure is tested with instrumented systems. Children with cerebral palsy cannot easily be measured with traditional manual muscle tests. Florence *et al.* (1992) give the Medical Research Council (MRC) manual strength test with the original 6-point scale as well as a modified 11-point scale.

However, these isotonic assessments can be used as guides together with other measures. The hand-held dynamometer quantifies isometric strength or the force required to break the active position held by a person against resistance given by the examiner. The procedure and reliability of hand-held dynamometer are confirmed by various authors (Taylor *et al.* 2004; Crompton *et al.* 2007).

Children under 4 years do not cooperate with either of these measures because they cannot understand the procedure, nor do they have the ability to isolate muscles for testing because of lack of selective muscle control. Furthermore, excessive co-contraction and impaired selective motor control in any person may interfere with the ability to produce agonist force (Damiano *et al.* 2002a).

Wiley and Damiano (1998) have strength tests for children who are able-bodied and in cerebral palsy. Their subjects are frequently older and less severely affected and can be classified in GMFCS Levels I, II or III (Palisano *et al.* 1997). Manual muscle tests are very difficult in adults and children with severe cerebral palsy classified in Levels IV or V. These individuals often have cognitive impairments which prevent them following test procedures. Ohata *et al.* (2006, 2008) recently investigated ultrasound sonography which might measure muscle strength and activity in these severely involved adults or in children at all levels of severity. They related atrophy with weakness.

Clinical assessment of strength. The observations are usually of muscle actions in motor functions, whether this is a holding action for postural stability or a moving action in voluntary motion or in rising (righting) and saving reactions. Long and Toscano (2002) also use observation of muscles in anti-gravity positions and assumption of positions, symmetry and any compensatory patterns rather than muscle testing in very young children. It has been found that muscle tests on the couch can differ from muscle actions in function, which include the actions in synergies and the postural mechanisms. For example, shoulder girdle muscles may work well in crawl position but not in a muscle test on the couch. Back extensors may be well activated in prone but not in sitting or standing. Extension of the elbow is greater when a child reaches out for a desired object than when tested with the conventional 'stretch your elbow' in muscle tests. Static and dynamic measures of lower extremity range of motion in the clinical examination are inconsistent with instrumental measures of gait (McMulkin *et al.* 2000).

Functional assessments such as sit change to standing and return to sitting assess both concentric and eccentric muscle actions (Shepherd 1995). Rising onto toes and standing on toes assess both concentric and isometric muscle action of plantar flexors. Rising from lying to sitting, crawl to sitting, and crawl to standing reveals strength of arms in weight bearing. Records of strength have depended on a therapist's judgement, such as a scale of: absent, present at initiation or throughout range or absent, trace, poor or strong. Such a scale indicates need for strengthening activities. But such scales can be questioned as being evidence-based physiotherapy. Voorman *et al.* (2007) within their research used a test of strength of legs by having children squat and stretch up eight times. Support for balance is allowed. The categories are:

- good strength for eight or more times
- moderate strength for fewer than eight or performed as part of the motion eight times
- poor strength if not able to squat and stretch out at all.

This test apparently also includes endurance as well as strength in ranges of flexion and extension of limbs. ROM was measured with goniometry in supine and in other tests. However, their test is scoring for impairment within function. This should motivate therapists to develop better scoring for evidence-based muscle actions in functional assessments in the future.

Spasticity

Slow passive range of movement demonstrates the muscle length or extensibility of the muscles. The slow passive ROMs are measured by goniometry and limitations of range show stiffness of spastic muscles, mobility of joints and tightness of soft tissues. The measurements of length limitations in slow ROM are not the same as measurements of range limitation in velocity-dependent spasticity or reflex response to quick stretch. To challenge us further, joint range may be full in very young children with stiff, spastic muscles, but muscle actions are *hypoextensible* and limit range of active movement. Clinical reasoning is available to select treatment options.

Clinical measurements of spasticity. The frequently used Ashworth scale and Modified Ashworth scales (MAS) have the examiner rate the amount of tone felt as a limb is passively stretched. In a scale from 0–5, there is an estimate of how soon in the motion and how much during the motion the resistance to stretch is felt (Bohannon and Smith 1987). It is also used in measurements for botulinum toxin A treatment of spasticity (see section 'Botulinum toxin A' in Chapter 11). However, it should not be the only measure.

There are questions about the objectivity of the MAS (Pandyan *et al.* 1999; Miller 2007). Damiano *et al.* (2002b) investigated the precision of the Ashworth scale by using isokinetic dynamometer measures of passive stretch together with electromyography (EMG), which shows muscle activity in response to the quick passive stretch. They show that slow passive stretch without muscle activation on the EMG is *stiffness due to muscle transformations and tight soft tissues*. This 'intrinsic' muscle stiffness has higher correlation with the original Ashworth test rather than the magnitude of resistance to quick passive stretch. The children in the study by Damiano *et al.* (2002b) were in less severe classifications (GMFCS Levels I–III), with most at Levels II and III (Palisano *et al.* 1997). Ashworth scales are weakly correlated with function measures. Damiano *et al.* (2002b) hypothesise that in future studies, measures with instrumented isokinetic dynamometers used with cases of severe cerebral palsy may demonstrate an influence of spasticity on function.

Scholtes *et al.* (2006) reviewed 13 clinical instruments to measure spasticity, having identified validity criteria from 119 references. They report on a number of 'Ashworth-like scales', the Tardieu Scale, a Modified Tardieu Scale (MTS), the New York University Tone Scale and other lesser known scales. They found most instruments to assess spasticity did not comply with the physiological definition of spasticity as a velocity-dependent response to passive stretch. This definition was used only in the Tardieu measures (Tardieu *et al.* 1954). Tardieu tests measure increased muscle tone at three different velocities of stretch and the joint angle at which the 'catch' or increased tone appears. However, the original Tardieu scales are time-consuming in order to carry out a comprehensive assessment and the speed of the velocities are not standardised. This is questioned, particularly the time-consuming aspect, for use with

Table 8.1   Modified Ashworth Scale

Score	Description
0	Hypotonic: less than normal tone, floppy
1	Normal: no increase in muscle tone
2	Mild: slight increase in tone, 'catch' in limb movement or minimal resistance to movement through less than half of the range
3	Moderate: more marked increase in tone through most of the range of motion but affected part is easily moved
4	Severe: considerable increase in tone, passive movement difficult
5	Extreme: affected part rigid in flexion or extension

Source: Modified by Hedberg *et al.*, see Ostensjo *et al.* (2004).

children. From their detailed studies, Scholtes *et al.* (2006) advise that clinicians make a comparison of 'the maximal ROM at a very slow passive stretch before and after treatment of spasticity and the joint angle of the catch at a fast velocity passive stretch before and after treatment'.

Boyd and Graham (1999) proposed a measurement of passive range by modifying the Tardieu Scale and calling it an MTS. They use goniometry to measure R1, the joint angle of the 'catch' after fast stretch, and R2, the maximum joint angle after slow stretch. It is suggested that if there is a large difference between R1 and R2, then there is a greater dynamic component, whereas a smaller difference would indicate that muscle contracture is greater than spasticity. As these measurements were essentially devised to plan BTX A treatment, they found that BTX A was useful for the dynamic component.

Fosang *et al.* (2003) investigated the reliability of clinical measures of Passive Ranges of Motion (PROM), MAS and an MTS. They did not use the MTS by Boyd and Graham (1999) as its reliability had not been assessed. They found that PROM and MTS measures can be reliable, provided the examiners were sufficiently trained with enough time for practice. Large changes as a result of intervention are needed to overcome error margins in test–retest and inter-rater results. Because of poor reliability the MAS, if used, should only be carried out by single raters for the same participant (subject/client).

Table 8.1 is an up-to-date Swedish modification of the Ashworth scale used in a careful research study by Ostensjo *et al.* (2004).

The *factors for reliable clinical assessments* are as follows:

(1) Standardise the posture for testing, the position of the other limbs and midline head position.
(2) Standardise the initial length from which the muscle group is stretched.
(3) Use the same maximal force for slow ROM (difficult to assess by researchers).
(4) Check that child/adult is relaxed, avoiding sensory stimulation by those present.
(5) Consider any fatigue of a child or older person.
(6) The time of day, temperature and any pain may influence results.

Selective motor control

Immature motor control does not activate the appropriate muscles but muscles and joint movements not needed for the specific action. This lack of selective motor control has also been called mass movement patterns or stereotyped movement pattern. The muscles in stereotyped patterns are so closely linked that an isolated movement is not possible. These patterns reflect a lack of fractionation in lesions of the central nervous system (Shumway-Cook & Woollacott 2001). A number of these patterns are described in cerebral palsy and considered abnormal movement synergies.

Measurement of the selective motor control by Voorman *et al.* (2007) is to ask a child to extend the knee and dorsiflex the ankle in sitting without feet supported.

For example, scoring for selective ankle dorsiflexion is:

Score 0 – no selective dorsiflexion, only synergy of hip–knee flexion with ankle flexion;

Score 1 – diminished selective movement. Selective dorsiflexion in the first part of the movement range. Later in the range there is no selective movement;

Score 2 – full selective movement, knee extension with ankle dorsiflexion.

The scores for both legs together vary from total scores 0, 1 or 2 for poor; total scores 3, 4 or 5 for moderate; and total scores 6, 7 or 8 for good selective motor control.

Boyd and Graham (1999) propose a different scale with a child tested in long-leg sitting.

Examination of deformity and ranges of motion

The therapist should obtain information on the following:

- *Structure of joints* in children over 3 years – especially subdislocation or dislocation of the hips, varus or valgus neck of femur, spinal vertebrae, knees and feet. The structure of all joints in the body is also important, especially as a child becomes older, adolescent and adult. X-rays are used for joints causing concern.
- *Inequality in the length of legs* but not so much in the arms, as far as function is concerned. Measure limb length from anterior iliac spine to medial malleolus.
- *Joint range.* There needs to be a flexible musculoskeletal system as far as possible for motor functional training. Passive ROM carried out slowly detects fixed or unfixed deformity. Limited range of deformity is due not only to joint problems but also to length of stiff muscles and to tightness of soft tissues (tendons, ligaments, connective tissue). Fixed deformity is a contracture which cannot be overcome in a passive range of movement and is present during sleep. Dynamic or unfixed deformity can be manually moved through full range and disappears during sleep. (Differ-

ent workers define deformity and contractures differently.)

- *Strength of short and overlengthened muscles* is assessed as they contribute to deformity.

See section 'Deformities and gait' in Chapter 11 in which different topographical types of spastic cerebral palsies are discussed.

Passive range (Table 8.2 and Figs 8.1a,b and 8.2)

Passive range examines any limitations or excessive joint ranges. Goniometers measure ranges, provided a standard procedure is used (see 'Factors for reliable clinical assessments' under 'Spasticity' above). Stuberg *et al.* (1988) and McDowell *et al.* (2000) question the reliability of goniometer measures. This can be improved if a single experienced examiner using standard procedures can control accuracy of measures, with care taken with proximal and distal segments for measures, standard force and single degree increases on the goniometer. Goldsmith *et al.* (1992) offer a measure for windswept position in the legs. Electro-goniometers are also used but not easily available. Ranges in paediatrics are not well documented (Long & Toscano 2002). The Test of Spinal Alignment and Range of Motion Measure (SAROMM) (Bartlett & Purdie 2005) measures deviations in symmetry of spinal alignment. It is reliable but still being tested for sensitivity to change.

Active range

Pre-operative and postoperative physiotherapy may require localised assessment to confirm that muscle groups which have been given the opportunity to act by the operation are in fact doing so. Active ranges and strength can clinically be observed in function as discussed under 'Clinical assessment of strength' above. Postural mechanisms need testing for strength of trunk and pelvic musculature pre- and postoperatively.

In Chapter 9, details are given of the motor patterns at each level of active developmental function in typical or normal children, which are delayed in cerebral palsy. Abnormal performances are also given in details of head, trunk, pelvis and limbs. These assessments need to be in Chapter 9 in order to immediately relate procedures which may improve them.

Table 8.2   Assessment of joint range.

Assess:
Passive joint range: to demonstrate joint flexibility, muscle length (extensibility, shortening), muscle and soft tissue tightness (spasticity, rigidity)

Test *slowly* for muscle and soft tissue tightness and with fast speed for true physiological spasticity. *Active joint* range for range and ability to move. Strength and the opposing degree of tightness affect active range.

Note: different positions may affect range of motion in some cases. Check in supine, prone and side lying. Observe postures in sitting and standing as well to see the effect of limited joint ranges. There is lack of consensus on paediatric ranges (Long & Toscano 2002).

Note any pain, especially in the hip ranges. Note associated pelvic and spinal positions during tests.

Hip flexor tightness – extension range
Supine. Bend one knee to chest, hold to flatten lumbar spine. The other leg will flex off the surface. Measure this hip flexion by goniometry angle between thigh and surface. Norm 0–20° age 2–5, 0° by age 12.

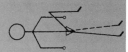

or
Bend both knees to chest. Hold one bent and see how far the other can be stretched down to the bed.

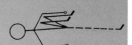

Prone. Both legs flexed at hip over edge of bed. Extend one hip towards midline as the other leg maintains flat lumbar spine.

Prone-lying hips and knees straight on surface. Single knee is bent from straight to 130–140 degrees. If the hip lifts into flexion, then there is shortening of rectus femoris. See test below for knee extensor tightness as short, stiff rectus femoris affects both hip flexor and knee extensor.

Hip extensor tightness – flexion range
Supine. Bend both hips and knees to chest. Note range and degree of extensor tightness. Ninety degrees flexion is for upright sitting.

Bend one hip and knee with thigh to touch abdomen, with the other held straight to fix pelvis. Full hip flexion is limited by hip extensor tightness or hip problems.

Hip adductor tightness – abduction range
Test in supine, knees over edge. Abduct hips with hips straight, knees bent to right angle. Each hip abducts to more than 30 degrees from midline with hips flat. Slowly extend knees in the abducted position. Tight gracilis reduces the degree of abduction in extension.

Abduct both hips with hips at right angles and knees flexed. Each hip is 45° from midline and there is 90° between them. These three procedures reveal tightness in different muscle groups and show any differences in range between each side. Another test is in supine with extended hips and knees. Abduct legs slowly then quickly and compare the measures of distance between them (knee-distance test).

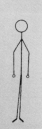

Hip abductor tightness – adduction range
Bring legs together and hips straight from *frog position* if present.

(Continued)

Table 8.2 (*Continued*)

Hip rotator tightness – internal or external rotation
Prone. Assess with hip extended and knee flexed to 90°. Fix pelvis with hand on buttocks. Hold lower leg and rotate knee and hip inwards. Rotate single knee and hip outwards. Full range is 90 degrees without defining internal or external range alone due to normal variations. Excessive rotation one way is detected.

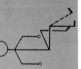

Supine. Hips are extended, knees over bed edge. Keep one leg in hip and knee flexion to fix pelvis. Rotate the other lower leg and hip inwards and then outwards. Supine hip and knee flexed. Assess internal rotation of both legs and exteranal rotation of one leg at a time. Keep pelvis fixed. Norm 45° between rotated lower leg and the starting position of vertical midline. Standing or walking is in midline between internal–external rotation.
Note: keep pelvis level for tests of abduction, adduction and rotation ranges.

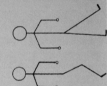
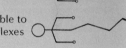

Knee flexor tightness – extension range
Supine one leg straight, bend one knee to be tested. With hip at 90° fully extend that flexed knee. Note popliteal angle between the tibia and the extended vertical line of the femur. Norm 30–40° from straight knee at 0 degrees. (Another convention is to measure the angle between the tibia and the femur itself. Norm around 140–150 degrees, with 180 degrees as the straight knee.)

Additional tests. Straight leg lift also reveals tight hamstrings (flexor tightness at knees and extensor tightness at hips). Norm 60°. Press knees straight in lying supine or prone (limited range may be detected). Observe long sitting with straight knees. Medial hamstrings flex and internally rotate knees with posterior tilted pelvis.

Knee extensor tightness – flexion range
Lying prone, flex the knee fully. If hip rises up into flexion, press hip down as far as possible to detect tightness of rectus femoris which decreases knee flexion range. Some ileo-psoas flexes hip. Short, stiff rectus femoris flexes hip and results in extensor knee tightness.

Another test is in supine. Flex knee with calf touching back of thigh. Limitation of knee flexion is detected.

Tibial torsion. Prone, bend each knee to 90 degrees with the hip held straight. Hold foot in normal position. Midline of foot is normally 10–20° turned out in relation to midline of thigh. Age 2–19.

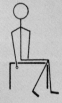

Sitting: flex knee for tightness of quadriceps.

Lying knees flexed over edge of bed. Bend one knee to counter lordosis and also eliminate hip flexor tightness (if present). Test quadriceps tightness with flexion of the other leg.

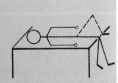

(Continued)

Table 8.2   (*Continued*)

Foot plantarflexion tightness – dorsiflexion range

Supine. Keep one leg straight. Bend the other hip and knee and dorsiflex the foot by grasping heel and *avoiding* passive dorsiflexion in mid-foot. Inversion redresses subtalar joint in equino valgus. Measure dorsiflexion with knee bent. Then hold dorsiflexion as knee is slowly and fully straightened. Measure dorsiflexion. Norm 10–20° beyond the dorsiflexed foot at right angles to the lower leg. Inversion increases range. Dorsiflexion with knee bent tests soleus and with knee extension tests gastrocnemius.

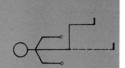

Foot: inversion, eversion, plantarflexion tested with knee straight. Test forefoot and toes.

Note: keep pelvis level (stop anteroposterior tilt, lateral tilt) during the leg assessments.

Shoulder flexor tightness – extensor range
Bring arm straight back.

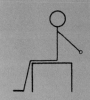

Shoulder flexor-adductor tightness – elevation range
Elevate arm forward and overhead.
Abduct and elevate arm.

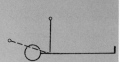

Shoulder rotations internal–external. Move lower arm.
Elbow flexor tightness – extension range
Slowly stretch *without* forcing elbow into extension with pronation and into extension with supination.

Carry out both tests with upper arm close to side of body.

Elbow extensor tightness – flexion range
Bend elbow with pronation and test with supination.
Elbow pronation–supination 180 degrees for full range pronation to supination.

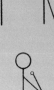

Wrist flexion–extension to 90 degrees.
Wrist deviation radial and ulnar
Finger and thumb adduction and abduction. Thumb touches base of fifth finger for full adduction.
Finger and thumb flexion–extension with wrist flexed and extended.
Remember to hold thumb at its base. Fingers extended only with wrist flexed or neutral are limited in range.

Head and trunk
Ranges assessed for torticollis or scoliosis.
In sitting spine bent, head between knees. The spine is in the centre, or slight deviation, rib-cage is normally equal on each side.

Note: Goniometry is measurement used for degrees of joint ranges of limbs.

Grade active range strength only as: present, weak, strong in young child or in the presence of intellectual impairment.

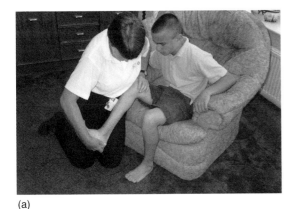

(a)

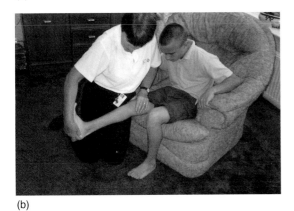

(b)

Figure 8.1 (a, b) Examining and explaining dorsiflexion with a person (see Table 8.2).

Examples of movement and functional observation of abnormally persistent postures in different positions are outlined below:

Head flexion, extension, rotation observed during head raise in prone, supine, sitting, standing developmental channels. Observe whether the head is held asymmetrically with too much extension or flexion.

Shoulder elevation, abduction, rotation, flexion and extension movements are observed during the functional examination of, say, creeping, reaching out and other arm movements involved in daily functions, play or music and movement. Shoulders may be held in abnormal postures.

Elbow flexion and extension observed during child's reach to parts of his body or toys. Forearm pronation or supination affects flexion and extension, and can be seen in isolation during daily actions or play. Elbows may be held in abnormal postures.

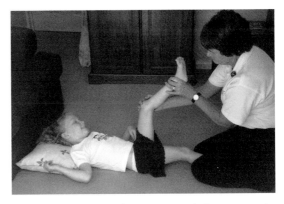

Figure 8.2 Examining hamstrings and knee extension (popliteal angle) whilst relaxing a child (see Table 8.2).

Wrist and hand will be observed during hand function developmental activities. Fingers may not function independently of persistent abnormal wrist postures.

Hip flexion and extension will be observed during all functions. Also ask the child in supine to bend his hip and knee to his chest and touch his foot, to sit or stand and bend to touch the ground, to sit on very low stools, or squat and come up to standing and sit/squat down again. There may be persistent posture of the hip(s).

Knee flexion and extension seen in sit-to-stand, as well as observing the child sitting using active extension to kick your hand or a dangling toy, and his knee extension in standing *tall*. There may be persistent flexion or hyperextension postures of knees.

Foot movements need to be tested separately, especially if there are abnormal feet. Playfully tip child backwards onto heels and forwards to toe standing for dorsi- and plantarflexion of feet. Observe persistent postures in sitting, standing and lying.

If the child cannot achieve a full active range, check:

(1) That it is not due to a decrease in the passive range of motion of the joint.
(2) That it is not due to weakness in associated stabilisers or synergists.
(3) That it is not due to interference of residual abnormal reflex reactions, abnormal selective motor control or lack of understanding by a young child or older person with cognitive or body image problems.

Functional measures

The GMFM (Russell *et al.* 1989, 2002). This assesses and measures changes over time in gross motor function in children from birth to 16 years. The motor skills are in the normal age range from birth to 5 years. This covers older individuals with cerebral palsy who are developmentally delayed and still functioning at these earlier normal developmental stages. However, the GMFM is not suitable for individuals who are very severely disabled and unable to achieve only a few, if any, of the test items. Other individuals who are mildly disabled, or become so, will be achieving skills beyond 5 years of the GMFM. The GMFM has 88 test items arranged in five sections or dimensions of lying and rolling, sitting, crawling and kneeling, standing and walking, running and jumping. Change in each dimension as well as a total score is calculated in percentage scores. The therapist can therefore use items as targets/goals for therapy from the dimensions which have the lowest scores or where change is expected from intervention. Results (outcomes) of therapy are measured on reassessment. The GMFM measures achievement of motor function but not the quality of performance, and does not assess hand function.

A GMFM with 66 test items (GMFM-66) exists (Russell *et al.* 2000) but it is complicated, needing more analytical skill and special software. It is not suitable for children whose only abilities are in lying, assisted rolling, minimal head control and supported sitting.

Generally, the GMFM score for an individual increases more in earlier ages than in later years. However, there may be various patterns with spurts of progress and periods of plateau. During these periods, the *quality of motor function* can be improving, especially if motor function is increasingly used in daily life.

Gross Motor Function Classification System (GMFCS) (Palisano *et al.* 1997, 2008). This describes the severity of functional disability, in a developmental picture, using age-dependent criteria. The descriptive features are reported at each level, saying what a child can do. The level of function decreases from Level I to V. The classification system can be used to compare individual children with each other at the same age. Therefore, children at different levels function differently at the same age. Children with hemiplegia, diplegia, quadriple-

gia, dyskinesia or ataxia are classified according to what they can do (Gorter *et al.* 2004). The quality of movement is not an important factor.

Classification of an individual child gives a shorthand description of a person with cerebral palsy and is particularly useful for communication between professionals and for generally relating therapy suggestions to a level of ability and disability of an individual. There are increasing levels of function for ages 1–2 years (before second birthday); 2–4 years (between second and fourth birthdays); 4–6 years (between fourth and sixth birthdays); and 6–12 years (between sixth and twelfth birthdays). The classification system has been extended in 2008 from ages 12–18 years. Classification levels are based on the highest level of mobility achieved by age 12.

For example, the walking levels are as follows:

Level I: Walks without restrictions; limitations in more advanced gross motor skills.
Level II: Walks without assistive devices; limitations in walking outdoors and in the community.
Level III: Walks with assistive mobility devices; limitations in walking outdoors and in the community.
Level IV: Self-mobility with limitations; children are transported or use power mobility outdoors and in the community.
Level V: Self-mobility is severely limited even with the use of assistive technology. Mobility only possible if the child can learn to use electric wheelchair.

Once a child has a level of function, he tends to remain in that level, but Gorter *et al.* (2009) found only about 60% of children classified at age 18 months were in the same level a year later. Morris *et al.* (2006) report that in several centres, doctors and therapists, as well as parents, are consistent in their identification of the level of a child.

Ontario motor growth curves (Rosenbaum *et al.* 2002). The motor growth curves (also called motor development curves) present a graph of GMFM-66 scores (on the vertical axis) by age (across the horizontal axis) for each of the five GMFCS levels. These smooth curves were meant to show how the *average* GMFM-66 score for children in each level increases with age before reaching a plateau. More recently, the Ontario group (Hanna *et al.* 2008) have subjected the data from Rosenbaum *et al.* (2002) to a new analysis, producing percentile curves for age

2–12 years. Except for Level I, the shapes of the median (50%) curves are quite different from the somewhat simplified curves fitted in 2002. The new curves give clear evidence that the average GMFM-66 scores for Levels IV and V reach a peak around 7 years and then decline.

The Ontario group (Hanna *et al.* 2009) has since extended their data to cover ages 16 months to 21 years. For Levels I and II there is no evidence of a decline (the curves reach a plateau), whereas for Levels III–V there is evidence that the average GMFM-66 scores reach a peak at around 7 or 8 years and then decline.

It is important to recognise that an *individual child's* score is likely to follow a much more erratic progress. This can be seen in the original graphs (Fig. 2 in Rosenbaum *et al.* 2002) where the points for individuals are widely scattered about the 'average' curves. For some children (in all GMFCS levels) the score continues to increase after age 8, whereas for some others the score may fall in the early teens. It is unclear how many children have scores that follow an 'average' pattern.

It is not apparent that the percentiles are useful in clinical practice, since Hanna *et al.* (2008) found that the percentile ranking of any individual child (in any GMFCS level) can rise or fall by 10 points or more over a year. Moreover, Hanna *et al.* (2009) state that 'children in Levels III–V are not "destined" to lose function in adolescence'.

The original motor growth curves (Rosenbaum *et al.* 2002) have been taken to predict a child's progress from 2 to 15 years of age, although each curve is an *average* and not a firm prediction for an individual. Unfortunately, there are professionals who might use these curves to give parents a prognosis for mobility in the long term. For example, Boyd (2004) considers the GMFCS and the motor growth curves to be predictive measures. Other physiotherapists consider the GMFCS as providing 'realistic expectations for clinicians to share with families' when planning long-term intervention. Such predictions certainly are not helpful in the early years when parents are often emotionally vulnerable and trying to cope with an unusual young child. However, there are parents who do ask 'Will my child walk and when?' A professional can discuss long-term prognosis in broad terms according to the child's *current* GMFCS level, which may change in future. There is more detail of this discussion in the section 'Prognosis for walking' in Chapter 9.

Gross motor performance measure (GMPM) (Boyce *et al.* 1995). This is a companion to the GMFM. It measures changes in quality of movement or performance of 20 items. Five components of weight shift, alignment, coordination, dissociated movement and stability are addressed. There are other components which are not considered and only 20 items of the 88 items in the GMFM have been included.

Specific functional items

The Sitting Assessment for Children with Neuromotor Dysfunction (SACND) is an assessment test of sitting (Reid 1995, 1997; Knox 2002).

The Functional Reach (FR) test (Donahoe *et al.* 1994; Niznik *et al.* 1995) is a performance-based test in standing to assess a postural response to voluntary reach with the arm horizontal. It is a dynamic balance test. It is measured by a ruler attached to the wall to show the maximal distance a child can reach forward beyond arm's length in the horizontal plane while maintaining a fixed base of support in standing, that is without moving a foot. It has been shown to have excellent reliability in children with spasticity (Niznik *et al.* 1995).

The Lateral Reach test (Brauer *et al.* 1999) examines ability to control the body sideways at the limits of stability while reaching with the arm horizontal and without taking a step or touching a wall. It was devised for adults. Bartlett and Birmingham (2003) use a Paediatric Reach Test for lateral and forward reach in sitting and standing in children from 5 to 15 years.

The Gillette Functional Assessment Questionnaire (FAQ) asks parents to assess the level of their child's walking ability on a 10 functional level scale (Novacheck *et al.* 2000). It has good reliability and validity of testing non-ambulatory and ambulatory children in communities and on different terrains.

Clinical tests also select items or specific dimensions (sections) in the GMFM. These may guide therapy and choice of equipment. However, such a selection does not fully measure a person's function. In addition, one does not learn the interaction between dimensions. There may be a gain in one dimension and a loss in another after therapy. It is valuable to test the levels and changes in all dimensions to increase understanding of what is happening in lying, sitting, standing and walking dimensions. However, in milder classifications (GMFCS Levels I–II, possibly III), using one or two dimensions has been accepted in specific research studies.

The Berg Balance Scale used for adults has been evaluated for children with cerebral palsy by Kembhavi *et al.* (2002) and Franjoine *et al.* (2003).

The Chailey Levels of Ability (Pountney *et al.* 2004). This is an assessment of abnormal postures in lying, sitting and standing with biomechanical details, so that appropriate positioning equipment can be selected. The biomechanical details are based on those observed in an infant from birth until walking. The assessment is tailored for older children in GMFCS Levels III–V. Such children are taller and heavier than a baby and have a different shape. The scoring is unusual in that the absence of a small detail of an ability can dramatically lower the overall score.

See Long and Toscano (2002) for review of tests in paediatric physiotherapy. Ketelaar *et al.* (1998) have carried out a systematic review of motor function assessments.

Measures of upper extremity and hand function

The upper limb cannot be assessed without assessing the postural mechanisms. The strength and ROM of arms and hands are involved in holding on, pulling up, using most walking aids as well as manipulation in activities of self-care and play (hobbies) gestures and communication. Measures of arm and hand functions in upper limbs are included in those given above, but with much less focus in the GMFM. Boyd *et al.* (2001b) have carried out a systematic review of hand and arm function studies.

QUEST – Quality of Upper Extremity Skills Test (DeMatteo *et al.* 1993), a measure, involves the child completing a series of movements with the upper limbs but also allows for some measure of quality of movement. The domains measured include dissociated movements, grasps, weight bearing and protective extension of arms. It uses a scale to rate hand function, spasticity and cooperativeness. An overall numerical score can be calculated. It is designed for children with neuromotor spasticity. It is a useful test for planning interventions. The 'dissociated movements' are fractionated movements such as shoulder flexion with elbow, wrist extension instead of mass flexion at all joints. Another example is isolated finger and thumb movements. The test is validated and reliable. It is recommended for use with the Peabody Developmental Motor Scales and Activity Cards (Folio & Fewell 2000) for accurate measures of fine motor skills.

The Assisting Hand Assessment (Krumlinde-Sundholm *et al.* 2007). A Manual is available. This is an assessment of the extent of how well both hands are used and monitors progress.

The Melbourne Assessment of Unilateral Upper Limb Function (Randall *et al.* 2001) is a reliable measure of biomechanical changes in upper limb function, assessing quality of movement. It was used in evaluating BTX A and training of impaired arms (Randall *et al.* 2001). There is detection of improvement to wrist dorsiflexion, supination and elbow extension during tasks.

The Manual Ability Classification System (MACS) (Eliasson *et al.* 2006). This system is a reliable way of classifying problems when using hands, in five functional levels. Good validity and reliability were found for children with hemiplegia, diplegia, tetraplegia, ataxia, dyskinesia and unspecified cerebral palsy between 4 and 18 years. Twenty-five parents as well as therapists were used in validation and reliability of this test. There were 168 children distributed in GMFCS Levels I–V. However, the MACS of fine motor function agrees with the GMFCS in only about half the children. This is also so with the Bimanual Fine Motor Function and GMFCS used by Beckung and Hagberg (2002). The MACS Classification leaflet can be downloaded in several languages from www.macs.nu.

Functional measures usually take place in the clinic and do not confirm what a child or older person actually does in their home, school or in their community. Measures of daily life activities and participation are needed for such confirmation.

Measures of daily activity and participation

Functional measures and measures of participation may show the child's ability or inability to perform items in the test. They do not usually record whether performance was abnormal or awkward when achieving the task. Other measures may be needed if the pattern or biomechanical elements are the aims of therapy.

The Pediatric Evaluation of Disability Inventory (PEDI) (Haley *et al.* 1992) measures adaptive functions from 6 months to 7.5 years. These functions are measured in three domains: self-care, including feeding, dressing, toileting; mobility, including transfers, indoor and outdoor locomotion, stairs with their speed, distance and safety; social functions, including communication, comprehension and peer interaction. The child is compared to normally developing children and his functional limitations are assessed. A parent interview can be used and a child can be tested in his own environment. It evaluates the improvement in independence following therapy. Nichols and Case-Smith (1996) validated the PEDI.

The Wee Functional Independence Measure for children (WeeFIM) (Msall *et al.* 1994) from age 6 months to 7 years. This is a measure of the degree of dependency of a child. This involves the 'burden of care' as it is scored to indicate how much assistance a person with a disability needs. There are 18 items in self-care, sphincter control, transfers, locomotion, communication and social understanding.

The above measures have been standardised with manuals of instruction and have been objectively tested for validity and reliability when used by the same assessor (intra-rater) or by another assessor (inter-rater). There are other functional measures of activities of daily living or motor function which are less relevant to people with cerebral palsy and their programmes of treatment. These other measures are designed for learning disabilities, strokes or developmental coordination disorder ('clumsy children').

The measures above are detailed and graded to show that a skill is being achieved or learned. It shows changes due to therapy interventions aimed at either increasing gross motor skills or increasing independence or decreasing assistance by carers as a child/adult becomes more independent.

The Canadian Occupational Performance Measure (Law *et al.* 1998) and the *Goal Attainment Scale* (Maloney *et al.* 1978) are examples of assessments used by occupational therapists to show whether management/therapy programmes are relevant to a child's function in the context of his or her own environment. These are very individual

measurements which are not standardised. Goal Attainment Scaling is unreliable, time-consuming and therapist-biased, but can be less biased if professionals are well trained to carry it out (Steenbeek *et al.* 2008). This assessment is then useful for joint goal setting and reporting outcomes with parents and child.

Harvey *et al.* (2008) review the following measures of activity limitation: GMFM, Activities Scale for Kids (ASK), Child Health Questionnaire (CHQ), Gillette FAQ, WeeFIM, PEDI, Pediatric Outcomes Data Collection Instrument (PODCI) and Functional Mobility Scale (FMS). They point out that the GMFM is a measure in the clinical setting ('what the child can do'), whereas parent and child measures, such as the ASK, give performance in their own environment ('what the child does do'). The review showed that GMFM and ASK are the most robust measures and that the other tools require further validation. Therapists rarely use the PODCI or the CHQ, which are more useful for doctors.

Quality of life measures are used by psychologists and social workers or occupational therapists. One example is the Lifestyle Assessment Questionnaire – Cerebral Palsy (LAQ–CP) (Mackie *et al.* 1998), which Kerr *et al.* (2007) have used in comparing gross motor function with restriction of participation. They found that better physical function correlated with a better quality of life; however, the GMFM assesses in a standard clinical environment and does not reveal participation when outdoors or in the community setting. They discuss that the relationship between function and participation is complex.

Another measure is PedsQL™ (Varni *et al.* 2005, 2006). Bjornson *et al.* (2008) found that walking skill or functional performance are not primary factors in self-reported studies on quality of life.

Norm-referenced measures of stages of child development

These measures compare a child with normally (typically) developing children. These measures and many other developmental assessments detect developmental delay and give a broad picture of a child or older person's stages of development but not quality of movement for cerebral palsy. Therefore, these developmental measures cannot show the details of progress in either function or in minimised impairment due to therapy.

- *Alberta Infant Motor Scale (AIMS)* (Piper & Darrah 1994) is a measure of motor development from birth to 18 months and observes child in supine, prone, sitting and standing. It is devised for 'at risk' infants, detecting developmental delay. It is not useful for children with cerebral palsy as normal quality of movement is expected. Therapists cannot obtain details of what needs to be treated in cerebral palsy.
- *Bayley Scales of Infant Development* (Bayley 2005) is a measure of developmental levels of mental and motor skills from age 2 months to 2.5 years.
- *Peabody Development Motor Scales and Activity Cards* (Folio & Fewell 2000) measure grossmotor and fine-motor skills of children from birth to 6 years.
- *Griffiths Abilities of Babies* (Huntley 1996, Luiz *et al.* 2006) is an overall development norm-referenced test for infants and young children.
- *The Denver Developmental Screening Test* (Frankenburg *et al.* 1992) measures fine- and gross-motor skills, personal social intellectual skills and language in young children.

Screening babies and children 'at risk' and detecting cerebral palsy. As this book deals with established cerebral palsy, the reader is referred to the work of neonatal physiotherapists. Assessment, intervention of posture and motility in preterm infants are discussed by de Groot (1993, 2000), Morris (1996) and Campbell (1999). They also give many references in this field. Prechtl (Einspieler *et al.* 2005) and other neuro-paediatricians are increasingly detecting cerebral palsy in very young infants but some of these abnormal motor patterns can resolve (Touwen 1978, 1987). Some examples of measures of infants' motor function are as follows:

- *Test of Infant Motor Performance (TIMP)* (Campbell *et al.* 1995). This is a measure for preterm babies up to 4 months to identify delayed motor development. It allows adjustments for prematurity. There are 59 items and the babies are presented with a variety of tasks and placed in different positions including prone, supine, side lying, and supported sitting and standing. It is said to be based on the systems theories of motor development, so looks for postural alignment or movement rather than the testing of reflexes, muscle tone or physiologic responses.
- *Neurosensory and Motor Developmental Assessment for Infants and Young Children* (Burns & MacDonald 1996) is an assessment for any child with neuromotor difficulties, including cerebral palsy. The assessment is for screening and follow-up of any infant from 1 month to 6 years.

Methods of observation of gait

Gait laboratories assist observations but are expensive and not always easily available. Some children are less natural in such assessments and cannot cooperate below 6 years (Mackey *et al.* 2003). Instrumented Gait Analyses have developed for the use of orthoses and pre- and post-orthopaedic surgery to evaluate spasticity, muscle contractions, force and skeletal malalignments. EMG, recorded joint movements and force plates are some of the tools used. These analyses are called 3DGA (three-dimensional gait analysis) and recommended by surgeons for complex gait deviations (Gage 1991, 2009). Dobson *et al.* (2007) have made a critical review of gait classification.

Clinicians depend on a visual assessment to evaluate children's gait patterns (particularly in young children) for therapy outcomes. There are a number of visual gait scales to assess a child before and after treatment with BTX A injections. These scales are similar to the Physician Rating Scale (PRS) (Koman *et al.* 2001), which assesses crouch (hip, knee, ankle flexion), knee recurvatum (hyperextension), equinus foot, hind foot, speed of gait and gait pattern. Videotapes are used for assessment. Corry *et al.* (1998) modified this test by removing equinus, hind foot and speed of gait, and adding change. They found a large disagreement in determining knee recurvatum. Boyd and Graham (1999), in their modified version, called the Observational Gait Scale, made further alterations for pre- and post-BTX A evaluations by adding sections to make eight sections. This test is more complex and more time-consuming (Mackey *et al.* 2003). Video gait analysis used by Ubhi *et al.* (2000) has a slightly different scale from the PRS concerning details of the initial foot contact after the leg swing.

There is reliability of foot contact in all the gait assessments mentioned and reliability in the first four sections in the Observational Gait Scale in their studies (Mackey *et al.* 2003). These are knee position mid-stance, initial foot contact, foot position in mid-stance and timing of heel raise in preparation for leg swing. The sagittal plane for observation by the workers in BTX A research was validated (Mackey *et al.* 2003).

There is also the Edinburgh Visual Gait Analysis (Read *et al.* 2003). Maathuis *et al.* (2005) commented on the PRS and Edinburgh Visual Gait Analysis in their study. They found excellent intra-observer reliability but poor inter-observer reliability for children with cerebral palsy and recommended one observer for longitudinal assessments.

Desloovere *et al.* (2006) found in their studies on gait analysis that strength and selective motor function had a higher degree of correlation with gait analysis than ROM and spasticity.

A clinical gait analysis is given in Fig. 8.3 based on the above discussions and on clinical experience (Levitt 1984). An easier functional observation is detecting a contact phase from heel strike to foot flat in mid-stance. Foot flat changes to heel lift at the end of mid-stance and toe off at the end of stance and beginning of swing. In Fig 8.3, there are more details which need an observation of the gait analysis in a slow motion video, so that repeated viewing for all the details can take place. Footprints of a child have been used to assess gait for step lengths, base and amount of weight bearing on each foot. Cadence is number of steps per minute and stride is the full gait cycle which equals two steps. The basic cycle of one leg is a step.

Fast walking is likely to activate the physiological stretch response. Fast walking is not common in the spastic type of cerebral palsy. In dyskinesia, individual children run headlong using momentum.

Grading in assessments

These are part of all the assessment measures given above.

The grading of motor scales is in tune with the way both able-bodied children and children with cerebral palsy develop. There are a variety of ways of grading in different centres. Joint setting of goals can include finely graded items of a function for short-term achievements. Parents, child and therapists are motivated by achievements which are more likely to happen sooner and easily observed – particularly in more severe cases (see Chapters 2 and 6).

The frequently used GMFM grades for scoring are 'cannot, initiates independently, partially completes and completes independently'. It is important not to have a 'yes' or 'no' grading which reveals no progress when a child has really achieved an active beginning of a new motor function or even a component. This also motivates parents and child and the older person with difficulties. The grading is used for individuals functioning without assistance to find out how a child copes independently. However, manual assistance by parents, carer or therapist or by equipment also reveals motor abilities in an individual. However, Haley *et al.* (1992) found assessment with handling less reliable than observation.

When assistance is used, this needs to be recorded as clear descriptions of *how much*, *where given* and *for how long* within the duration of the motor act. Progress is then shown as the assistance decreases. The MOVE Europe programme (MOVE Europe 2001) is an example of how assistance called 'prompts' is recorded when given and when decreased according to the child's achievement of a motor function. It is a programme structured for teachers and carers. Therapists will have a greater variety of methods of manual assistance to offer in training carers, parents and others. Records of all such grading in manual assistance by those assisting a child need to follow training and sharing of methods with parents, carers, teachers and others involved with a child. Use videos or photographs of effective methods of assistance. Show these to anyone who is working with a child. Invite comments from people caring for a child at home, school or in a respite home.

Abnormal performances of motor functions are difficult to grade and record due to their individuality. This can be recorded in videos and sequential photographs or still photos. It still depends on a therapist's experience as to what abnormalities of motor performance are observed and which are given significance. Grading is reliable only if there is a broad category of a 'near normal pattern' as opposed to a 'very abnormal pattern' recorded on a chart or checklist. Gait analyses convey more details about quality of walking (see Fig. 8.3 for gait analysis).

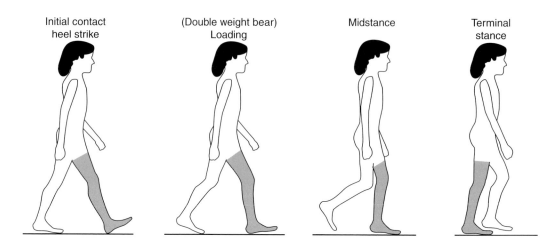

	initial contact strike loading	midstance to terminal stance
Head	Erect arrest forward/down shift	Erect
Trunk	Erect lateral shift to right	Erect lateral shift to right
Pelvis	Forward rotation right Lateral tilt up right	Level Lateral tilt up right
Hip	Flexion 30°	Extension
Knee	Full extension, semiflex on loading. 5°	Full extension
Ankle	90°	90°. Increase dorsiflexion 10° midstance
Arms	Right back swing, left forward swing.	Midway
Examples of abnormal gaits	Toe contact, whole foot contact; swivel on toe while loading. Forward shift abnormal, continues as *run* or backward lean. Unstable. Hip flexion – hyperextended knee. Hip flexion – knee flexion. Hip flex – lordosis – pelvic tilt. Pelvic retraction; abnormal rotation.	On toe; pronation, equinovarus. Hip, knee flexion: overflexed ankle. Hyperextended knee. Excessive hip internal rotation/external rotation; adducted/abducted pelvic retraction. Excessive pelvic tilt up. Antero-posteriorly tilts excess. Unstable. Fleeting stance phase. No lateral shift.

Note In all phases of gait kyphosis, lordosis, scolioses, abnormal head position, abnormalities of arm postures/swing may be present.

Figure 8.3   Right leg gait analysis (child over 2–3 years of age).

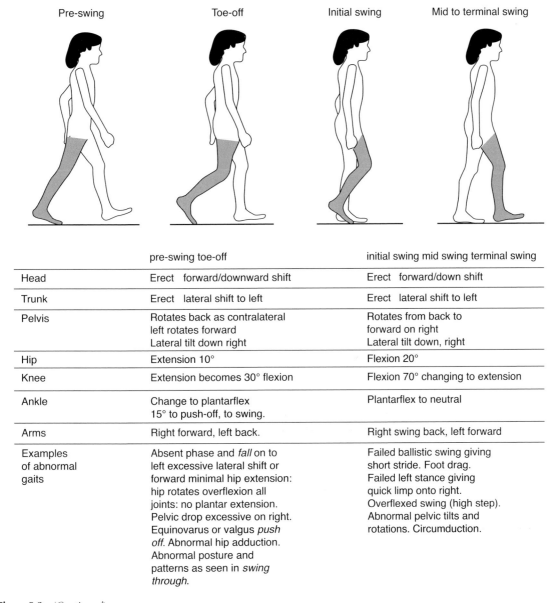

	pre-swing toe-off	initial swing mid swing terminal swing
Head	Erect forward/downward shift	Erect forward/down shift
Trunk	Erect lateral shift to left	Erect lateral shift to left
Pelvis	Rotates back as contralateral left rotates forward Lateral tilt down right	Rotates from back to forward on right Lateral tilt down, right
Hip	Extension 10°	Flexion 20°
Knee	Extension becomes 30° flexion	Flexion 70° changing to extension
Ankle	Change to plantarflex 15° to push-off, to swing.	Plantarflex to neutral
Arms	Right forward, left back.	Right swing back, left forward
Examples of abnormal gaits	Absent phase and *fall* on to left excessive lateral shift or forward minimal hip extension: hip rotates overflexion all joints: no plantar extension. Pelvic drop excessive on right. Equinovarus or valgus *push off.* Abnormal hip adduction. Abnormal posture and patterns as seen in *swing through.*	Failed ballistic swing giving short stride. Foot drag. Failed left stance giving quick limp onto right. Overflexed swing (high step). Abnormal pelvic tilts and rotations. Circumduction.

Figure 8.3 (*Continued*)

Reactions and reflex responses

These are summarised in Table 8.3 so that a therapist recognises them as possible compensations by a child trying to function. They are not measures for the hierarchical reflex model, which were previously emphasised in some developmental therapy plans. Each of the reflex reactions in Table 8.3 need not be routinely examined by the therapist except as an academic exercise. The postural mechanisms and voluntary motion for motor control are assessed in more detail within the developmental functions in Chapter 9. Treating and developing these components within motor functions will simultaneously modify or eliminate infantile reactions or reflex responses.

The measures of function rather than reflexes are a more relevant demonstration of change following

Table 8.3 Reflex reactions. A reflex conveys a stereotyped response to a stimulus. As responses vary in children, the term reflex reaction is used.

Reflex reaction	Normal until	Stimulus	Response	Therapy
Sucking	3 months	Introduce a finger into mouth	Sucking action of lips and jaw	Train correct feeding
Rooting	3 months	Touch baby's cheek	Head turns towards stimulus	
Cardinal points	2 months	(1) Touch corner of mouth	(1) Bottom lip lowers on same side and tongue moves towards point of stimulation. When finger slides away, the head turns to follow.	Desensitise face by child's own touch and other stimuli by therapist
		(2) Centre of upper lip is stimulated	(2) Lip elevates, tongue moves towards place stimulated. If finger slides along oronasal groove, then the head extends.	
		(3) Centre of bottom lip is stroked	(3) Lip is lowered and tongue directed to site of stimulation. If finger moves towards chin, the mandible is lowered and head flexes.	
Grasp	3 months	Press finger or other suitable object into palm from ulnar side	Fingers flex and grip object. (Head in midline during this test.)	Weight bearing, stimuli over whole hand, hand opening in development of hand function
Hand opening	1 month	Stroke ulnar border of palm and little finger	Automatic opening of hand	
Foot grasp	9 months	Press sole of foot behind the toes	Grasping response of feet	Weight bearing in development of standing
Placing	Remains	Bring the anterior aspect of foot or hand against the edge of a table	Child lifts limb up to step onto table	Use in provoking early step
Primary walking (automatic walk: reflex stepping)	2 months	Hold baby upright and tip forwards, sole of foot presses against table	Initiates reciprocal flexion and extension of legs	Weight bearing in development of standing
Galant's trunk incurvation	2 months	Stroke back lateral to the spine	Flexion of trunk towards side of stimulus	Train trunk stability in development of sitting and standing
Automatic sitting	2 months	Pressure is placed on the thighs and the head is held in flexion. Supine position.	Child pulls to sitting from supine	Train child's own rising in development of sitting

(Continued)

Table 8.3 (Continued)

Reflex reaction	Normal until	Stimulus	Response	Therapy
Moro	0–6 months	Baby supine and back of head is supported above table. Drop head backwards; also associated with loud noise	Abduction and extension of arms. Hands open. This phase is followed by adduction of the arms as if in an embrace	Train vertical head stability, use grasp, use prone position, use flexion position, shoulder fixation with grasp or hand support
Startle	Remains	Obtained by sudden loud noise or tapping the sternum	Elbow is flexed (not extended as in the Moro reflex) and the hand remains closed	Desensitise to noise by warning and experience
Landau	From 3 months to 2.5 years, strong at 10 months	Child held in ventral suspension, lift head. When the head is depressed	The head, spine and legs extend. Extend arms at shoulders. The hip, knees and elbows flex	Used in therapy to activate extensor muscles
Flexor withdrawal	2 months	Supine; head mid-position, legs extended-stimulate sole of foot	Uncontrolled flexion response of stimulated leg (do not confuse with response to tickling)	
Extensor thrust	2 months	Supine; head, mid-position, one leg extended, opposite leg flexed – stimulate sole of flexed leg	Uncontrolled extension of stimulated leg (do not confuse with response to tickling)	Weight bearing, joint compression, knee splints and calipers in development of standing
Crossed extension	2 months	Supine; head, mid-position; legs extended – stimulate medial surface of one leg by tapping	Opposite leg adducts, extends, internally rotates and foot plantarflexes (typical scissor position)	
Asymmetrical tonic neck (ATNR) reaction	6 months, usually pathological	Patient supine; head in mid-position; arms and legs extended – turn head to one side	Extension of arm and leg on face side, or increase in extensor tone; flexion of arm and leg on skull side or increase in flexor tone	Use both arms together and train head in midline, use prone position, only encourage in severe older child
Symmetrical tonic neck (STNR) reflex	Rare and usually pathological	(1) Patient in quadruped position or over tester's knees – ventroflex the head. (2) Position as above, dorsiflex the head	(1) Arms flex or flexor tone dominates; legs extended or extensor tone dominates. (2) Arms extend or extensor tone dominates; legs flex or flexor tone dominates	See Prone development Correct weight bearing on hands and knees. If correct abnormal posture in all development then usually ignore the STNR

Reflex reaction	Emerges at	Stimulus	Response	Therapy
Tonic labyrinthine supine	Pathological	Patient supine; head in mid-position; arms and legs extended. Test stimulus – is the position	Extensor tone dominates when arms and legs are passively flexed	See Development in supine; development of sitting. Overcomes excessive extension
Tonic labyrinthine prone *Reaction to prone*	3 months	Turn patient prone – head in mid-position. **Test stimulus – prone position**	Unable to dorsiflex head, retract shoulders, extend trunk, arms, legs	See Development in prone. Overcomes excessive flexion
Positive supporting	3 months	Hold patient in standing position – press down on soles of feet	Increase of extension in legs. Plantarflexion, genu recurvatum may occur	See Development of standing. Excessive anti-gravity response
Negative supporting	3–5 months	Hold in weight bearing position	Child 'sinks' astasia	See Development of standing
Neck righting	5 months	Supine, rotate head to one side, actively or passively	Body rotates as a whole in same direction as the head	See Development of rolling in supine Stimulate body rotative reactions
Associated reactions	Pathological	Have patient squeeze an object (with a hemiplegic, squeeze with uninvolved hand)	Clench of other hand or increase of tone in other parts of the body. Abnormal overflow	See Development of hand functions

Reflex reaction	Emerges at	Stimulus	Response	Therapy
Rising Labyrinthine head righting Vestibular righting (decrease of head lag)	2–6 months	(1) Hold blindfolded patient in prone position, in space, as head drops (2) As above in supine position	Head rises to normal position, face vertical, mouth horizontal Head rises to normal position, face vertical, mouth horizontal	For all reactions, see all sections on developmental training in Chapter 9
	6 months	(3) Hold blindfolded patient in space – hold around pelvis, tilt to the side	Head rights itself to normal position, face vertical, mouth horizontal	

(Continued)

Table 8.3 (*Continued*)

Reflex reaction	Emerges at	Stimulus	Response	Therapy
Optical	6 months	As above, no blindfold	As above	
Amphibian	4–6 months	Patient prone, head in mid-position, legs extended, lift pelvis on one side	Automatic flexion outward of hip and knee on same side	
(a) Body righting, (a) derotative	4–6 months	Supine – rotate head or one knee one side, passively	Active derotation at waist, i.e., segmental rotation of trunk between shoulders and pelvis	
(b) Rotative	6–10 months	Rotate hip and knee or arm or head actively	Active segmented rotation (hyperactive at 10 months, cannot lie supine)	
Lift reaction (*not* the pathological lift reaction (Tardieu))	5–6 months	Lift body through space	Head rises (lifts)	
Shoulder/pelvic girdle righting	3–6 months	Fix distal part(s) of limb	Rise up on to limb	
Postural fixation counterpoising (see the sections on developmental training in Chapter 9)				
Tilt reactions (a) Supine and prone	6 months	Patient on tiltboard. Arms and legs extended, tilt board to one side	Lateral curving of head and thorax, protective reaction in limbs accompany trunk reaction	

(b) Four-point kneeling	7–12 months	Patient in quadruped position, tilt towards one side	Lateral curving of head and thorax. Abduction–extension of arm and leg on raised side and protective reactions on lowered side may accompany this	See Chapter 9
(c)		Tilt forward and back (antero-posteriorly)	Forward – head and back, flex. Backward – head and back, extend	
(d) Sitting	9–12 months	Patient seated on chair – tilt patient to one side. Tilt forward anteroposterior back	Head and thorax curve abduction–extension of arm and leg on raised side, other protective reactions may accompany this	
(e) Sitting		Tilt forward / Tilt back	Child extends head and back / Child flexes head and trunk	
(f) Kneel-standing	18 months	Patient in kneel-standing position, pull or tilt patient to one side	As above	
(g) Standing	12–18 months	Patient in standing position. Tilt sideways. Tilt anteroposteriorly	Trunk as above	
Staggering reactions (see 'Saving from falling' below)	12–18 months	(1) Move to left or to right side push or holding upper arm	Hopping, or step sideways to maintain equilibrium	
		(2) Move forward	Hopping, or step forwards to maintain equilibrium	
		(3) Move backwards	Hopping, or step backwards to maintain equilibrium or dorsiflex feet going on to heels	See Chapter 9
Saving from falling	5–10 months	Prone – sudden tip downward / Sitting – sudden tip downward / Standing – sudden tip downward	Immediate extension of arms with abduction and extension of fingers to save and then prop the child	
	6–9 months	Standing – sudden tip sideways – one arm		
	9–12 months	Standing – sudden tip backwards – both arms		

Note: Motor patterns of the responses may be abnormal. This is *not* a chart for testing a child, but as background information for observation in function.

therapy and management (see Chapter 1, section on 'Abnormal reflexes').

Speed of performance

One of the problems in cerebral palsy is a delay in initiation and especially in completing a movement for a task (Shumway-Cook & Woollacott 2001). This is due to inadequate force generation (weakness), limited range of motion and poor anticipatory postural stabilisation. There may also be poor understanding and remembering of the movement required.

Independence of a child and older person with disabilities is not fully achieved if they cannot move fast enough for the particular needs in a specific environment. To help the children fit into regular (mainstream) schools or later normal work situations as well as live with people in society, they need to be trained to function at reasonable speed. This could be slower than normal but not *very* slow. It is easy to assess when a child is very slow and therapy is adjusted accordingly. Other speeds have to be assessed if they are relevant to the child's life, and whether people are likely to wait for a person whose movements and walking are slow. Able-bodied people do learn to adjust their speed to that of the person with a disability, and if not then this needs to be suggested.

Assessment of speed includes time taken to walk a specific distance. The 6-minute walk is such a test. The 1-minute walk test (McDowell *et al.* 2005) is more appropriate for severely involved children. Pirpiris *et al.* (2003) compare two assessments of walking speed. The assessment of speed of a task depends on the precision needed for it. For example, lifting a tiny object with a hand demands more coordination and so takes longer than lifting a larger object. Timing for assessment is best carried out unobtrusively to avoid increasing anxiety in some individuals. Assessment for electric wheelchair will also be associated with the problems of speed as well as distance and terrain that need to be managed by a person with disability.

Additional assessment required

Sensory examination. Loss of sensation in the cerebral palsies is rare, having only been described in hemiplegia (Tizard *et al.* 1954). Also, it is difficult to assess sensation in babies and young children with disabilities or older children with severe multiple impairments. Perceptual disorder or agnosias are much more common and various assessments are available and done by neurologists, psychologists and specialised occupational therapists and teachers. Lack of body awareness and other perceptual problems may be lack of *sensory experience*. Poor sensory awareness is common in people with severe multiple disabilities due to immobility or poor mobility. Sensory unawareness can lead to pressure marks and pressure sores as well as from a child's or older person's inability to move or turn in any position.

Assessment of daily activities. Assessment of feeding, dressing, washing, toileting, play and hand function must be made when planning therapy in collaboration with parents, carer and child (see Chapters 2). These assessments and measures overlap with the assessment of motor developmental channels, especially hand function (see Chapter 9 and 10). The PEDI and the Canadian Occupational Performance Measure (above) are used by occupational therapists for daily life.

Assessment of equipment includes the selection, the measurements and the assessment of the child in or using the particular piece of equipment.

Chapter 9 relates items of equipment within development of lying, sitting, standing and walking, and hand function so that more detail is best given in the context of daily life activity. Therefore, equipment is not separated from opportunity for a child's own potential for exploration and activity.

The general principles for assessment of equipment are given.

Select equipment according to the following considerations:

(1) *Assessment of the child's disabilities and abilities*, especially emerging 'unreliable' abilities to decide if equipment is necessary, and if so, then which items remain appropriate over time. The correct amount of aid makes it possible for him to carry out tasks otherwise impossible, but too much aid prevents his own active participation and development of emerging ability.

(2) *Assessment of the child's deformities* or threatening deformities. Ranges of movement need to be adequate for equipment or allowing stretch within child's current potential. Good alignment in any apparatus and correction of

abnormal postures must be maintained during the use of the equipment. For example, standing may be correct in a standing frame, but become abnormal on hand function in standing; sitting may be upright in a push-chair with special modifications but become abnormal when the chair is pushed.

(3) *Good design* of equipment takes account of adjustments for child's growth, removal of supports with increasing ability, a variety of modifications for different children in a clinic/school, is as portable as possible and looks as 'normal' as possible. Simple designs easily adjusted by busy parents and staff are desirable. Continue to check measurements of the child as he grows so that equipment is not too small. Continue to reassess equipment in relation to achievements gained in therapy and daily care. Once again, equipment must facilitate independence, not substitute for it.

(4) Assess that special equipment provides a variety of additional motor experiences in different positions. Equipment needs to give individuals appropriate support so that they can participate in communication, eating and drinking, social and educational activities as well as have assistance for desirable mobility to access these and other functions.

(5) Assess that equipment can be transported and stored and have manoeuvrability so that they can be used in different environments in a person's life.

(6) Monitor different items of equipment for a variety of postures throughout the day and night as part of the prevention and correction of deformities. Consideration of night-time postural management is detailed in Chapter 11, as part of the 24-hour postural care programme to minimise deformities.

(7) Check for any pressure points on bony prominences during use of orthoses and equipment.

Assessment of a child and family needs.

(1) The ability of parents and carers to use equipment correctly needs ongoing supervision, education and support by each child's therapists. Their acceptance of equipment in their home needs collaborative discussion and self-reported questionnaires by patients and their families

(Goldsmith 2000). Encourage their views so that ideas on equipment can be developed for better practice.

(2) There may be problems such as equipment being too cumbersome in a home or school; isolating the child from a family group too much; proving too fragile and requiring expense, time and worry on the part of people caring for the child; and other considerations of a similar kind. Home and school visits are a great help in discovering these problems as some parents may not report these difficulties after 'all the efforts made' by staff to assess, provide and check the equipment in a clinic.

(3) Respect cultural views such as not using lying on the floor or use of crawling apparatus and preferred use of floor seats rather than special chairs in some social groups.

Provision of equipment, designs and new ideas change with research and general progress in helping children with disabilities and this may help the particular child at the reassessments.

Daniels *et al.* (2004) and Polak *et al.* (2008) have surveyed standing frames and night-time positioning equipment available in the United Kingdom.

Assessment of techniques required

As the assessments are made, the therapist collects her aims of therapy and daily care and selects techniques from any source to carry these out. In addition, the selected techniques will be assessed during use. Assessment of techniques chosen *must* take place, as one cannot always predict the individual child's response. There must be an *active* response or participation or whenever possible an active initiation on the part of the child with any technique. A change in a component/ability of function needs to be detected after using a method by the end of a session. If not, it should be discarded within the first or first few sessions, and another method found. Passive correction of deformities is included as part of the therapy programme. Most passive procedures should in any event *not be totally passive*. They must be assessed to see whether the passive correction manually, with plasters, splintage, orthoses or equipment makes it possible for an *active* participation of other parts of the child's body or of the particular part of the body being corrected. Always assess how a child is positioned in special equipment and how he uses any walking and/or mobility aids to decide on their effectiveness.

Assessment of parents' or carer's abilities to manage techniques and their opinions are sought as these are significant (see Chapter 2).

Records

Considering the approach in this and the last chapters, records are made of the following:

- *Background information* of medical history, general health, drugs being used, assessment of individual's other abilities and disabilities, general development and family background. These are mostly taken from records of other professionals as parents are unhappy about being 'asked the same questions by many professionals'.
- *Developmental history.* Additional details for therapy not in other professional records.
- *Priorities of child/older person, parents, teachers or carers.* These include motor function and daily living activities. Other professional records are used for priorities of social, financial, housing and any priorities other than motor function. The therapist must be informed about them as such priorities may be more pressing for parents at different periods.
- A *daily living activity or task.* Priority of an activity of daily living such as eating, drinking, washing, dressing, toileting and mobility of a child/older person given independently and that of parent/carer assisting the person with disability. Consider these daily tasks in home, school or community.
- *Current motor functions* of child/older person for the chosen task.
- *Current abilities/components* of motor function already achieved by individual.
- *Impairments constraining task* such as deformities, joint range, strength, selective motor control.

- *Functions and component abilities a child still needs to achieve.*
- *Outline of methods, equipment, orthoses* and other resources.

Reassessments records

Outcomes of developmental functions and components with improved abnormal performance. Records of impairments. Videos, films and photographs, either static or sequential (Holt *et al.* 1974), are useful for records of assessment and outcomes (evaluation of progress). The viewing of a child needs to be the same each time he is assessed to enable accurate comparison. Kraus de Camargo *et al.* (1998) use a video-based system.

Measures are chosen which can provide specific records for many of the headings above.

See Appendix 1 for clinical grading of physical ability for aims of treatment.

'*Goals*' need to be clarified from the above records as:

Ultimate aims. Child's goals; parents' goals; and individual family members' goals. These may be annual goals.

Short-term goals. Therapists' and individual's joint goals together with goals of others involved with them. A goal needs to specify the function, how it is performed and, if possible, time expected for achievement. These goals are related to accomplishment of the 'ultimate aims'. These may be set for a few weeks or up to 3 months. Short-term goals are 'what a child needs to learn or achieve' and they include a motor function with functional components specified. A goal may also specify which impairments will be diminished either within function or separately. Both aspects are important.

Some therapists have set goals for the end of a treatment session and achieve these immediate goals. However, although encouraging and even used in many studies to suggest the value of a therapy approach, this is non-scientific as results may not be maintained that day or later.

Outcomes or results. This leads to modifications or changing of short-term and, in time, of long-term aims and goals as well as selection of methods to implement them.

Select measures according to *child's functions and impairments* given in this chapter.

Record clinical progress when any supports, equipment, walkers or orthoses are no longer needed.

Summary

(1) Assessment is essential for a therapy plan which is relevant to each child.
(2) Assessment methods must be selected in *direct* relationship to techniques of treatment. Such a practical approach is outlined in this book.
(3) Objective, valid, reproducible measures still need research, though many more are now available and increasing.
(4) The measures of function and impairments relevant to function and deformity outlined in this chapter are selected according to the individual child's or older person's goals. A practical developmental functional assessment of postures and movements in Chapter 9, together with examination of deformity in this chapter, alerts a therapist as to which measures may be selected.

(5) The practical assessment which is directly related to functional training includes a developmental functional assessment (developmental levels), examination of deformity (threatening or established), daily living activities and assessment of equipment. These assessments can be used for checking progress but are not all precise enough. Some of these practical assessments need to be used when suitable and sensitive measures are not yet available.
(6) Additional assessments by other professions are needed. They are concerned with communication, perception, cognition, social behaviour and health problems.
(7) The way in which you approach a child in assessment affects the information obtained.

Note: See Appendix 1 for the detailed clinical physical ability assessment guide and the developmental levels' illustrations.

Treatment procedures and management

9

Motor training

Motor training in this chapter includes 'hands-on' treatment procedures called *physiotherapy suggestions* and therapeutic activities by anyone daily involved with a person with cerebral palsy, called *management*, or *treatment and management*. The therapist needs to select and supervise methods for others assisting a person, according to what is relevant to their situation and skills. As discussed in Chapter 2, a therapist clarifies what a child and parent or carer want to achieve, what are the joint therapy aims and methods, with joint evaluation of which methods are appropriate. Selection of aims and methods by a therapist is based on the assessment framework discussed in Chapter 8.

Aims and methods are for the following interrelated aspects:

(1) The motor functions needed for the individual's chosen daily task. There are methods for specific delays in motor function and stated below as *delays*. These are the functions that he or she cannot do. However, there are functions that an individual can do. In this case some items given in *delays* are not observed in these individuals. Generally an individual has achieved motor function at earlier developmental stages than their chronological age. This depends on his or her severity and experience.

(2) The components (specific abilities/ prerequisites) of the motor functions needed for the individual's chosen task. These are various postural mechanisms and voluntary movements. Methods include activation of these abilities at each developmental stage. In this chapter, the absence of these component abilities accounts for particular motor compensations or continuing use of motor abilities at an earlier developmental level. Examples are given under the subsection '*Abnormal performance*'.

(3) The impairments which either prevent achievement or can create abnormal performance may be weakness, hypertonic stiffness, limited joint ranges, hypotonia, involuntary motions, abnormal movement synergies, residual infantile responses and limited repertoire of movements. A child or older person either uses the impairments or avoids use of more impaired body parts in motor compensations. These are also included in *abnormal performance* at each developmental stage of motor function.

(4) Associated factors in motor function. Although this chapter concentrates on the motor problems, they are not isolated from other influences. The methods of motor training are interwoven with visual, hearing, sensory and perceptual experiences. Understanding is needed for some functions such as walking safely or following instructions for some techniques. Motor

training is shared with parents, any family members and carers in *management* in the style described in Chapter 2, and then views of these people add emotional, social and cultural influences on motor training. The child's own views also influence selection of methods. When a child learns motor function in group treatments (Chapter 12), this too adds emotional and social influences from a person's peer group.

The direct training of developmental motor *functions often simultaneously minimises the constraints by impairments*. It is the *appropriate* selection of methods for direct training of active motor function with its components that can increase strength, improve joint ranges, decrease stiffness of hypertonus, modify hypotonus, reduce residual infantile responses and some involuntary movements. As motor training increases a child's repertoire of movements and postures, there is less need to use abnormal performances.

Therefore, the emphasis on motor function and simultaneous improvement of performance in this chapter does not separate treatments of impairments from training of function. They can be integrated. However, this does not imply the disappearance of the cerebral palsies but rather an improvement of function as much as is possible for each child.

Chapter 11 on deformities suggests treatments of specific impairments which are not adequately modified by functional methods. This is particularly needed in severe conditions when active function is very poor or absent. There are also treatments of secondary impairments.

Motor training in daily life activities

Although this chapter concentrates on the motor problems and locomotion for daily life, there are also preparation for other activities in a child and older person's lifestyle. In Chapters 2, 10 and 12, motor training is more explicitly presented as part of training daily life activities. Chapter 10 further summarises the motor functions trained in this chapter in the context of feeding, dressing, washing, toileting and playing. Reviews are given of motor function and perception and motor function in communication, speech and language. Occupational and speech and language therapists specialise in these aspects, and collaboration with them is essential.

Learning motor function only in these whole daily life activities and contexts can be too complex. Motor function needs to receive specific concentration on the deficient motor apparatus. Similarly, perceptual problems, speech and language difficulties and special problems of hearing and severe visual impairment need to have structured separate sessions of specialised treatment and teaching. However, as Neistadt (1994) points out, the specialised training of perceptual problems does not transfer to other contexts. Like motor training, they apparently need to be trained in different contexts as well.

Thus, therapy and management have four main related procedures:

(1) Techniques which integrate motor function with communication, vision, hearing, sensation, perception and understanding in the contexts of whole daily life activities.
(2) Methods for motor function which are relevant to an individual's home, school and community.
(3) Specialised techniques for specific motor abilities and functions to initiate dormant motor control to augment existing function, minimise abnormalities and generally increase motor activity for quality of life.
(4) Methods which parents, carers and teachers are able to manage in changing circumstances.

Developmental levels and techniques

The therapist will use the developmental channel most appropriate to the posture in which a child might manage to carry out the chosen daily activity. This might be standing for transfers, sitting for eating and socialising or lying for bed mobility and getting out of bed. The therapist's assessment of the developmental stages of a child's postures reveals which each child can use independently or with appropriate support.

The following are important points for the developmental motor training:

(1) Different positions for the chosen activity may be used by a parent or carer to assist their own management of an individual. This posture may not necessarily be developmentally challenging for a child or older person. For example, lying may be used for dressing a child, when this child is capable of supported or even

unsupported sitting. A child may be able to help with dressing in a different posture. Lying may be used 'to save time' or as a habit from the period when a child was less able. A mother's intuitive handling of her able-bodied baby includes accurate timing of when to give less support and when to expect more advanced skills. A baby with very different motor behaviour demands more learning about handling from a mother. Furthermore, there needs to be recognition that learning to change any existing habits is not always easy. At appropriate times, a therapist explains, demonstrates and negotiates the value of another posture based on assessment of a child. At the same time, a therapist gives sensitive consideration for comfort and support of a mother, or carer (Chapter 2).

(2) Therapy plans become involved with *simultaneous* use of each developmental channel of prone, supine, sitting, standing and hand function. There is also crossing of channels when a child goes in and out of various postures. It is most unwise to first train stages in lying before stages in sitting and standing.

(3) We cannot assume that obtaining a functional component *in one channel will transfer* to another channel, as muscle work, joint positions and gravity are not the same. Each component needs practice within each channel. Most of the postural mechanisms in prone do not necessarily transfer to upright postures and walking.

(4) Gravity can be used to activate and strengthen particular muscle groups. For example, using side lying makes arm reach or leg movement easier along a surface. A child in supine can use gravity to allow abduction and external rotation from bent hips and knees during changing of nappies or dressing. In bed mobility a child in prone pushes himself to the end of a bed/plinth and his legs drop to the floor. He then pushes up against gravity with arm supports and back extension.

(5) Abnormal postures are modified or corrected by use of specific functions. Any preference shown by an individual for particular motor patterns of, say, flexion will need methods to emphasise motor functions with extension in each developmental channel and vice versa. Such emphasis attempts alternatives to the individual's preferred motor patterns in cerebral palsy. In different channels different muscles are strengthened. There is, therefore, prevention and minimising of deformities together with learning of a variety of movements for all muscles and joints.

General plan of the developmental programme

Initially therapy plans start with the developmental sequences in prone, supine, sitting, standing and hand function as guidelines. Typical components of functions and whole functions are developed in these sequences. As a therapist gets to know each child, modifications may or may *not* be needed. With experience of a child's needs, together with careful observation of each individual, modifications become obvious. The developmental sequences are therefore flexible and not a dogmatic scheme.

Using the assessment findings of what individual children can and cannot do, plan a programme to:

- Establish motor functions already achieved, so giving a person confidence that there is something he can do. Build on these motor functions in the next developmental levels.

- Attempt motor functions at the next developmental levels not just current level of child. This is to check any flickers of response to assess readiness of a child to try a more advanced motor item(s). Parents are encouraged to report when their child seems ready for a more advanced developmental motor function. These are also called 'transition stages' and thought to be the times when intervention is most beneficial (Bodkin *et al.* 2003).

- Consider any developmental omissions/gaps as possible contributions to compensations, resulting in abnormal performance. Omissions are not always important owing to individual variations.

Age of child and techniques

Select techniques according to a child's next developmental level and *not* according to chronological age. Use a similar approach when treating deformity. For example, asymmetry or persistence of prone flexion is normal for a child developmentally delayed to levels 0–3 months. Select methods for 3–6 months. Commence *functional training* of feeding, dressing, washing for a baby and for a severely and profoundly affected child, adolescent or adult using whatever developmental prerequisites of sensation, understanding or motor abilities that an individual may have, no matter how minimal (see Chapter 10). Communication to babies, children and older persons with learning disabilities have to be given according to their level of understanding (see section 'Motor function and communication, speech and language' in Chapter 10).

It is unfortunate that some workers still think physiotherapy should be cut down in older children and more time given to education as motor progress is no longer expected by them. In some individuals, motor controls may only mature much later and unless stimulated will remain dormant. There is controversy and different views on the need for training walking (see subsection 'Prognosis for walking' in this chapter).

Different environments. For any age group, an individual's teachers and other personnel in their life need to be shown how to include motor activities so that precious school time is not lost from their education. The physiotherapist at the child's school can work out ideas with teachers and classroom assistants for motor activities appropriate for classroom, playground or in physical education. At all ages, school children and older people with cerebral palsy need to be kept as physically fit as possible. Extra effort also needs to be made by a therapist to maintain contact with a school child's or adolescent's parents (see Chapter 7 for adolescents and adults).

Onset and techniques

Response to therapy sometimes seems much quicker if the onset is sudden on a previously normal nervous system. However, ultimately spontaneous recovery and motor development in acquired brain lesions may be as unpredictable as in babies born with apparent brain damage. Children with either congenital or acquired lesions warrant appropriate therapeutic procedures given in this book so that the potential of any of their nervous systems is given every chance to reveal itself. There are more be-

havioural problems in many children following a traumatic brain injury, which may interfere with therapy. Psychologists need to be consulted for advice concerning these problems. Expectations of better results in children who have 'already known normal movements' may be more of a frustration than a help. It is not so much the memory and experience that matters but the amount of damage *and* the capacity of any particular damaged system to compensate for the abnormalities.

Diagnosis and techniques

The techniques are not devised for particular diagnostic types but for motor problems of developmental *delay* and *abnormal performance*. Different diagnostic types of cerebral palsies may have similar functional levels and some similar abnormal performances described in this chapter. Other diagnostic conditions causing only motor delay may exhibit abnormal performance also seen in cerebral palsy, for example rounded backs, hyperextended knees or pronated feet. This is especially so if abnormal performance is a compensation for delayed balance (postural mechanisms).

Application of techniques

These should be carried out by qualified paediatric physiotherapists and occupational therapists and for daily management jointly selected with anyone caring for the child or with an older person with motor dysfunction. Selection depends on an individual's abilities, time and changing family situations.

Repertoire of techniques in this book cannot possibly include all those available. Firstly, not *all* individual problems and different situations could be included together with possible techniques. Secondly, it is difficult to describe techniques without demonstration and only those techniques which could be described have been included. Thirdly, those techniques which have been frequently used have been selected. There are many more. Techniques in this book are thus *suggestions* not *recipes*.

Lack of response to any technique given in this book indicates the need to try others in this book or in other publications or preferably from clinical colleagues. Check that if the child scarcely responds to any technique, it is not due to:

(1) Inaccurate assessment of the child's level of development.
(2) Inadequate knowledge of the child's non-motor areas of function, such as vision, understanding, perception and emotions which interfere with motor function.
(3) Lack of skill of the therapist with the particular technique.
(4) A need to modify or change the initial aims and goals of therapy.
(5) A need to review the collaborative aspects between parent, carer and therapist. See Chapter 2, particularly the points to check, near the end of that chapter. The lack of reinforcement of therapy by anyone involved with an individual needs to be considered, as professional therapy is not enough without others involved with a child.

As visual impairment has a significant impact on motor function, this is now discussed in more detail.

Motor development and the child with severe visual impairment

Motor delay will occur because of the visual impairment in otherwise normal children. When cerebral palsy is also present, the delay will be augmented. Intellectual disability may be present or only appear to be present as the child is limited by the multiple disabilities. The therapist should learn what influence the visual problems have on motor development as they do not only delay but also create unusual patterns and sequences of motor milestones. Abnormal movements or *blindisms* such as hand flapping, waving over light sources, eye poking, rocking and other bizarre patterns are seen in children, especially in some of the children referred late for training and parental advice. These will need special methods advised by psychologists, paediatricians or specialist teachers for children with visually impairment.

The methods for motor developmental training in this book can be adapted for children with severe visual impairment provided that the following factors are kept in mind.

Hypotonia, motor development and the postural mechanisms

As discussed throughout the book the postural mechanisms are undeveloped in children who are hypotonic (see the subsection 'Postural mechanisms' in Chapter 1 and the subsection 'Hypotonicity' in Chapter 11). Blind as well as sighted children who are immobile may be hypotonic. Jan *et al.* (1977) discuss floppiness or hypotonia associated with lack of movement in blind babies. Assessment and development of the postural mechanisms in the visually impaired baby and young child have been studied by the author and found to be delayed. As vision is an important factor in detecting the vertical in the child's world and in appreciating any tilt of his world, it is not surprising that the blind baby's postural control is absent or poor (Sonksen *et al.* 1984). Blind babies prefer to lie safely on the ground and avoid the challenges of gravity. The development of the postural mechanisms is the story of motor development against gravity and changes in gravity. Their absence inevitably delays this gross motor development. Motor development is discussed below. The visually impaired child, with or without cerebral palsy, will need careful assessment and training of the postural mechanisms using auditory, tactile and increased proprioceptive and vestibular stimuli.

Postures such as rounded backs in sitting and standing, hyperextended knees and flat feet are common in young hypotonic children, particularly in visually impaired babies and children (Fig. 9.1). The specific delays in postural stability, counterpoising, forward tilt and posterior saving reactions are often observed to accompany the presence of round backs and shoulders (Levitt 1984).

Vision stimulates and monitors the postural mechanisms. Sugden (1992) reviews the various studies on this aspect. It is the exciting object or person that a typical baby catches sight of that provokes him to look up. This then stimulates the head righting and postural stability of the head. It is also the effort to understand the visual stimuli that further activates exploratory movements and increasing postural control whilst exploring. Methods to develop the postural mechanisms or the motor functions cannot be isolated from a child's total development (Zinkin 1979; Sykanda & Levitt 1982; Levitt 1984, Chapter 14; Sonksen *et al.* 1984).

Total child development and motor training

Mother–child relationships. The shock and stress felt by the mother who does not even receive the *primal gaze* from her blind baby (Goldschmied 1975), as well as his unusual reactions to her feeding and cooing, must be understood by any therapist attempting to help. All motor developmental training needs to be designed to build up mother's and father's confidence in parenting their child. Many of the gross motor activities in play help enormously in creating bonds with the child. The techniques in this book should all be adapted to take place on mother's lap, close to her body and face so that her kisses, touch and stroking and talking to the baby not only help motor development but also body image, movement enjoyment by the baby and demonstrate to the baby love and security which he needs so much. Clinging to mother in an unknown or puzzling world should be allowed for longer than in sighted babies and children. The weaning of the child with visual disability to a physiotherapist needs to be carefully done after mother–child bonding and confidence is established. Introducing more than one therapist or developmental worker may be disconcerting to the child and even the parents. Other disciplines advise one therapist rather than all handle a child themselves. Such a child is particularly sensitive to touch and voice, and needs to be handled by a few familiar people until confidence is established. Family participation in helping and especially in enjoying the motor programme with a child who is visually impaired is planned by therapists. If mother is under stress, it is important not to overload her with exercises, but rather use corrective movements and postures within the daily living activities of the child. Social workers and other counsellors work closely with therapists to help the family (see Chapter 2).

Motor function and the child's daily life (Chapter 10) is usually the priority in the developmental motor training programme for a child with visual disability, not only from the parent's viewpoint but also from the child's viewpoint. The purpose of motor function needs to be emphasised when conveyed to each baby and child (Fig. 9.2). If not, he or she could be trained in basic motor patterns but never use them. He or she cannot *see* their purpose!

The assessments of the child's developmental stages in feeding and other self-care, play or sensorimotor understanding and in exploration of the world must be obtained in order to introduce the corrective motor patterns appropriately. There are special stages and sequences for severe visual impairment (Reynell & Zinkin 1975; Kitzinger 1980).

Use of compensatory stimuli for motor development. As vision is not available, it seems obvious to use auditory and tactile stimuli to facilitate motor development. However, it is vision which normally teaches the baby what makes sounds, where they come from in direction and in distance, how humans communicate and the association of sounds with situations such as mealtimes, bath times and so on.

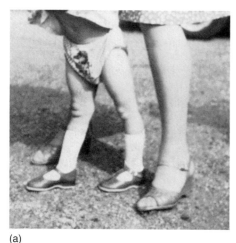

(a)

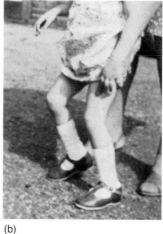

(b)

Figure 9.1 Hyperextended knees (a) being corrected (b) by training pelvic control (postural stability and counterpoising).

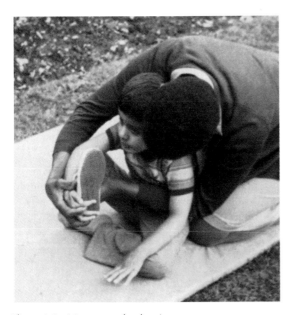

Figure 9.2 Movements for dressing.

Therefore, first train a baby what sounds mean before they can really motivate him to move. Also use existing movements to confirm what sounds mean.

Auditory development is followed as observed in the normal child (Sheridan 1975) but with special adaptations for the visual impairment (Sonksen 1979). First, the baby is trained to listen, then to turn to sound and after that to reach for sound. A very young child will first localise the source of sound near his or her ears horizontally and then above and below the head. Each child is helped kinaesthetically to search for the sound *kept stationary* nearby. Developmentally this will be at ear level, horizontally, above, below and then behind the child. The child will *only* achieve reach for sound when his conceptual development includes *the permanence of objects* and their sounds. It is at about these stages that reach and move towards a sound will only be worth using to stimulate roll over, creeping, crawling or bottom shuffling. Until the permanence of objects is conceptualised, help the child locate sound and move towards it by providing tactile and kinaesthetic stimuli. Reaching for an object making the sound is easier if a child's hand moves along a surface on which the object is placed.

Similarly the appreciation of tactile stimuli, localising and searching for them, has to be developed. Linking tactile with sound stimuli is carried out.

Encouraging a child to create sound independently is also included as he bangs a mobile, rattle, tambourine or a surface with hands or feet. The motor programme cannot be planned without these aspects that are devised by teachers, psychologists or developmental paediatricians together with the therapist.

Mother's voice and her touch rather than the therapist's will be more successful in the early stages. Vibration, smell, taste and air currents can be introduced and associated with real objects, and situations link sound, touch, proprioception and vestibular stimuli. All these aspects are part of the child's conceptual development (Sonksen *et al.* 1984).

Body image development. Poor body image is related to poor motor experiences and not seeing body parts static or moving. Use of tactile stimuli on a baby's body helps to develop the body image. However, it is the baby's parent's hands as well as the baby's hands that are best to do the touching first. Hands of the baby are notoriously slow to move and explore because of many reasons, not least of which is the absence of *hand regard*. Help the baby bring his hands together in midline, *pat-a-cake* hand to hand, touch hand to mouth, to face hand to body and hand to feet (see Fig. 9.3). Later use as many other stimuli to his body such as rubbing with towels, soap, creams and powder at bath time. Use vibrating toys, bells and playthings placed for him to find on his tummy or limbs and invent similar ideas. The sections on stages of hand function development in this chapter and section 'Motor function and perception' in Chapter 10 offer ideas for the sighted child in this book. For the child without sight, these stimuli offered in play activities need to be emphasised and also *presented more slowly* and stage by stage. Do not bombard the baby with too many stimuli at once. Confusion or fear could be aroused if stimuli are not sensitively given. Thus, carefully introduce different surfaces for the child to roll on, creep, crawl and walk on with bare feet.

Always give a child time to experience tactile and auditory stimuli and allow the child to reach and find out about toys and objects with such stimuli and as independently as possible. Create opportunities for movement so that a child can feel his own body movements and how he actively produced them. If a child cannot or does not move alone, parents can move him and change positions for him. A child enjoys feeling his mother move about by being slung close to her body in a baby pack. Body image depends on proprioceptive and vestibular function.

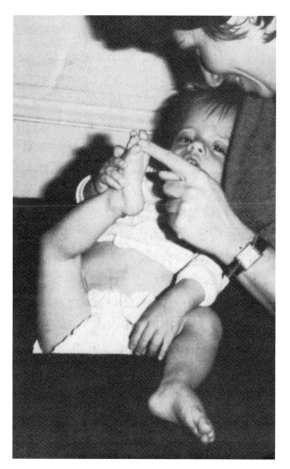

Figure 9.3 Body image development.

Proprioceptive and vestibular function. These aspects are also part of total child development. They are compensatory stimuli for visual impairment and also develop body image. All the postural reactions are dependent on these stimuli in a developmental context discussed in this book. Touch, pressure and resistance can be correctly given to stimulate movement giving clues as to direction and degree of muscle action. Opportunities are also given for a child to lift, push and pull objects of different weights, which also increases proprioception and strength.

However, as with all therapy methods, give a child time and observe whether the child understands and is not confused by what is expected of him. Do not use therapy techniques with handling, pressures or other stimuli from behind him as he may well lean back or use his extensor thrusts to reach the stimuli or the familiar voice behind him!

Visual development. Not all blind babies are totally blind. Even reaction to light only can be used and perhaps developed to the child's full, if limited, capacities. An assessment of the developmental *use* of residual vision is given by the developmental paediatrician and specialist teacher and relates to vision available for exploration and learning. This guides the therapist in her motor plan for the individual child. The therapist needs to learn how large an object can be seen by the child, how far away, whether it can be seen if stationary or moving and which visual fields are present. The therapist also needs to know whether there is equality of vision in each eye and the acuity as well as any other special visual defects which may affect a child's motor development and use of therapy methods. The development of a child's visual potential is easily integrated with the methods for head control, hand function and all balance and locomotor activities discussed in this book. The appropriate level of visual ability needs to be related to a child's motor programme. There are times when one may have to accept unusual head position and other patterns which make it possible for the child to use residual vision. There may then be muscle tension or aches to be treated with exercises and massage.

Language development. It is important to talk and clearly label the body parts used and the motor activity if this does not distract a child's attention on body image and motor training. A child may also not yet be able to understand words. Delay is *normal* for a child who cannot yet understand the meaning of sounds, words and conversation as he cannot see what they mean, cannot see gestures and cannot link the stimuli from the external world. Psychologists and teachers work closely with the therapists to plan the language and speech programme. This enables therapists to give general encouragement of language development and be advised on communication systems for a child and by a child with severe visual impairment.

Hand function development. The development of hand function is obviously the most important area for the child whose hands are his eyes on the world. The chapter on hand function in this book should be adapted to use compensatory tactile, auditory and proprioceptive stimuli before motor actions can be expected to follow the normal rate of development. Do not force objects into the child's hand but train him to search for the nearby rattle, to orientate his hand to take it and to develop a variety of searching actions or finger moulding and feeling actions. Bilateral hand function will take more work than with a sighted child. Encourage both hands together in midline, holding and especially exploring both sides of a cup, bowl, ball or toy and transfer of toys. Train losing the toy and finding it. Offer toys which involve a child having to take them apart, and constructing them again. Also, find objects and toys which activate crude and fine voluntary grasp and release. Offer playthings which depend on hand and fingers pressing a switch to activate a sound, music or vibration or fan blowing air, the latter supervised by an adult.

All these actions do not only promote motor development but integrate with concepts of cause and effect, object permanence and other intellectual development of the child. Remember that index finger pointing and associated index/first finger grasp is very much a visual conceptual skill and will be delayed. Offer toys and food to promote finger actions as mentioned in the chapters on hand function, motor function and play, feeding and other self-care activities.

Gross motor development. Prone development is not popular with the baby with visual problems as there is no interest there, sounds cannot be heard as easily and he may be far removed from family and especially mother. There are no visual lures to provoke him to look up and progress to creeping and crawling. It is often noted that crawling is not used by blind children and that they prefer shuffling on their bottoms and then walking. It is, however, possible to train prone development on mother's lap, on a soft cushion with attractive noises, especially that of mother's or father's voice with their gentle stroking of their child's back. The advantages for a child having activities in prone are increased head and back muscle strength due to head and back extension. When a child pushes up on hands, this adds strengthening of shoulder girdles for arm and hand function. Balance on hands and knees leads to additional exploratory skills of crawling through space, feeling the ground and gaining additional body image experiences. The round backs and shoulders often seen in children with visual impairment benefit from stronger back extensors together with additional postural training in upright sitting and by using the arms to reach up for toys and especially to play with father or mother's face and hair.

Crawling is not of course essential for the acquisition of walking, as bottom shufflers demonstrate.

However, creeping, crawling, rolling or any mobility across space helps spatial learning and especially that *the floor is continuous.* This enables a child to be less afraid and be more motivated to walk alone. Walkers with wheels all around the child should be avoided as he will not develop his own postural and locomotive reactions. The child often sits or leans onto these walkers, stepping his legs but not learning to take weight through his legs and so learn to walk. Baby bouncers and rocking chairs are also undesirable if used for a long period when someone is not present. A child can withdraw into a rocking or bouncing world which engenders disinterest in the environment. Baby bouncers may provoke abnormal leg patterns, excessive 'on toes' postures (*blindism*) and increasing spastic shortening and dyskinetic patterns. Short supervised sessions in any equipment do often produce more desirable results, especially if parent–child interaction is happening.

Blind babies without other disabilities develop stationary postural control slightly later or within the ranges of sighted developmental levels (Fraiberg 1977). However, there is more of a delay of moving into, out of or forward from these postures. Thus, this book on developmental levels should be used as guidelines and neither as rigid rules for developmental ages nor as strict sequences for severe visual disability. The postural mechanisms of stabilisation, counterpoising, tilting and saving (protective) reactions and the methods given are in the sections on motor training of developmental functions below, but delays and modifications will be required according to a child's particular vision and hearing development and his or her emotional and social situation.

As fears are common, the techniques should be adapted to build confidence and provide fun and a sense of adventure. Large balls, rolls and swings should only be used *after* confidence has been established in relation to the levels of development of the postural mechanisms present or just commencing in the individual child. Rising reactions will require extra care as all workers in this field demonstrate how much visual lures promote posture changes. All other motor developmental training from 0 to 5 years presented in this book should be offered and learned by a child to decrease the frequent clumsiness associated with visual impairment. Coordination exercises, balance tasks, music and movement, dance, games and physical education are of great value to children with visual disabilities. The older child will also be receiving mobility training from those employed for this work by the Royal National Institute of the Blind (United Kingdom). Teachers for severe visual impairment will integrate their work on this and other aspects with the therapists, as there is a need to create a whole programme for each child and family.

Prone development

The following main features need to be developed at the individual's developmental stages:

Postural stability of the head (Fig. 9.4a–d) when lying prone (0–3 months), on forearms (3–5 months), on hands (4–6 months), on hands and knees (6–9 months), in half-kneeling hand support (9–11 months) or on hands and feet (12 months). Head held in alignment with spine (4 months), with chin well in (5–6 months).

Postural stability of the trunk. At first a baby in prone is often in flexion with hips off the surface and then tips over into side lying with weight bearing continuing forward on cheek or side of face and shoulders (0–3 months). Weight then shifts towards the legs. As head, shoulder and trunk stability develops the child can control side lying and symmetrical prone lying (6–9 months). The back becomes straight and then slightly extended on forearms (3–5 months) becoming fully extended on hands (6–7 months). In 'pivot prone' (5–10 months) the trunk stabilises well in extension. When a child is on forearms, he shifts his weight backwards and forwards and to each side (3–5 months) and similarly when on hands (6–7 months). Weight shifts are later used if creeping along the floor. When on hands and knees, weight shifts continue with a straight back held against gravity and adjusting antero-posteriorly for rocking, then using this with lateral and diagonal shifts during crawling.

Postural stability of the shoulder girdle (Fig. 9.4a–d). When taking weight on forearms (3–5 months), on hands with elbows semi-flexed (4–6 months) and elbows straight (6–7 months), weight bear on hands and knees (6–9 months) and in prone lying with arms held stretched forward along the ground to hold a toy (5–

6 months) or later when holding an object in the air (6–7 months). There is 'pivot prone' (begins 5–6 months and established 8–10 months) with weight on abdomen and pelvis with extended trunk and legs in the air as well as with arms held abducted-extended in the air to stabilise shoulder girdle ('high guard' position). Shoulder girdle stability is promoted with trunk stability in extension. In other positions, stability develops further during half-kneeling or in upright kneeling, leaning on hands (9–12 months) and during grasping a support, within all prone developmental stages, especially around 9–12 months.

Postural stability of the pelvis (Fig. 9.4d) on knees with hips at right angles (4 months), on elbows and knees (4–6 months) and on hands and knees (6–9 months). Stability of pelvis and hips on the surface (6–9 months) enables on hands with straight elbows, stabilises in half-kneeling and upright kneeling with support (9–12 months) and without support (12–18 months).

Postural stability and counterpoising of limbs are closely related.

Counterpoising of the head takes place in activities which include head partial raise and turn (0–3 months) and head movements whilst

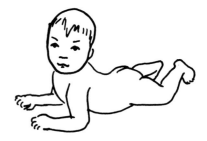

Figure 9.4   (a) Postural stability of head and shoulder girdle (on forearms).

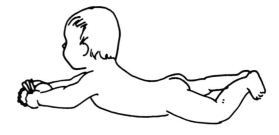

Figure 9.4   (b) Postural stability of head and shoulder girdle.

holding the head up against gravity (3–5 months). Free head movements are counterpoised in prone-kneeling postures (6–12 months).

Counterpoising the arm movements in prone abdomen on the ground, creeping actions (3–5 months), when weight bearing on one forearm whilst reaching with the other (5–7 months) or leaning on a hand reaching with the other (7 months) (Fig. 9.4c). Reach in all directions increases counterpoising abilities. All reaching is preceded by weight shifts in all positions in base and then away from moving arm, later towards a reach well out of base. Arms are counterpoised in crawling (9–11 months) and on hands and feet (12 months).

Counterpoising leg movements takes place in prone lying during creeping actions (3–5 months), leg movement on knees with upper trunk and arms being supported (5–6 months), leg lift when on hands and knees (6–8 months). Weight shifts precede leg movement first within base laterally and in rocking forward and back, leading to counterpoising limbs for crawling. This is together with the counterpoising of arms in crawling (9–11 months) and in bear-walk (12 months). Stand lean on hands on low table (modified bear-walk position), weight shift laterally develops to allow counterpoising of leg lifting and also prepares for cruising at low furniture. This overlaps into the development of cruising in standing at normally 9–12 months levels in this chapter.

Rising from prone (Fig. 9.5). Head (0–3 months), on to forearms (3 months), on to knees (4 months), on to forearms and knees (5–6 months), on to hands and knees (6–7 months), to half-kneeling hand support (9–12 months), prone to standing (12–18 months). Change to other postures from and to prone position, involving rolling, sitting or squatting (6–10 months) and from 'bear-walk' posture to standing (9–12 months). There are hand supports and grasps which assist rising. Children assume many other positions with later motor development.

Tilt reactions in prone (Fig. 9.6). Reactions seen on tilting the surface on which the child lies at about 6 months, on hands and knees at about 9–12 months and in upright kneeling around 15–18 months.

Saving from falling reactions (Fig. 9.7) in the arms at 5–7 months downward-and-forward 'parachute', followed by arm propping. Arm saving sideways and forward can also be seen when a child is on hands and knees, if the child is suddenly pushed sideways or if pushed forward from a heel-sitting position, or from supported upright kneeling. Leg reactions also occur on pushing the child over sideways, forward or backward when he is on hands and knees. Arm and leg reactions accompany the tilt reaction, especially if the trunk reaction is particularly poor.

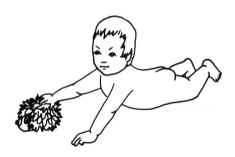

Figure 9.4   (c) Postural stability and counterpoising arm reach.

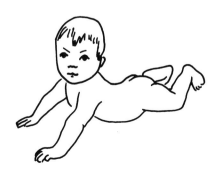

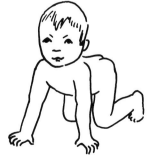

Figure 9.4   (d) Postural stability on hands and on hands and knees.

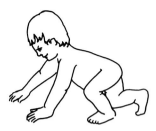

Figure 9.5   Rising from prone.

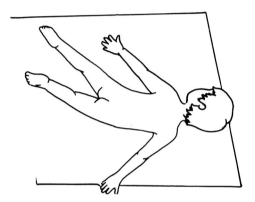

Figure 9.6   Tilt reaction in prone.

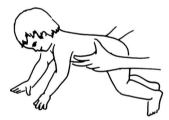

Figure 9.7   Saving reactions in the arms.

See *Stages in Prone Development* in Figs 9.8–9.22.

Treatment and management at all developmental levels

Rolling and rising

As rolling development takes place from supine to prone, prone to supine or a complete roll with side lying as an initial transition position, techniques are all outlined in the section 'Supine development' below.

In this section, strategies are presented for rising directly from prone onto arms, onto knees, onto hands and knees and eventually into various sitting and standing postures in the prone developmental levels. The active and active-assisted sequences of rising strengthen muscles, stretch and increase ranges with a minimising of the tightness of hypertonic muscles.

0–3-month normal developmental level

Some common problems

Dislike of prone position. This may be due to early breathing difficulties, inability to turn the head and free the nose, inability to lift the head up, excessive flexion creating discomfort in prone, post-gastrostomy, severe visual impairment or even lack of opportunity given to lie on the stomach. Later a dislike of prone may be due to a child's inability to use the hands in prone.

Delayed development of head control and on forearms (on elbows) posture. There may be no head raise or partial head lift and even no turn to free nose and mouth. Head turn is initially associated with body turn and later head turns keeping the body still. Head control may be poor when rising up on forearms and taking weight on forearms.

Abnormal performance (Fig. 9.23). Many of the motor patterns of a normal neonate and baby of 1–3 months may persist as abnormal performance in older children. This includes flexion posture or persistence of asymmetry in lying, with or without a Galant's reflex on one side. There is abnormal asymmetrical head raise, rising on only one forearm, asymmetrical stabilisation on elbows. There may be more flexion–adduction in one leg than the other as the hips lift off the surface into flexion. Only one leg may flex and abduct into a forward creeping pattern with hips flexed or flat on the surface. Children with bilateral or hemiplegic impairment can begin to creep flexing the better or unaffected side whilst the other affected leg is less active in extension and internal rotation. This is seen especially when the child raises his head and turns to the less affected or unaffected side. Creeping pattern is limited without head control and use of arms.

There may be excessive flexion and adduction of both or either of the arms, with shoulder retraction, pelvis and hips in posterior flexion rather than lying

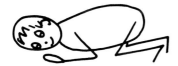

Figure 9.8 Flexion posture decreases. Head turn (*0–3 months*).

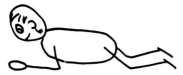

Figure 9.9 Head raise and hold (*0–3 months*).

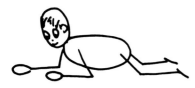

Figure 9.10 Head raise, weight on forearms (*0–3 months*).

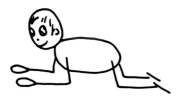

Figure 9.11 On forearms and/or weight bearing on knees (*3–6 months*).

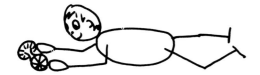

Figure 9.12 Stretch forward to reach; stretch legs. Lean on one forearm and reach with the other arm (*3–6 months*).

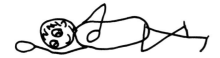

Figure 9.13 Roll from prone to supine (*3–6 months*).

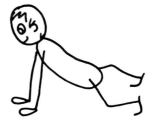

Figure 9.14 Weight bearing on hands (*6–9 months*).

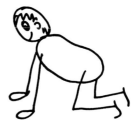

Figure 9.15 Weight bearing on hands and knees (*6–9 months*).

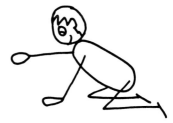

Figure 9.16 Lean to one hand reach with the other (*7 months*).

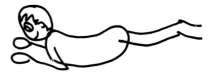

Figure 9.17 Extend head, shoulders, hips pivot in prone position (*8–10 months*).

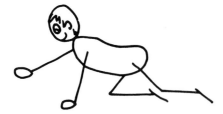

Figure 9.18   Hands and knees, lift arm, leg or both (*8 months*).

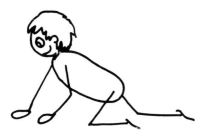

Figure 9.19   Crawling. Rise into crawl position (*9–11 months*).

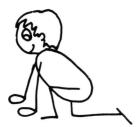

Figure 9.20   Half-kneeling lean on hands (*11 months*).

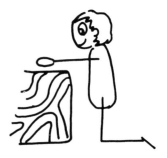

Figure 9.21   Kneeling supported (*11 months*).

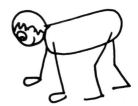

Figure 9.22   Bear-walk (elephant walk) on hands and feet (*12 months*).

flat. There may be flexion of the trunk or legs, or all of them. The head may be overextended with chin poking in lying and when raised. Extensor thrusts may persist. The child's weight is taken onto his face, chest, knees and sometimes on feet when flexion is less. On head turning weight may not shift to the opposite side and body weight does not shift towards legs due to lack of head raise and flattening of pelvis. Weight shifts are needed for creeping along surface.

In hypotonia, particularly in very young children there is flexion–abduction of arms and legs with flattened pelvis into the *frog position*. In hypertonia, independent head raising in individual children may be associated with overflexion of stiff arms, stiffness of legs in extension–adduction–internal ro-

tation. This persists into the next level when abduction and external rotation is normally expected.

Treatment suggestions and management

Acceptance of prone position. Accustom the child to prone by placing him slowly on his stomach and on soft surfaces, such as sponge rubber, inflatable mattress, over large soft beach ball, over your lap (adding a cushion if your knees are bony!). Check that his nose is over the edge. Rock and sway him to a song.

Gently roll the child from side lying towards prone either on the soft surface or suspended in a blanket. Roll him back and forth slowly, keeping his nose free and observing whether he accepts going towards prone. Try using the incentives for head raise and turn, given below, to make prone lying more acceptable.

Severe conditions in older people. Prone is more acceptable in prone standers (*Prone standing frames*) in which the angle of the forward incline can be adjusted according to the person's ability to just raise, hold or turn his head. The rest of the body is well supported by the frame so that head control can be trained. Interesting mobiles, television and social contact are among ideas to make this

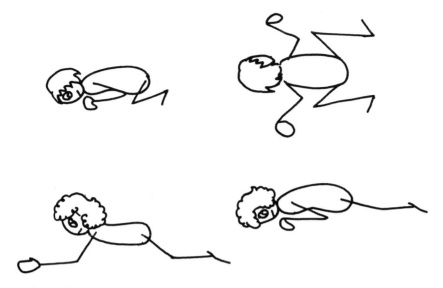

Figure 9.23   Some abnormal postures in prone.

position worth doing by the person with cerebral palsy (see discussion on 'Aims of standing equipment' below). The aims are primarily for head control at this developmental stage.

Note: Some children continue to strongly refuse to go prone and should not be made to do so. They may be like those able-bodied children who are *rollers* or *bottom shufflers* and a few others who do not use prone development in their motor development (Robson 1970). Cultural influences may affect use of prone.

Head control. Train the following aspects of head control:

- Raising the head (righting).
- Holding the head steady (postural stability).
- Turning the head from side to side (counterpoising the movement).

Suggestions are as follows:

(1) Place the child in prone with his arms elevated across a sponge rubber roll, a large therapy ball, a pile of pillows or across your lap. Also hold both a child's shoulders back and inwards towards the spine to keep him stabilised symmetrically as this assists active head raise and hold. Rock a child forward and backwards over the edge of the roll/ball or your lap to activate raising the head. Vary the speed to a song. He achieves both stability and head action when

motivated to look at a familiar face, bubbles in the air or a mobile. In prone lying on a table/couch, a child may be assisted or encouraged to reach out, elevating both his arms to someone's face or object of interest. Sit on a seat so that you are at the child's eye level. When using both arms symmetrically, the child keeps his head and body in the midline. It is easier if he reaches downwards to a toy, with the help of gravity, or horizontally along a ball's smooth surface. If a child can reach horizontally towards his object of interest, his head often raises as well. Stiff arms may first have to be grasped near the shoulder joints and turned outwards as they are extended forwards over the edge of your lap or apparatus.

The child's legs may be abnormally bent or stiffly extended, turned in and held together, before or only during head raise or turn. In such cases, turn his upper legs out keeping them apart *while* he is initiating head control (Fig. 9.24). This helps him learn postural control without excessive leg tension.

A table with a smooth surface placed against a stationary ball or roll also enables arm reach forward enhancing head raise. Instead of your stretching his arms, he may manage active reach with some assistance. Later he may be able to push a heavy object down an inclined surface followed by a push along a horizontal surface. These activities stretch out bent arms and strengthen them together with the shoulder girdle which enables more functional activities that you can offer the child.

(2) If a child has preferred head turning to one side, then extend the shoulder girdle on the opposite side to activate head raise and turn to the other side (Fig. 9.25). Draw his attention to someone he knows or objects of interest on the opposite side. Head raise and turn are components for later learning to roll.

(3) When training head control, continue to present him with interesting objects such as mobiles, Christmas decorations, mirrors, moving toys on springs or mechanically controlled, sounds from musical boxes and from toys. Place objects below, in line and above him. First use visual and auditory stimuli in the centre and progress to having them at each side of the child and move them slowly from centre to the side and

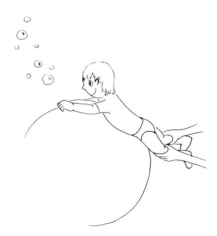

Figure 9.24

from side to side. These stimuli also develop visual and auditory attention together and tracking together with training of head control. Later eye movements are learned without head movement.

(4) Place wedge on a table or platform so that the child can see someone's face when he looks up. A friendly person obtains eye-to-eye contact by sitting in the centre and opposite the child, and sings or speaks to him and then gets him to move his eyes from side to side to follow her face. Rhythmically tapping under the chin or at the forehead of a child, gives momentum for head lifting, provided a child accepts having his face touched.

(5) Keep wedge on the floor or in a sandpit or in front of a trough of water where other children are playing so that social interaction can be facilitated. Adjust angle of the incline on a wedge to enable better head control or use of child's hands and arms for play.

(6) Place a child in prone on an inflatable mattress, water bed or trampoline and gently bounce him to stimulate and enjoy his active head control. Tip the child from side to side to activate head turn. These are some of the early components for learning to roll towards supine.

(7) Swing a baby in prone over adult's arms or large child on a horizontal tyre suspended from a tree. Help a child to go down a slide while lying prone on a cushion. Place a child on a wedge on wheels or on a trolley with a roll of towels between his body and upper arms.

(8) Weight bearing on forearms will also activate a child's head control (Figs 9.26 and 9.27). Give adequate support with a small roll of towels

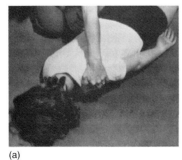
(a)

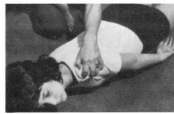
(b)

Figure 9.25

between his chest and upper arms to prevent shoulder hunching or pulling his arms down against his body. Check that a child's forearms are well away from the body, with elbows at right angles and beneath the shoulders and, if possible, hands open. Keep the head and trunk centre, legs apart, straight and, if possible, turned out from hips.

(9) Motivate a child to raise his head and look down with chin held in, at a book or a toy in order to avoid hyperextension of the head (Fig. 9.28). Help him with gentle manual pres-

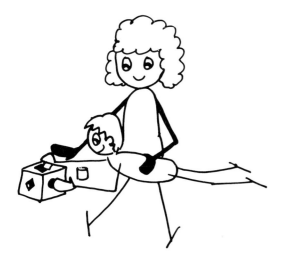

Figure 9.26

sure down on a rounded back. Press his pelvis down for symmetrical weight bearing when he is placed on forearms. A small roll under his chest and between his shoulders overcomes hyperextension of head and body and helps to bring forearms forward to counter retracted shoulders. Reverse a child's position on the wedge so that he kneels over the edge with his body fully supported in order to decrease lordosis and elongate a rounded back or lateral spinal curve (Fig. 9.29). Lying across your lap with his legs over the edge, feet flat on the ground, also corrects spinal postures as he practises head control during play on a low table.

Equal weight on forearms. Weight bearing is often better on one side.

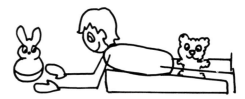

Figure 9.27 Head control and weight bearing on forearms (on elbows). Prone, on forearms over low wedge, roll cushions. Keep legs apart and turned out in those cases where legs press together and/or twist inwards. Use a pommel, toy, small wedge or cushion for legs.

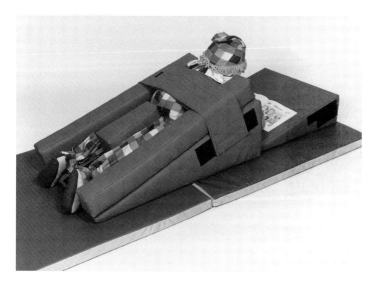

Figure 9.28 Wedge with lateral supports, adjustable strap to prevent twisting of trunk, sliding or rolling off wedge. Abduction block to separate adducted legs. (With permission from Jenx, Sheffield, UK.)

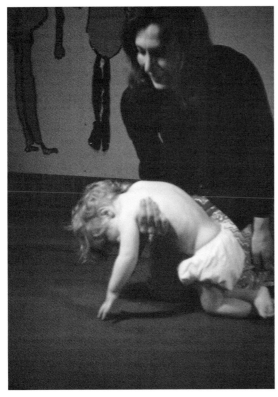

Figure 9.29 (a) Child needing head, shoulder and trunk control.

(1) When the child is in prone lying over a roll, pillows or wedge, gently press down at the top of his head carefully aligning it with his spine. Train a *long neck with chin held in.* Use joint compression through upper arms or by pressure at the top of his shoulders for more muscle action (as shown in sitting in Fig. 9.99).

(2) Encourage weight bearing on the more unstable side by placing a toy near the other arm for visually directed reaching. Gently push and hold the child over the weaker weight-bearing forearm, whilst he is preoccupied with play. Press down on the shoulder with elbow directly beneath it. Use this motor pattern during feeding, other play activities and functions in supported sitting and standing.

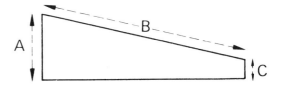

Figure 9.29 (c) Measurements for wedge for prone lying, arms over edge 'A'. 'A' represents measurement from axilla to wrist, 'B' represents measurement from axilla to 2 in. (50 mm) above ankle and 'C' represents length to top of foot.

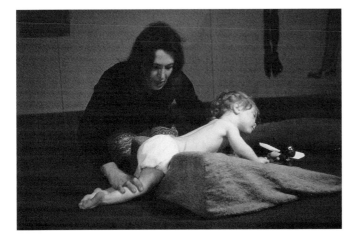

Figure 9.29 (b) Use wedge for weight bearing on knees. Straps may be needed to hold the child on the wedge. Also note child attempting head raise and a forearm support with pelvis support.

(3) Hold a baby with his full weight through his forearms and gently shift his weight from side to side, or playfully lift a child up from side lying onto one forearm and then repeat onto the other side. Emphasise weight bearing more onto a hemiplegic side. An older child can do this if you hold his legs up in the air while he takes weight on to his forearms. Shift his weight from side to side which may elicit stepping on forearms. Hold thighs to keep stiff legs apart, turned out with straight hips and knees.

Remember: Always try removing any supports given by your hands or equipment to check whether the child can lift the head or take weight on forearms on his own momentarily or reliably.

Physiotherapy suggestions

Abnormal postures. These are corrected within the treatment suggestions above. Physiotherapists select methods that parents or carers can manage and find relevant to their situation. Special methods and equipment for deformities may be needed (see Chapter 11).

(1) *Activate symmetrical head raising and holding upright.* Assist a child to move both arms into elevation, abduction–external rotation behind the plane of a child's head. For a child who understands, use your manual resistance, asking him to push his elevated arms back against your hands pressed against his upper arms. Keep his elbows as straight as possible. This activates associated head raising. He then tries to maintain arms in elevation against your manual resistance ('stay there', 'don't let me push your arms down'). Help him keep the chin in with long neck posture. The head holding is also activated by appropriate manual resistance carefully given between the ears at the lower occiput ('stay there').
(2) *Facilitate head raise and turn* by lifting the child's elevated arm on one side back and behind the child's head as in the creeping pattern (Fig. 9.30a). An older child can have arm on a cushion to actively practise holding the elevated arm stable and then practice active head turn.

Creeping patterns. It is difficult to describe these patterns without demonstration. Some aspects will

be described as these techniques are particularly helpful to decrease flexion in prone, for muscle strengthening, lengthening and for activating early creeping on abdomen. Babies or severely involved older children are most responsive and may use the automatic actions under their own control later.

The *face arm* is elevated into shoulder abduction–external rotation (Fig. 9.30b). The *occiput arm* is brought down into shoulder extension–adduction–internal rotation (Fig. 9.30c). The child may lie flat on the surface or over the edge of a roll, small pillow or wedge.

(1) Assisted active changing of the arms, so the opposite arm is elevated whilst the face arm moves down. These arm actions facilitate head raise and turn, back extension and, when on a surface, leg creeping movements.
(2) Use of stretch-rotation and appropriate manual resistance will activate the creeping movements of limbs with body-pelvic rotations.
(3) The child may continue active creeping on his own and so acquire one form of locomotion beginning at this level of development.
(4) Rising onto forearm can be stimulated by having the elevated *face arm* held stationary by your hand. You stretch the *occiput arm*, giving manual resistance to the rebound creeping action response. If the child understands, ask him to pull his arm forward and above his head. An automatic rising reaction on to the forearm of the face arm occurs. As the child rises, he also raises and turns his head. His sense of rising is an experience he can draw on later.
(5) Using action of leg for creeping involves single leg flexion–abduction–external rotation, preferably with pelvic rotation backwards. The other leg is held in extension–adduction–*external* rotation. Legs should be held at the thigh and knee using stretch-rotation and resistance according to the young child's reaction (see also Fig. 9.30a).
(6) Active leg creeping may stimulate arm creeping actions. If the child understands, ask him to bend his hip and knee up and out against your hand on his thigh to have full pelvic rotation backwards. Offer him enough resistance to augment his movement so that an associated arm action to creep is gained.

This creeping technique is useful for activation of more affected arms or the hemiplegic

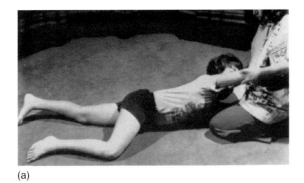

(a)

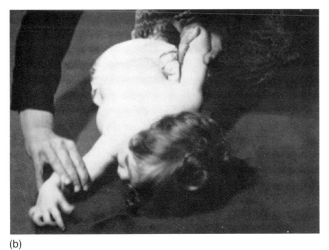

(b)

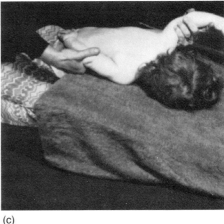

(c)

Figure 9.30   (a–c)

arm of babies or severely affected children. Movement and/or rising are initiated.

There are many possibilities for automatic rising reactions and other stabilising and movement reactions with Vojta's creeping techniques in addition to my own modifications. However, they are best demonstrated and supervision given by physiotherapists experienced in this approach.

Modified creeping over mother's lap or down a slippery wedge/incline is enjoyed by children. Once automatic creeping is experienced by a child, he needs to use it actively to reach an object or person he wishes to touch.

Train active rising on to both forearms or later hands at the same time. Hold the child's head by spanning his occiput between his ears. Ask him to raise his head up against your manual pressure. This pressure and sometimes manual resistance facilitates rising on to his forearms or hands and teaches him to initiate rising with head action.

Augment head holding and forearm support by asking a child to maintain head posture as you gently push his head. Encourage child to pull his chin inwards getting *a long neck*. Also give manual nudge or push to front, side, back of shoulders, as child is told to 'stay there' or 'don't let me push you down' or simply 'hold it'.

Note: Use of resistance is particularly recommended for stabilising and strengthening the child with dyskinesia, ataxia and hypotonia. In all types of cerebral palsies, manual resistance needs to be appropriately given so that there is no abnormal overflow such as increase of involuntary movements, extensor or flexor spasms.

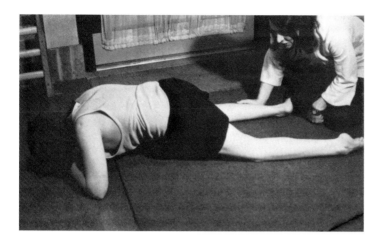

Figure 9.31   Rising onto knees and arms.

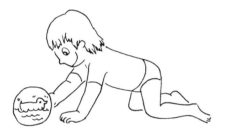

Figure 9.32   On hands and knees unsupported (*6–9 months*).

4–6-month normal developmental level

Common problems

Delay in acquisition of rising on knees, rising on to hands with extended trunk and flat pelvis. Weight bearing on knees, knees and forearms and on one forearm; reaching for objects; inability to lie prone with both or one of the arms stretched out to reach overhead; unable to roll over to supine or unable to creep on abdomen, on elbows or using a variety of creeping movements of both arms and legs.

Abnormal performance. Asymmetric, abnormal positions of limbs, clenching hands during the activities, beginning *mermaid crawl* (see 6–9-month level), asymmetric weight bearing.

Abnormal rising patterns in prone such as abnormal rolling patterns within rising. A child may use either excessive hyperextension of head and trunk, or flexing hips and knees under the abdomen on forearm support, then pushing up onto the hands or only rising onto the knees, leaving head, arms,

hands and trunk fixed in flexion. Some children cannot use the arms at all or a child manages to push up on semi-flexed arms with hunched shoulders and then sits back on heels with legs bent inwards (*W sitting*).

Although useful for a child who has struggled to achieve these rising patterns, more mature and less effortful patterns can be trained.

Treatment suggestions and management

Rising on to knees, forearms and knees. Encourage the child's rising onto knees instead of your lifting the child each time. Place one leg in creeping position and hold firmly or fix the foot against a heavy box, tip the child's *opposite* hip and pelvis up and back with a slight touch and wait for active rise on to knees, first on to the one that is fixed. The other leg creeps forward on to its knee. Carry this out without giving the child a *tip-up* at his hip, *if he can manage alone* as shown in Fig. 9.31. Use instruction 'Knee forward and get up!' Rising onto forearms, and later, hands are usually activated as well.

Weight bearing on knees, on forearms and knees (4–6 months), on hands and knees, on hands with abdomen on the ground, or on hands over a wedge (6–9 months) (Fig. 9.32). Place the child on his knees, knees and forearms, hands and knees or on his hands with straight elbows with abdomen on the ground, according to what he can manage at his level of development.

(1) If there is tightness of hips and knee flexors, use *on hands* support with back, hips (buttocks) and legs straight. Press both sides of his pelvis

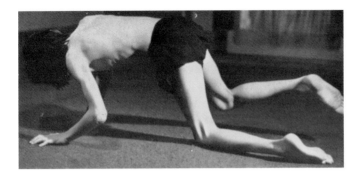

Figure 9.33   (a) Unstable shoulder and pelvic girdles with excessive action of elbow and knee flexors to maintain balance (postural control).

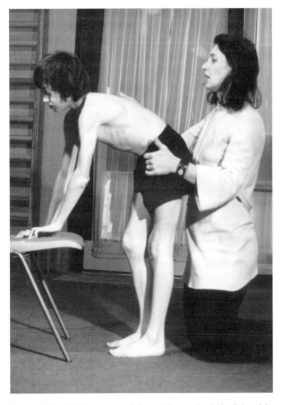

Figure 9.33   (b) Training stability with weight shift of shoulder and pelvic girdles in four-point standing – a modification of developmental sequence.

down and invite him to do this alone when he can.

(2) Use your lap, wedges, rolls, pillows, suspension in blanket, sponge rubber shapes or big soft toys for support until the child can balance alone.

(3) Use interesting toys, balls, sand and water play in these positions.

(4) Have hips at right angles when he takes weight on his knees. Active use of the hands also increases greater weight bearing on knees for stability.

(5) Press down on the child's lower back and buttocks to increase his weight bearing on his knees, and prevent sliding of his knees during his play with his hands, or *shoot out into extension*, or sideways into *frog position*.

(6) Use elbow splints to help weight bearing on hands with straight elbows so that shoulders develop stability during these weight-bearing activities.

(7) Open the child's hands by pressing his weight through the heels of his hands; by gently bringing the thumbs out from their bases and not from their tips. Press palms flat with joint compression through the length of the arm. Keep elbows straight. Do this while a child watches television or mobiles for interest so that he maintains the position for a period. Avoid distracting a child from his interest.

Unstable weight bearing through the arms. Use joint compression through the top of the shoulder or the upper arm with straight elbow to develop stability on hands in prone, in sitting or standing positions (Fig. 9.33a,b). A low table is used for training arm-propping support. Keep the arms in straight alignment with the line of pressure through shoulder or elbow. Have a child's weight through posterior 'heels' of the hands to avoid finger flexion. Arms are placed on a surface below the child, so the weight of his body adds to the joint compression, for example, a child may enjoy being held upside down for 'standing or *walking on hands*' with his elbow splints, for similar effects. Use a variety of floor textures to increase tactile experience.

Motor control actions for daily activities. These can also be learned in four-point standing and in prone stander with table.

(1) Weight bearing on one forearm, reach with the other. Weight bear and shift from forearm to forearm. Encourage reach with one arm on floor, then above his head and in different positions to obtain objects.
(2) With the child bearing weight on both forearms give him toys in each hand to grasp and play with. Let him grasp the ends of a bicycle pump, concertina, plastic bottle, transparent cylinder with coloured water or marbles inside, grasp two balls or blocks to bang together or push a ball from hand to hand. Toys should move or make a noise if touched, patted, pressed or grasped. Remove any supporting wedge and hold the child on one of his forearms while he actively uses the other arm in play. Whenever possible remove adult support altogether (see the section 'Development of hand function' in this chapter).
(3) Child in prone lying on forearms on thick soft sponge, inflatable mattress, water bed, trampoline, press the surface down on each side so that the child tips on to his elbow. Also help him shift weight back and forward. Use a song or rhythm to develop weight bearing and weight shift for the methods in point (4).
(4) Place a child on a low platform or low wedge on wheels with the legs held in abduction with abduction splint or a pommel. The child will move backwards or forwards by push or pull forearm actions. If he is on a bed and wishes to get off, he could then move himself backwards so that his legs come off the edge of the bed, his feet take the weight and he can stand up leaning on elbows and progress to supporting himself on his hands with his body against the bed (see Chapter 10 for uses of forearm support).

Note: Avoid creeping on forearms on a pronetrolley or a 'forearm drag' along the floor in those cases where there is a strong tendency to tightness of elbow flexors and shoulder hunching, and motivate other forms of locomotion. Also practise a child's forearm weight bearing on one side whilst the other arm stretches out for toys. Try stretching both arms well forward to toys or to push a big ball away.

Arms stretched overhead and forward: arm saving reactions: arm propping.

(1) Encourage a child to reach forward and overhead for toys, to push away a ball, balloon or toy on wheels. Older children can walk their hands up a wall or wall bars as far as possible (Fig. 10.1). Use a small bolster or wedge to help him stretch his arms out *and* up towards toys on a box or suspended above him. Arm elevation activates head raise and hold.
(2) Place a child over a beach ball or large roll with his arms over the top. Tip the ball forward and encourage him to reach for the ground in preparation for saving himself from falling. Encourage him to prop himself on his hands by first placing his hands on the ground and then gradually increasing his weight onto them, whilst you hold his body safely on the ball. You can hold the body of a young child and tip him upside down near a surface, for example a table, and encourage him to put his arms out to save himself and then to take weight on them (Fig. 9.24). Provide different tactile surfaces for hand propping.
(3) Place a child on his abdomen on a large cushion with his arms stretched forward, and help him to go safely down a slide head first.

Note: The therapist needs to check whether positions of arms and legs are as correct as possible during all the activities above so that a child learns them in the best possible posture. For example:

- Shoulders and hips bent at right angles in weight-bearing positions.
- Knees pointed outwards without a *frog* position.
- Extended hips and knees as straight as possible, apart, and if able turned outwards.
- Shoulders and arms turned out rather than in excessive internal rotation.
- Hands open and palms down if weight bearing.

It is important to recognise that *all the training* of weight bearing on elbows, one elbow, on hands may be done in *sitting* or *standing*, leaning forward or down onto a low table or box. This reinforces the prone development *or* if prone is occasionally not indicated for a particular child, these activities can and need to be trained in these other positions (Fig. 9.33a,b).

Rolling from prone to supine. See subsection 'Physiotherapy suggestions for rolling and roll-and-rise'. Weight shift from side to side with arm and shoulder, or leg and pelvic rotation to enable achievement of rolling from prone.

Physiotherapy suggestions

Facilitate rising for assumption of four-point position which becomes more independent in the next developmental stage.

(1) Fix one of the child's legs in creeping position manually (Fig. 9.34). Press down through his buttocks. Alternatively, hold his other leg above or below the knee and stretch it into extension–adduction–external rotation which

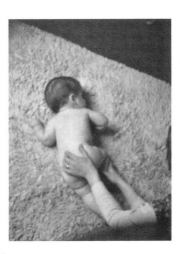

Figure 9.34

stimulates leg forward creep and rise onto the other knee. If the child understands, he should be instructed to *bend* a hip and knee. The child can then rise onto hands with or without chest support.

(2) When a child is actively able to commence or even complete rising up on to knees and forearms, but is weak, manual resistance is used to reinforce his efforts. Apply manual resistance at the pelvis in a diagonal direction (Fig. 9.35) for better muscle activation and avoidance of stimulating spasticity.

Augment holding of posture on hands and knees

(1) The child attempts to maintain this position as the therapist slowly and quickly pushes him and later uses manual resistance to push child out of position, advising child to 'stay there'. Push child as in the following ways:
   - Laterally at each hip or each shoulder.
   - Forwards and backwards at hip or shoulders.
   - At opposite shoulder and hip.
   - At shoulder and hip on the same side.
(2) Manual resistance carefully given to occiput with chin in and to shoulders advising child to '*stay there*' assists stability. Similarly use resistance for hips when child is only on knees with chest and arms supported by roll or wedge.

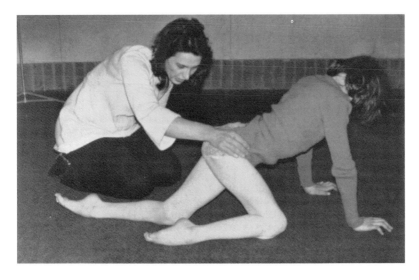

Figure 9.35

6–9-month normal developmental level

Common problems

Delay in weight bearing on hands and knees, in lifting one or alternate limbs, weight bearing on one hand and reaching for objects in all directions, crawling with only hands or only knees, pivot prone position and absence of rising from prone to hands and knees.

Abnormal performance of motor abilities, over-flexed hips, knees or feet, internally rotated legs or arms, lack of reciprocation in crawling, *bunny hopping* both knees forward in heel sitting and asymmetrical weight bearing. Persistence of *mermaid crawl* or *commando crawl*, which is motion by pulling forward on flexed arms with the legs stiffly extended, adducted and internally rotated. The hands may clench with each *pull* forward and often the legs adduct strongly with this pull.

Lack of postural stability of the pelvis and hips creates creeping on the abdomen rather than on all fours and can mask a child's ability to take weight on hands with a flat stabilised pelvis.

Absence of reactions normally expected are saving reactions in arms now forward and laterally and tilting reactions in prone. For persistence of any early reactions, see 0–3-month level.

Treatment suggestions and management

See Figs 9.32 and 9.33 and add the following:

Weight bearing on one hand, reach for a toy and on hands and knees lift one arm or leg or both. Place the child on hands or on hands and knees over rolls or your arm and when possible expect independent balance to develop stability and counterpoising. Other ideas are for example:

(1) Lift individual limbs whilst he maintains balance to a song or counts.
(2) While child takes weight on his hands or hands and knees, encourage him to stroke different textures on the ground, such as carpets, tiles, grass and sand. Let him feel cool, warm, scratchy and smooth surfaces.
(3) While balancing on hands and knees, he might scrub the floor, reach for a dangling toy, roll balls, move small toys on wheels, dig into the sandpit with one hand or spade, on the grass

he could pick flowers, handfuls of grass and so on. He can stretch a leg to kick tinkling bells, or playfully touch a person.

These abilities are augmented with counterpoising exercises, with and without resistance, given below.

Crawling. This can be trained with the child suspended in a blanket. Hold each end of the blanket and tip the child in it so that his weight is taken more on one side, releasing the other side for a 'step' forward. Guide the moving knees or arms only according to a child's ability.

Note: It is important to avoid the use of crawlers and the training of crawling in children who prefer other means of locomotion and especially those who have tight hip and knee flexors. In these cases, use a wedge on wheels or prone-trolley with roll of towels under a child's chest so that shoulders stabilise on straight elbows with the hands crawling on the floor. The legs are extended on the prone-trolley. Play 'walking-on-hands' or 'wheelbarrow' with adult supporting child's legs in a straight hip–knee position. Weight shift from hand to hand develops counterpoising of trunk muscles. In cases of severe knee and elbow flexion, splintage of these joints should be used as the child gets about on his platform on wheels.

Rolling. Encourage rolling on grass down a slight incline, on sponge rubber, on an inflatable mattress down a mound and on different surfaces.

Physiotherapy suggestions

Flexion or lack of postural stability of head, shoulder girdle and hips in extension positions may be treated with techniques on wedges (small and large) already mentioned and with pivot prone. Pivot prone or Landau position is activated by a head raise to extend body and legs with legs held in abduction.

- This can be carried out on a large ball or roll.
- Also elevate-abduct-externally rotate arms behind plane of head to stretch spine and arms.
- Older children using pivot prone and action of arms can strengthen shoulder girdle stabilising muscles and trunk by pulling against weights over pulleys opposite to them.
- Pivot to each side is taught to a child for some mobility on the floor. Weight shift on the body and pelvis is developed and also overcomes

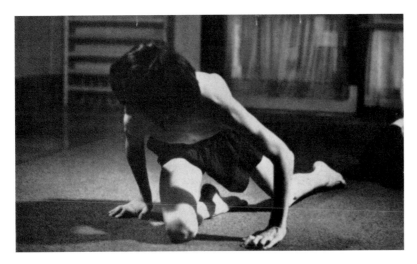

Figure 9.36 Instability of pelvic and shoulder girdles and a poor counterpoising. Unstable crawling and stationary four-point posture.

abnormal weight bearing on only one side. Pivoting to each side is unlikely to transfer to standing, owing to different gravity conditions.

Note: The extension in pivot prone is not enough for standing. It is in the vertical position that postural stabilisation of the head, trunk and hips must be trained (see the section 'Development of standing and walking').

Counterpoising exercises. Child maintains balance on hands and knees and carries out arm or leg patterns to achieve counterpoising. See Fig. 9.36 for person with instability needing the counterpoising (postural adjustment) exercises.

Leg pattern. Ask the child to bend one knee up to the ceiling; manually resist his knee flexion forward and outward. Then reverse to hip and knee extension with adduction and external rotation (Figs 9.37 and 9.38). Resistance given to leg pattern will also increase stabilisation at the shoulder girdle and opposite hip at the same time.

Arm pattern. Use creeping pattern of child's arm from extension–adduction–internal rotation behind his back, facilitated to elevation–abduction–external rotation as described at the earlier levels (Fig. 9.30). Other arm patterns are arm flexion adduction across chest, change to abduction–extension–external rotation with trunk rotation backwards. As the child moves his one arm against resistance, he increases weight bearing or stabilisation on the other three points. If he is on his hands only, abdomen on the floor, shoulder stabilisation and counterpoising are stimulated as follows: he balances on the one hand as single arm pattern of

movement is carried out actively or against correctly given resistance.

(1) Continue pivoting in extension or other active limb and trunk extension activities to counter the persistence of any flexion patterns. This helps to avoid flexion deformities.
(2) Continue rising on to hands *and* knees as above or roll-and-rise (see Fig. 9.65a,b in supine development).
(3) Child crawls against resistance given to his knees. Grasp his knees and guide them outwards as you resist each step forward (Fig. 9.39).
(4) Augment holding the hands and knees posture against nudge or manual resistance. Concentrate on pelvic girdle stability for children who hop with both knees together in 'bunny hopping' crawl. Suggestions to discourage bunny hopping are given below.

Points (3) and (4) overlap into the next stage of development.

9–12-month normal developmental level

Common problems

Delay in rhythmic independent reciprocal crawling, maintaining half-kneeling position hands on ground, on hands and feet and other more advanced postures. Absence of rising from hands and knees

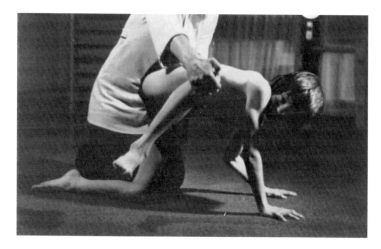

Figure 9.37 Counterpoising exercises.

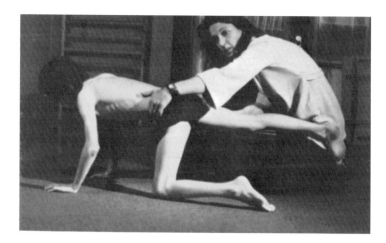

Figure 9.38 Counterpoising exercises. Positions of therapist's hands. Child's leg flexion against hand on thigh or pull against hand on tibia. Leg extension against hand on tibia.

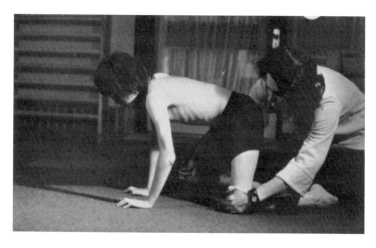

Figure 9.39 Crawling against manual resistance of therapist – guidance or resistance of knee into external rotation avoids adduction and offers a wider base for balance.

often through half-kneeling to standing whilst holding a support. There is delay in ability to change from prone to sitting, prone to squatting, prone to supported half-kneeling while grasping support or hands on floor. Changes of posture are poor.

Abnormal performance. A child may crawl with abnormally externally rotated knees. He may use excessive adduction–internal rotation of hips in crawling, in half-kneeling and weight bearing on hands and feet. If the child can *bear-walk* on hands and feet, he has his heels off the ground and/or excessive flexion of the knees with hips internally rotated and adducted. When pulling himself up to standing using his arms and hands, he drags excessively extended and adduction legs with feet on toes.

If he is tipped either forwards, sideways or backwards, then he may not save himself in either one or all these situations. Strengthening exercises for head and back extension normally use extension action at this level, but this may be very weak.

Treatment suggestions and management

Half-kneeling. Seat the child on the side of your lap when you sit on the ground. Bring his outside knee on to the floor, he is then kneeling on one knee, hold the other knee forward and outward. Remove your lap and place his hands on the floor for support. Encourage him to play in this position by moving a car or rolling a ball under the *bridge* of his knee, round his foot, or spend time in tying his boot laces, count his toes, paint his toe nails and so on. Later, he should grasp horizontal bars at various levels and place his hands flat on the wall, low tables or your flat hands. Half-kneeling position should be maintained with the front knee pointing outward. Hold his knee out with his foot pointing out and placed out to the side. This is often difficult. Ask the child to press his front knee outwards against your hand and also maintain balance. Augment his balance by offering manual resistance to his hips at the side, shoulder girdle at the side and shoulder and hip girdles at the same time.

Whilst on hands in half-kneeling and also in upright half-kneeling, grasp a support. Manual resistance may also be used. In addition, head lift against resistance applied between his ears across the lower occiput helps to augment the stabilisation.

Rising from prone to standing. At first, children normally pull themselves up to supporting themselves on their arms in kneeling upright and then up to standing by stretching their legs and going onto their toes. This pattern persists if a child uses spasticity to extend the legs. Train half-kneeling in a more mature transitional position on the way to standing up. The half-kneeling position is assumed with child's hands on the ground (like a normal toddler) from hands and knees position or then grasping supports and pulling himself up to standing via the half-kneeling position. Assumption of half-kneeling takes place using the exercises shown in Figs 9.37 and 9.40. The therapist is helping the child place his foot flat on the ground. Figure 9.41 shows how to hold the knee and foot steady as the child rises. Another method is to hold the child's body under his chest whilst he controls his limbs in rising. You may also ask the child to rise against your hand, pressing his lower back and pelvis or resisting the knee extension as shown in Fig. 9.41.

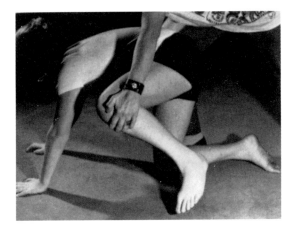

Figure 9.40 Assumption of half-kneeling against the manual resistance or guidance of a therapist.

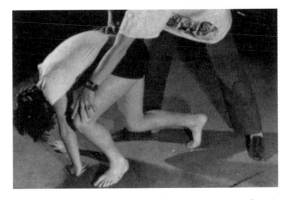

Figure 9.41 Assumption of standing against manual resistance or guidance of a therapist.

Note: The application of manual resistance must be done by physiotherapists as careful control of any overflow of undesirable activity depends on the appropriate degree of manual resistance.

See also other patterns of rising from prone in Fig. 9.179. Children have their own strategies which are acceptable provided that they avoid recurring motor patterns associated with deformity.

Weight taken on hands and feet, and bear-walk. The child may place his hands on a low stool if he cannot easily reach the ground. Stabilisation together with gentle passive stretching of tight hamstrings is carried out in this position. In addition, the counterpoising exercises and activities of play, dressing or other tasks can be done in this position using a low table and are illustrated in the development of standing at the 9–12-month developmental level (Fig. 9.33b).

Stepping with support on hands and counterpoising legs and plantigrade feet can be carried out using a stool on wheels, sliding a low chair, with a sledge or stable wooden toy on wheels. Hold the child's thighs and knees straight and turned outward if there is any excessive flexion–adduction–internal rotation on weight bearing. Give manual resistance for flexion–abduction to the stepping leg whilst holding the knee of the other leg straight, to stretch tight hamstrings or increase the action of the stabilisers of that hip. Wearing knee gaiters for the bear-walk or for slow upright stepping prevents the overuse of knee flexion which compensates for pelvic instability. Keeping the knees straight, or as straight as possible, can activate the stabilisers of the pelvic girdle. Joint compression through hips or knees of the standing leg also helps active stabilisation, so knee flexors do not need to overact to maintain balance.

There are able-bodied children who automatically bear-walk when there is rough or cold ground which are not pleasant for bare knees during crawling. There are also able-bodied children who never bear-walk, but this is desirable in cerebral palsy for stabilisation of shoulder girdle and pelvic girdle, stretching of tight hamstrings, stretching of tight heel cords (heels kept flat on the ground) as well as for counterpoising of each limb as a step is taken.

Hyperextended knees may also be treated in the bear-walk (see Fig. 9.169). Increasing stability of the hips may be associated with a decrease of hyperextension of the knees which is another compensation for lack of postural stability of hips and pelvis.

Balance on hands and feet with one foot lifted onto a low wide box prepares a child for climbing stairs on hands and feet.

Tilt reactions and saving reactions in limbs on hands and knees may be stimulated on a rocker board, inflatable mattress, trampoline or thick soft sponge rubber (Fig. 9.42). However, they are not as important in prone kneeling as in the upright postures, but do activate muscles in cases of weakness.

Changes of posture from prone kneeling (on hands and knees) to sitting and back again, to prone lying and back again, to half-kneeling and back again, and many other changes as in the righting reactions should be trained at this level of development. See the development of sitting at this level. These activities overlap into all the other channels. They have been initiated at earlier levels in prone (see above).

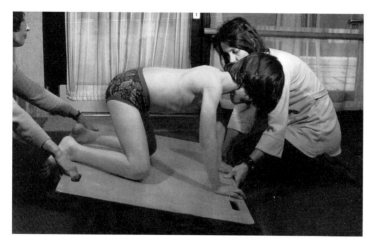

Figure 9.42 Tilt responses activated on a rocker board.

Use of bunny hopping. Reciprocal crawling rather than the continual bunny hopping of both knees forward is expected at this developmental level. Unstable pelvis, excessive tightness of hip and knee flexors and also habit prolong bunny hopping and aggravate these problems, as well as adding deformities of the feet. A child who bunny hops may well have no other way of getting around. Therefore, offer other means of locomotion such as the prone board on casters for prone lying with hips and knees straight, a tricycle, pedal car and preferably appropriate walkers, with knees in gaiters, if necessary. Training children to *bottom shuffle* is also a good alternative and easily trained and learned by many children. The child sits with feet in front on the ground. He leans on his hands at his sides, presses his feet flat on the ground and stretches out his knees and moves along the ground, backwards or forwards. Avoid bottom-shuffling in side sitting to prevent any hip subluxation or persisting asymmetry in a child with hemiplegia.

Encourage crawling on all surfaces, sand, grass, carpets, tiles, as well as using crawling on to a large step made with mattresses, wood or firm sponge rubber, and climb in and out of boxes, cubby holes, through play tunnels or a blanket over the backs of stable chairs and under tables. Teach a child how to avoid bumping his or her head for spatial and body image experiences.

Crawling up stairs. This can be started on the hands and knees or hands and feet onto a low wide bench and then on stairs. Normally these crawling abilities are established at developmental levels around 20 months.

Discourage crawling in children with tight or short hip and knee flexors and plantarflexed feet. Practise other forms of locomotion with extension of legs. Older people with cerebral palsy usually prefer not to learn crawling activities. There are children who do not prefer to crawl anyway.

Training upright kneeling. This is discussed here as the child rises from prone positions to this position. Kneeling upright holding on to a support is expected at the age of about 9–12 months whilst kneeling alone only at about 15 months in normal child development (Gesell 1971). Supported upright kneeling activates trunk on pelvic stabilisation or vertical stability, before or at the same time, as supported standing with straight knees and plantigrade feet. Treat equinus, knee flexors and hips for a desirable upright standing position.

Avoid excessive use of upright kneeling position in children who persist with hip flexion, lordosis or hip–knee flexion with dorsiflexion in this position. However, these postures may be controlled by giving pressure to buttocks to extend hips whilst keeping the knees at right angles. The back is held straight by the child if he leans his body against a sofa with the arms placed well forward to reach and grasp toys at the back of the sofa seat. A child may balance next to a low bench, leaning on hands below or at waist level. Avoid the arm support at shoulder level or above as this may throw his weight backwards, resulting in heel-sitting. However, to control a child's deformities, use a variety of positions, such as half-kneeling on the floor supported at one side of your lap with your hand supporting his chest, to control lordosis. Sway supported child forwards to stretch plantar flexors of the front foot in half-kneeling.

Use upright kneeling for dyskinetic (athetoid) and ataxic types of cerebral palsy and if postural abnormalities associated with hypertonus can be controlled. Weight shift at this lower base is easier than in standing. Later train weight shifts while holding on, followed by knee walking sideways, forwards and backwards. Independent kneeling upright develops after standing alone and knee walking as well as kneeling on a rocker board may be useful in some children.

Kneeling upright, holding on, leads to half-kneeling holding on and then removal of hand grasps to balance alone in these postures. Kneeling is used as a transition posture in rising to standing.

Supine development

The following main features should be developed according to an individual's developmental stage:

Postural stabilisation of the head (Fig. 9.45). The normal neonate's head is in midline with physiological flexion but on the side by 1 month. The body is tipped to the same side as the face, as there is no postural control yet and neck-righting response is active. Head stabilisation in midline is (4–5 months normally) on a surface and with head held off the surface (5–6 months). This develops from any chin poking to chin in midline and then pulled in to look down. If a baby is held suspended horizontally in supine, he holds his head alone in midline. Full head control is raising and holding of the head as well as head turning. Head turn to look keeping body midline or with pelvis to the opposite side (4–6 months). Head raise (4–6 months) is part of the rising reactions discussed below.

Postural stability of the shoulder girdle as the child holds the arm up to face in midline or when hands are held in midline (4 months) for hand to mouth and for *hand regard*, which overcomes the shoulder retraction of 3 months. The arm is then held in the air for reach, reach and grasp, and hand–eye coordination (4–6 months) including visually directed reach to raised foot for touching and 'mouthing'. There is anticipatory mouth opening to 'mouth' at 5 months. One hand reaches to foot on the same side and then to the opposite side whilst the other arm and shoulder often stabilise to hold the leg up for reach and grasp (see the subsection 'Basic arm and hand patterns for all levels of development' and also Table 9.4).

Postural stability of the pelvis with posterior tilt in being pulled to sit (4–6 months, Fig. 9.50) and as the child holds legs in the air with feet touching in dorsiflexion-supination (5 months), there is also one leg up in the air (4–6 months) in order to grasp a knee and then a foot and foot to mouth. There is then anterior pelvic tilt and stability (5–7 months) when a child *bridges* his hips in extension with feet on the surface. Repetitive change from posterior to anterior pelvic tilt develops pelvic mobility (Fig. 9.52). This enhances ability to shift body from head to toe, which is used in some back shuffles along the floor.

Postural stability of head, trunk and pelvis is closely related to counterpoising of limb movements. See discussion on head and trunk symmetry in Note below.

Counterpoising the limbs in the air (Fig. 9.43). Children cannot do this tipover when they are on their backs in water. Thus, holding a limb up in the air with absence of a hard surface increases a demand on the musculature for counterpoising and reveals developmental inadequacy. Counterpoising involves weight shift on trunk and pelvis, mainly laterally. There is activation of limb muscles together with neck flexors, pectorals, serratus anterior and abdominals (5–7 months). There is associated elongation of short neck and trunk extensors in any early chin poke and back arching. All this happens when normal babies flex and hold their limbs steady in the air. Pivoting on the back using weight

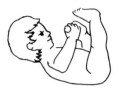

Figure 9.43 Postural stability and counterpoising of the limbs.

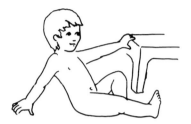

Figure 9.44 Rising from supine.

shift to each side counterpoises lateral arm and leg movements so that a child can move in circles (9–10 months).

Rising reactions and actions (Fig. 9.44). These are probably the most important reactions or actions to be trained in supine development. Many abnormal postures and abnormal reactions are particularly obvious in supine, and a child is particularly helpless in this situation. Training the child to get out of supine involves counteracting most of these problems. This training seems to be as important if not more so as spending time training the child's correct position in supine. Supine, *head rising* (righting) and the *overcoming of head lag* (4–6 months) prepares rising out of supine. Various rolling and *rolling-and-rising* sequences of motion enable a child to rise out of supine. If these cannot be achieved, other strategies need to be found as, say, that used by the athetoid child (Fig. 9.70) and pull to sitting or standing using hand grasp. Rising patterns also contribute to a child's learning to get out of bed and turn at night.

Note: Normal asymmetries in supine lying are from 0 to 4 months, becoming symmetrical in 4–5 months. Persistent asymmetry can lead to deformities. Abnormal asymmetries in the postural mechanisms against gravity from 4 months onward need therapy, as this is associated with asymmetrical arm and leg function. However, when postural control is symmetrical, there is more opportunity for a variety of normal symmetry and normal asymmetry

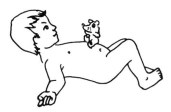

Figure 9.45 Postural stability of the head and head raise.

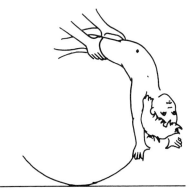

Figure 9.46 Arms saving (parachute) reaction from supine.

patterns of hand, arm and leg function for perceptual, cognitive and communication development.

Tilt reactions and *saving reactions* (Fig. 9.46) are less important in supine than in sitting and standing. They may be used only laterally for trunk strengthening exercises and for correcting a postural scoliosis. Saving and posterior tilt correct round backs and strengthen back extensors.

See *Stages in Supine Development* in Figs 9.47–9.56.

Treatment and management at all developmental levels

Supine rise to sitting and development of head righting (rising)

From 0–6-month normal development level. Help the child learn *to overcome head lag* using all or some of the following suggestions:

(1) First, have the child lying half-way down against a back support or wedge, and encourage him to come up to sitting. Gradually lower the back support so that eventually he raises his head and trunk from supine to sitting.

(2) At first you will also have to hold his shoulders well forward, then later his upper arms and, as soon as possible, have him grasp your hands with his elbows straight. In these ways pull the child up to sitting, *waiting* for his own active head raise and later head and trunk (righting) raising. Some children bring their heads up first, their trunks follow. In others, trunks may come up first and stimulate the head next (head-on-body righting; body-on-head righting). Hold the pelvis to stabilise it so that 'the lever' of head and body can be raised more effectively. This pelvic control develops later.

Note: Carry out methods (1) and (2) slowly from supine or half lying to sitting and lower the child back from sitting to supine without a collapse. Muscles are then activated well.

In methods (1) and (2) observe a child's legs. If his legs stretch, press together or twist inwards, then hold them apart, turn them outward on either side of a small wedge or on your lap (Fig. 9.58).

Hold a child's arms with straight elbows and turn arms outward if there is a strong tendency for them to twist inwards from the shoulders or bend tightly to his body.

Children who continue to bend their knees excessively, when hip flexion is needed, or if there are tight hamstrings, then hold knees straight or use knee-pieces during methods (1) and (2) for rising actions.

(3) Many children only manage to raise their heads if pulled to sitting in diagonal directions and not straight up against gravity. This diagonal direction is often preferable, as this is how the child will first manage to pull himself up to sitting. This is normally seen at about 9 months. Bring a child's shoulder or arm diagonally across body to the opposite side (Fig. 9.57). Help or wait for him to half rotate his body and lift his head as he is brought up to sitting. As the child comes up to sitting, he may automatically lean on a forearm or may require your pressure on his shoulder to help him take more weight onto this forearm. If he cannot use his forearm for support, you may hold both his hands, arms or shoulders and pull them across and over to one side of his body as he comes up to sitting in this diagonal direction.

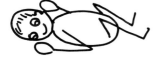

Figure 9.47 Flexion: asymmetry of head (*0–3 months*).

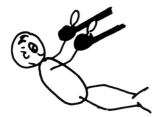

Figure 9.48 Head lag (*0–3 months*).

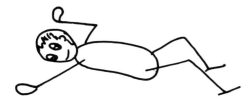

Figure 9.49 Asymmetrical postures (*0–3 months*).

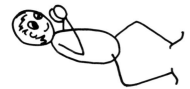

Figure 9.50 Head, hands in midline (*4 months*). Symmetrical weight bearing on head and body.

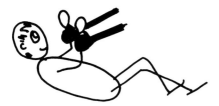

Figure 9.51 Decrease head lag. Lifts head when about to be pulled up (*3–6 months*). Stabilises pelvis.

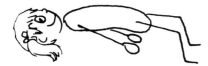

Figure 9.52 Bridging hips (*5–7 months*).

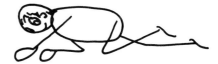

Figure 9.53 Roll over (*6 months*).

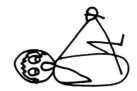

Figure 9.54 Grasp feet (*7 months*).

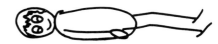

Figure 9.55 Lying straight, symmetry (*8 months*). Head turn isolated from trunk.

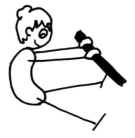

Figure 9.56 Pull self to sitting. Dislikes supine (*9–12 months*)

Head control is associated with weight bearing on forearm and also onto the leg.

(4) Rising to sitting may also be trained from the side-lying position, particularly in those children who are excessively extended in the supine position, have very poor head raising from supine or require additional action of the shoulder girdle muscles, back extensors or arm elevation pattern (Fig. 9.59). Child in side lying, hips and knees semi-flexed, head forward, chin in and arm underneath the head with bent elbow. Gently lift the child's upper arm behind his occiput, turn the arm outward from the shoulder, as far as is comfortable for him, then wait

for his own active participation as he is being assisted up towards sitting with support of his upper arm. At first he leans on forearm and later let him rise to side sitting, leaning on his hand instead of on his elbow. Check that his palm is down on the ground, his head is lifted up and sideways and his shoulder girdle, arm and back are actively rotated backwards with extension. Avoid side lying with any subdislocated hips or when excessive hip flexion–adduction is present in the top leg. Avoid pulling upper arm back to protect shoulder joint.

From 6–10-month normal developmental level. Help the child *to rise* to sitting on his own in the following ways:

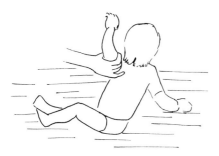

Figure 9.57   Supine rise to sitting.

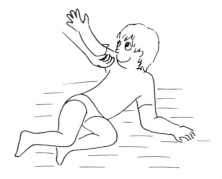

Figure 9.59   Rising to sitting from side lying.

(1) Encourage his own head raise in supine by holding him firmly just over the edge of a roll, your lap, a bed or in lying down the incline of a wedge. At first hold the child behind his shoulders and later hold the upper arms. Place bells or toys on his tummy (Fig. 9.45) or feet so that the child is motivated to look up at them or at his toes (painted red if necessary). Call him to raise his head to look at you.

(2) Supine to sitting can be carried out by helping a child to grasp a rope, a horizontal bar or to reach across his body to grasp a fixed vertical bar with one hand. He then pulls himself to

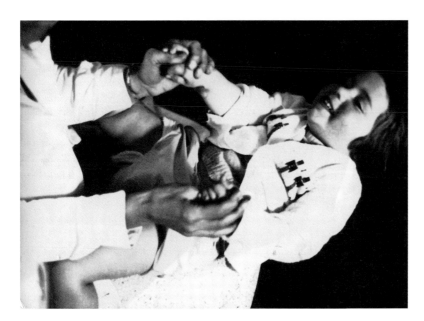

Figure 9.58   Rising to sitting with the child's legs on either side of the therapist.

sitting in a diagonal direction with half-rotation of his trunk. He props himself on the other forearm or hand.

(3) Supine to sitting can be accomplished by a child if he holds a short pole or stick, held by you as well, so you help him to sit up. Train him to avoid hunching his shoulders and excessively bending elbows and wrists to do this. You can press his wrists down during his grasp, so overcoming palmar-flexion.

Remember: The able-bodied child of around 9 months will first come up alone to sitting from supine in a diagonal direction with a half-roll to one side, leaning on one arm. He will only come straight up to sitting, independently and without his own support much later, in an advanced pattern at around 4 years.

Motivate lying to sitting with your ideas or use a song or the verbal rhythm of 'Up you come', then 'Down you go'. This perception and language may only be understood later.

Physiotherapy suggestions for rolling and roll-and-rise

Rolling techniques will help the child to roll to side lying where his hands might meet and he can see them. Well-chosen rolling methods correct the abnormal positions of the legs and arms and can also stimulate head righting, simultaneously decreasing infantile neck righting and activating various body derotative and rotative patterns. He is then, in effect, using his body to turn in order to rise from supine. Some children need rolling for locomotion and exploring space. Some of the many methods available are as follows:

Reflex rolling or primitive reactions. Turn the baby or child's head to one side and hold his jaw firmly. Press down and across the fifth intercostal space towards the *opposite* site. A reflex rotation will begin at the pelvis causing both knees and then one knee to flex up and over to the side of the child's occiput. This technique initiates rolling in very young children and in the presence of severe impairments, also actively corrects leg adduction–extension, arm flexion, hand fisting and abnormal *roll-en-masse* (Fig. 9.60), and *frog position.*

Side lying. Rotate the child's shoulder girdle forward while rotating his pelvis back. Change to rota-

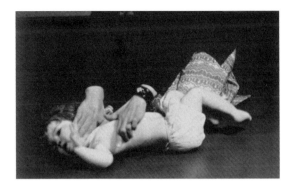

Figure 9.60   Reflex rolling.

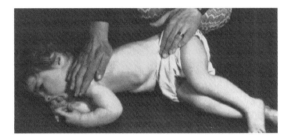

Figure 9.61   Rotation of the shoulder girdles and pelvic girdles. Knees can be flexed and rotated to the opposite side.

tion of the shoulder backward and pelvis forward, and vice versa (Fig. 9.61). If speed is correct and the rotary stretch on the trunk adequate, these *counter rotations* stimulate an active response in the child's shoulder or pelvis or in both areas. This also treats the rolling *in one piece* as seen, say, in the neck righting reaction. If rotation of the shoulder girdle is possible against some manual resistance, there is often an associated head raising with the rotation. Rotation of the girdles, pelvic/shoulder, not only facilitates rolling but also initiates arm movements and leg movements. Train shoulder rotation backwards as a preliminary to pulling the arm out from underneath the body in those children who get their arm caught in rolling over.

Supine. Leg patterns

(1) Bend both the child's knees across to the opposite side whilst rotating and holding his upper shoulder back. Release his shoulders and an active roll of the upper trunk follows. This roll might be manually resisted at the shoulder as well, but check that the correct amount of

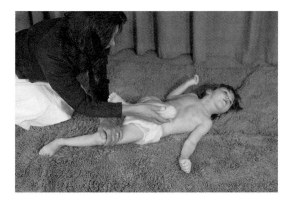

Figure 9.62   Supine, leg patterns.

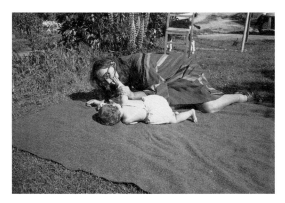

Figure 9.63   Supine, arm patterns.

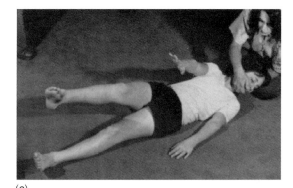

(a)

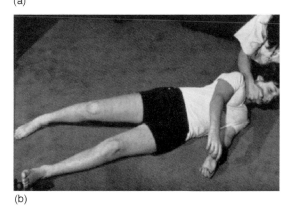

(b)

Figure 9.64   Head pattern to stimulate rolling. *Note* limb action (a) and (b).

resistance is given so that a full flexion spasm does *not* occur (Fig. 9.61).

(2) Stretch one of the child's legs into extension–abduction as a stretch stimulates this leg to move to flexion–adduction to the opposite side. Wait for his upper trunk to roll over bringing the arm across (Fig. 9.62). A retraction of the shoulder often delays or even prevents the arm coming over within the child's roll from supine to prone. If possible, augment leg flexion–adduction against manual resistance given at the knee and thigh. This shows him an active leg pattern, which he can learn to use later.

Arm patterns

(1) Bring the child's arm from his side in shoulder extension–abduction–internal rotation and across his body to flexion–adduction–external rotation (child's palm must be towards his face) (Fig. 9.63). Wait for him to turn his head, trunk

and legs. The therapist may guide the movement, activate it using stretch and resistance. A child actively reaches for a toy on the opposite side of the moving arm during this activity or as a result of this training procedure if he has no active reach.

(2) Bring one arm across to the other side to touch his mother's face as you give manual resistance to pelvic rotation forward which follows this action.

(3) If the underneath arm gets caught, initially hold it straight above his head.

Note:

(1) Prone-to-supine rolling: use a pelvic rotation backward to turn.

(2) During rolling over, various leg patterns are themselves stimulated, that is leg flexes over with the roll from supine to prone in some children. In others the child may use the leg to *push off* in an extended–abducted pattern (Fig. 9.64). During the roll from prone to

supine, some children extend and abduct the upper leg. Other children flex the upper leg as they roll. Similarly arm patterns vary. The therapist must select the technique according to the action she wishes to obtain and which a child is most able to begin to do on his own.

(3) Combinations of head, arm and leg patterns also vary.

(4) All rolling patterns relax a stiff child and are enjoyed when repeated rhythmically supine to prone and reversed.

Head patterns. Gently raise the child's head into flexion rotation, and wait for him to follow with rolling towards the side to which his face is rotated. Hold his head lightly as he rolls. You may have to hold his chin up as he reaches prone. Resisted head flexion rotation may be used as well in children who have good head control and respond with rolling in their waist and not in a total body action. Prone-to-supine rolling is carried out with head raise to extension rotation. The arm patterns above may also activate associated head patterns. Some children may use an arm to push off together with head patterns (Fig. 9.64).

Rolling to instructions. The facilitation patterns of either head or limbs need to be imitated as experienced for active learning by a child. Instructions used for, say: *prone lying* 'lift your head and one (right) arm up and back as far as possible', 'roll over'; 'lift your leg up and back, over to the other side', 'roll over'.

Supine lying. 'Bend one knee right across to the other side as far as it will go', 'roll over'; 'grasp your hands and stretch your elbows – bring both arms over to one side as far as possible', 'roll over'; 'lift your head and look over to one side as far as possible', 'roll over'.

A child selects the rolling pattern that he can actively manage. A carer works together with child and therapist in practising selected patterns that can be managed (see below).

Treatment suggestions and management for rolling and rising

Rolling

(1) Place the child on his back, on his side or on his stomach (keep his face and nose clear if in prone) on a blanket. Hold each end of the blan-

ket – two adults may be needed – and suspend the child in the blanket just off the ground. Tip the child gently from side to side, waiting for him to complete his roll over. If he cannot do this himself, you can roll him in the blanket until he picks up the rolling motion himself. *Do not* do this with a child who needs to arch his back or overextends in order to tip himself over from prone position. However, training sideways rolling with a child suspended in a hammock or blanket prevents arching. This is because a child's head, shoulders and hips are bent in a hammock to counter extensor thrust or arching.

(2) Child in supine lying. You bend one hip and knee well over to the opposite side and wait for him to complete the roll over (Fig. 9.62). Use this for his participation during washing and dressing.

(3) Bring one of his arms over to the opposite side with the palm of his hand towards him and reaching out to your face, or to a toy he likes on the opposite side (Fig. 9.63). Offer him a toy to encourage his independent rolling from side lying and then from supine.

(4) Child in prone lying. Use his active head raise and turn to initiate a roll. You bring his hip and pelvis, or his shoulders, backwards and towards the opposite side and with his legs flexing; this encourages rolling. If there is excessive hip and pelvic extension, give the hip and pelvis additional flexion during rotation. Some children may push off on one hand to help roll from prone to supine, or rise on to their lower arms underneath their bodies.

(5) Child in prone or supine on a soft thick sponge rubber mattress or inflatable bed. Press down on one side of his body so that he tips over towards you and rolls. Rolling on such surfaces is often easier as he does not get *stuck* with his arm caught under his body. At first it is necessary to place the arm, which gets caught underneath, above his head.

(6) Encourage rolling on all surfaces, floors, carpets, grass and sand. Make an incline with a pile of mattresses or sponge rubber, or place the child on the top of a slight mound of grass or sand and let gravity help him roll downhill on his own.

(7) If a child can roll over *wait* for him to do so. In addition, train him to roll over from his back to his stomach and then to get up on

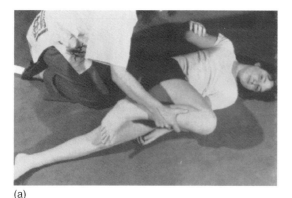

(a)

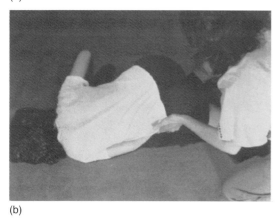

(b)

Figure 9.65   Roll-to-rise onto hands and knees. *Note* many methods exist for this but must be demonstrated clinically.

to his hands and knees (as described in section 'Prone development', 3–6-month level or Fig. 9.65a,b).

0–3-month normal developmental level

Common problems

Delay in gradual overcoming of head lag on pull to sitting. Inability to lift hand to mouth in supine but able to do so in infantile half side lying.

Abnormal performance (Fig. 9.66). Excessive extension of either head, shoulder girdle, back and legs or all of them (opisthotonus). Some arch into opisthotonus in infancy but become floppy later. Babies who are floppy (hypotonic) may have intermittent extensor spasms of head, spine and hips. They may also lie in 'frog' positions with the legs flexed–abducted–externally rotated, arms limp at

their sides or in shoulder abduction, elbow flexion, hands open or closed. Apparently normal flexion positions may also be present in babies who later show spasticity. Kicking of legs begins and has abnormal patterns. There may be abnormal asymmetry such that the one leg flexes, abducts and sometimes externally rotates while the other flexes, adducts and sometimes internally rotates, or one may kick more vigorously than the other. This asymmetry may become so great that the legs look *windswept* to one side, especially when kicking stops. Later hip dislocation is threatening in the adducted–internal rotated leg. Persistent head turning to one side may occur. Pelvic obliquity and scoliosis may appear early or in later stages (Fig. 9.68a).

Hands have grasp reactions with frequent clenching normally at 0–3 months, but abnormal if still present in an older child. The child may startle with Moro responses and remain in asymmetry including that of these asymmetrical tonic neck responses, later than the normal baby. This delay may result in the use of various infantile reactions for function or during motor function in the older child with cerebral palsy. On passively pulling the child to sitting, his legs first flex adduct and by the next 3–6-month level, flex abduct. A response of extension–adduction of the legs is abnormal. Some cerebral palsied children even extend the hips so much that their hips come well off the surface. Individual children cannot stabilise the pelvis against a surface and slide easily on it.

Physiotherapy suggestions

See subsection 'Physiotherapy suggestions for rolling and roll-and-rise' as very young or very severely impaired children can only respond on an automatic level at this early stage. Continue into next stage of development and then add more advanced methods, which need active learning by individuals.

Treatment suggestions and management

(1) See subsection 'Supine rise to sitting and development of head righting (rising)', from 0–6-month level.

(2) Bring a child's arms well forward and turn them out from his shoulders so that his both hands touch your face, or make him touch his own

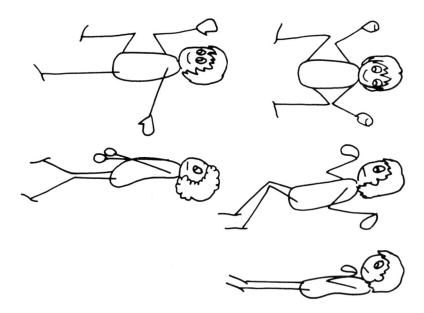

Figure 9.66 Some abnormal postures in supine.

hands, mouth, chest or abdomen naming these body parts. Stimulate visually and with noises in the centre to encourage his head holding in the centre whilst hands make contact with bells or musical toys dangling in the midline.

(3) Eye-to-eye contact with your eyes parallel to his, at first in the centre. Keep your face close to the face of a child with severe visual impairment. Stimulate him to follow sounds, lights and mobiles from side to side (see development of hand function in Table 9.4).

(4) *Abnormal performances* are modified as follows:

■ *Discourage* supine if the child has marked asymmetrical tonic neck reaction (ATNR) after 4 months, excessive Moro after 6 months or has extensor spasms or leg withdrawal reactions. It is better that the child functions first in prone, side-lying head supported with chin in or selected sitting positions with and without support according to a child's level of development. Positioning in sitting is discussed below in the section on sitting. There needs to be training of the head in midline and this may be too difficult in supine. If supine is inevitable during periods in the day, hold the child's head up with chin in into some flex-

ion in the hollow of a special neck cushion, use a hammock (Fig. 9.67a) or special supine lying frames/equipment (Figs 9.67b and 9.68b) (see Appendix 2). This overcomes the head falling or pressing back into extension. Head flexion often diminishes the ATNR, Moro or extensor thrusts. In this position, have the shoulders well forward to counter retraction. Motivate symmetrical arm movements to a parent's face, with toys, mobiles and use your own ideas. For the *windswept posture* (Fig. 9.68a) use special lying frames (Fig. 9.68b–d).

■ Excessively extended children should be flexed at head, shoulders and hips in side lying or supine. The severely extended child, with arms in abduction, shoulders retracted and elbows bent or stiffly extended, needs to be positioned in side lying with firm support from pillows or in *side-lying* equipment (Fig. 9.68c,d) so that his hands will be able to meet and he can see them, and they can touch his mouth and later reach for toys in front of him (5-month level). Place a toy between his hands that can easily be grasped. In later stages, train him to lie on his side, showing the child how to balance in side lying with one leg on

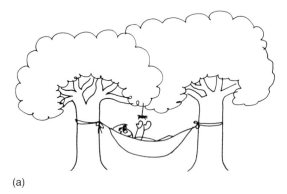
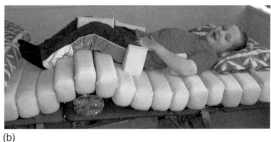

(a)   (b)

Figure 9.67 (a) A hammock counteracts excessive extension, so the head and arms can be used functionally. Supervision is essential. A blanket held well strapped to the four corner posts of a child's cot is wider and safer for some young children. (b) Example of a sleeping or resting on adjustable bed to correct persistent extension. Different lying positions can be used for other abnormal postures. ('Dreama' reproduced with the permission of Jenx, Sheffield)

top of other, as well as one in front of the other.

- For a child with abnormally straight legs, pressed together and turned in, use abduction splints or lying equipment (Figs 9.67b and 9.68b–d). Keep the child's legs apart and steady the hips as you assist a child to rise to sitting to activate head and later trunk control (Fig. 9.58). For 'frog' position use sandbags to keep the legs together or lying equipment as well as manually stabilising the pelvis with legs together as you train rising to sitting or play with the child in supine. Long trousers or pyjama pants that are well stitched down the centre can be used to bring the legs together in cases when hypotonic legs can easily be positioned.
- Persistent head turning to one side needs motivating a child to look the other way. A child's bed should be on the opposite side of the room. You offer toys, communication activities and, in sitting, food from the side towards which the child rarely turns. Carry the child so that he can also look to the side which is not usually preferred. The physiotherapist needs to make sure that the child does not have a congenital torticollis which requires stretching or orthopaedic advice about an operation. Plagiocephaly may accompany head turning. This strong head turning or preference has been ob-

served in some babies who subsequently developed normally without therapy (Robson 1970).

- See therapy for development of grasp in supine following the stages of hand function development in the section 'Development of Hand Function' given below. A child's hand function levels may differ from supine levels if arms are less affected than legs. Development of reach up against using gravity may be difficult and delayed in supine. Moro, startles, leg withdrawal or extensor patterns are simultaneously modified in positioning in sitting or in fully supported prone standing frames in children who tolerate them. Rolling techniques (leg patterns, arm patterns and side lying) simultaneously modify any residual neck righting or extensor thrusts seen in supine.
- Abnormal synergies, such as persisting leg extension–adduction–internal rotation, are best corrected in the creeping patterns in prone development. If prone development is not indicated in a particular child, train reciprocal leg movement in supine with head raised on pillow if necessary. Carry out active-assisted full range of reciprocal motion to a slow song. Hold the child's knees and bend one hip and knee up and out, holding the other leg straight and turned out. Change the motion by bringing

the bent leg down as you move the straight leg up into flexion. This also maintains joint ranges and existing muscle lengths. Reciprocal leg motion is not shown to be directly relevant to upright stepping. Reciprocal kicking continues, though supported reciprocal stepping has stopped (Thelen *et al.* 1987).

4–6-month normal development level

Common problems

Delay in acquisition of symmetry, in keeping head in the centre, in bringing the arms together and in hand regard. Delay in the disappearance of head lag and in acquiring ability to raise the head off the bed. The child is unable to *bridge* his hips off the floor, unable to reach for a toy (see hand function in Table 9.4).

Abnormal performance. Flexed legs now abnormally extend, adduct and internally rotate in many children lying supine and when brought from supine to sitting position. Normally legs flex, abduct and externally rotate at this level. Presence of clenched hands (see discussion on arm function). Abnormal absence of isolated foot movements or knee movements, as these only occur as part of 'mass patterns'. Abnormal anterior pelvic tilt (see Fig. 9.68a).

Reflex reactions. May not be developing body derotation. Reflexes of 0–6-month level may not be disappearing.

Treatment suggestions and management

(1) See hand function (Table 9.4) and section on methods.
(2) See rise up to sitting and rolling techniques.

Physiotherapy suggestions

Arm reach. Child in side lying and progress to supine. Train arm patterns with assistance or against your manual resistance according to child's ability. For example, use the flexion–adduction–external rotation with straight elbow and also with bent elbow so that hands reach across a child's body or to touch a child's mouth or face. Carry this out in side lying and with both limbs in supine (see Fig.

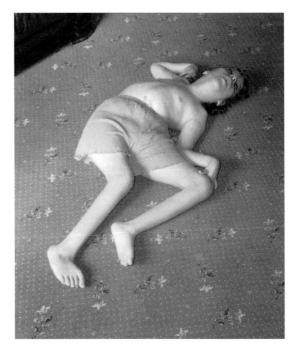

Figure 9.68   (a) Windswept posture, scoliosis and arms flexed.

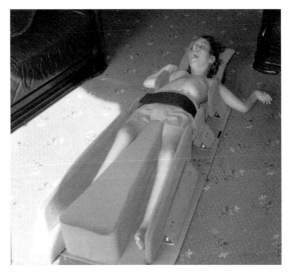

Figure 9.68   (b) Position to correct postures in supine.

9.68c,d). Place attractive objects in positions, near a child, to encourage his own activation of these and other arm patterns. A lack of shoulder girdle stability may cause compensatory shoulder hunching, but your manual guidance is given to help control this.

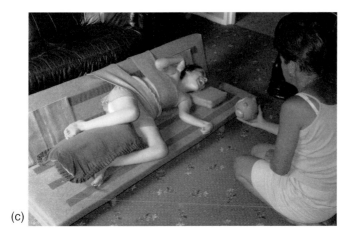

(c)

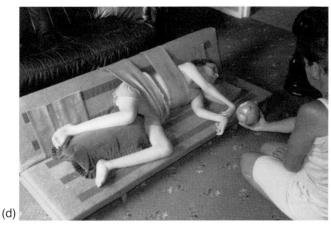

(d)

Figure 9.68   (c) and (d) Correcting posture in side-lying board. Her active arm reach for ball adds correction and communication.

Bridging (Fig. 9.69). Hold the child's feet flat on the floor. He raises his hips to let a toy go *under the bridge*. Check that this is *not done* by using a lumbar lordosis instead of hip extension. Check that arms do not flex up excessively but remain straight. He might grasp the sides of bench/plinth to keep arms straight. Hold the 'bridge' steady while the wind tries to 'blow it over'. The child tries to maintain the stability of the 'bridge' as far as possible as the therapist gives appropriate manual resistance at the side of the child's pelvis, on the anterior superior iliac spines, or one hand in front and one behind to rotate his pelvis. A pillow under his hips may help initially as he learns to maintain control against your manual pressure and resistance.

Note: Semi-bridging and moving backwards is a form of locomotion used by some children with dyskinesia (athetosis) and more rarely by other

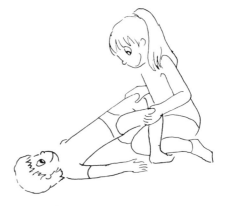

Figure 9.69   Bridging.

children with cerebral palsy. However, this is often abnormal as it includes excessive tense or hypertonic arching of head and back and retraction of the shoulders. If excessive, this should be discouraged by training other forms of locomotion which are satisfying. Equipment on casters such as wedges or corner seats and well-supporting special tricycles may be useful.

6–9-month normal motor developmental level

Common problems

Delay in grasping feet with legs in the air. The child is unable to roll over or pull himself towards sitting.

Abnormal performance. He cannot lie straight with arms and legs extended, with legs extended or with legs abducted–extended–externally rotated. A variety of abnormal postures may be seen including asymmetry of head, trunk or limbs, or all these. Normally, the pull to sit should provoke extension–abduction of legs. Anterior pelvic tilt may persist abnormally.

Abnormal rolling patterns may be persistence of normal early extension of head looking over shoulder, with trunk arching to obtain a roll. The child may lead with head and arms but with legs stiff and straight or relaxed and passive or may roll using legs but upper arm bent and retracted at the shoulder. Some roll using an action of *flexion into a ball*. In most abnormal patterns there is no rotation at the child's waist, only a rolling action in one piece using the total flexion or extension. There may be rolling to one side only, especially in hemiplegia. The roll is towards the affected side only using the unaffected side to carry out the roll over, or in tetraplegia or diplegia using the less affected side to carry out the roll. An inability to roll may also be due to weakness of limbs of head raise and of trunk muscles.

Treatment suggestions and management

(1) See rising to sitting, 6–10-month level, rolling techniques (see particularly sections on rolling to instructions and Treatment suggestions and management). Use arm and leg patterns against manual resistance to augment roll, when this is possible, at this stage. See also Table 9.4 for a child's development of hand function. At this stage a child may show his own strategies of rising (see Figs 9.70 and 9.71). See also the section in Chapter 6 on 'A child's own goals and strategies'.

(2) Have the child in supine and help him to hold one or both his feet. Turn his pelvis with hips and knees outward, bending a leg so that his foot touches one or both of his hands. He can then look at and also grasp his feet and hold them. You may need to bend his hips and lift his bottom off the bed if he is unable to reach his feet. The child needs to actively bend his hip and knee to his chest so that the full hip flexion is attained. Ask him to 'kiss his knee', 'to pull his sock or shoe off his toes' or to 'hug his knees to his chest'. When you hold his legs up above his face, he may enjoy playing 'peek-a-boo' as he opens and closes his ankles and feet. All these actions help overcome abnormal pelvic tilts and activate abdominals. When you gently stretch his knees for him to reach further to the feet, there is also stretching of hamstrings.

Note: No further training is needed in supine lying, as from 10-month developmental stages onward the child normally *dislikes* lying supine and persists in rolling out of this position or pulling up to sitting.

(3) Practise rising to sitting with half-rolling and also use rolling over in order to get out of bed. Also train rolling to prone and then rise into crawl position and later into standing using arms to push and support.

(4) Having trained the child to rise from supine to sitting *does not mean he can sit*. See development of sitting (Figs 9.77–9.90) which should be trained at the same time as supine development. Levels of development of sitting stages may differ from rising to sitting stages. The postural mechanisms differ.

Development of sitting

The following main features need to be developed as far as possible:

Postural stability of the head or vertical head control with trunk being externally supported. Head bobs and steadies, set forward, and then erect (0–3 months). Chin may sometimes first poke, then held in and be pulled in (retracted) to look down.

Postural stability of the shoulder girdle is activated with arm and hand propping or hand grasps for sitting with decreasing adult support (4–6 months). Arm props provide a larger base, protract

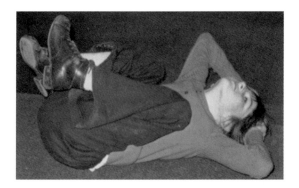

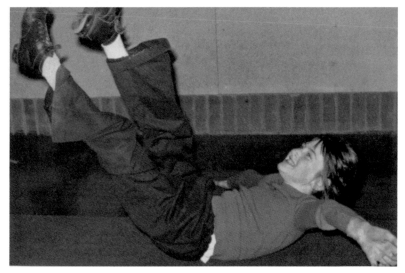

Figure 9.70 Individual using her own method of rising (bend knees to chest and swing up to sitting, or grasp clothes and pull up to sitting).

the shoulders and are part of a forward lean with legs apart as natural biomechanics for sitting alone. Later, use of the hands also activates shoulder girdle stabilisation and vice versa.

Postural stability of the head and the trunk (Fig. 9.72). Head and upper trunk with upper trunk ex-

tension (3–5 months) develops to full trunk extension and sitting alone (6–9 months). The trunk extension of stabilisation counteract a normal round back (C-curve). At first, arms are up in 'high guard' retracting scapulae with rhomboids to augment stability (5–7 months) and the wide base of abducted

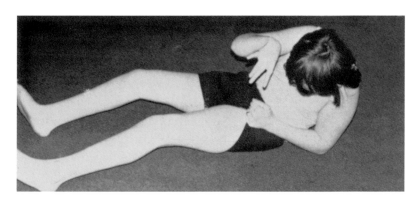

Figure 9.71 Individual using his own method of rising to sitting. He grasps his clothes and pulls himself up alone.

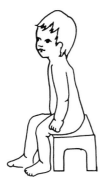

Figure 9.72 Postural stability.

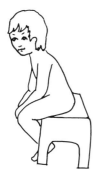

Figure 9.73 Rising to upright sitting and reverse.

externally rotated legs continue with weight bearing on the lateral sides (3–6 months). Nevertheless, the child cannot risk using arms and hands, which disturb the sitting balance. A baby chair is needed for support (4–6 months). Counterpoising hand use begins later as does a smaller base used for weight shifts with arms reaching up to shoulder level (7–9 months, see below). Cervical and lumbar lordosis develops (7–9 months). The variety of sitting postures on the ground increases from ring sitting to half ring to long sitting. There is a smaller base with less leg abduction–external rotation and knee flexion, reflecting increasing stability. There is controlled asymmetry in half ring (6–9 months), later side-sitting postures with growing independence and reliable stabilisation of trunk on pelvis during sit and turn (9–12 months).

Postural stability of the pelvis. Pelvis position depends on the head and trunk stability. The normal neonate has a perpendicular pelvis with a round back and not a posterior tilt and remains so until sitting alone with anterior tilt (Aubert 2008). The pelvis tilts anteriorly with trunk extension and then

posteriorly during forward leg lift with arm support (6–9 months) and without support (9–12 months). The pelvis becomes more mobile to foster balance with body weight behind, laterally or in front of the base (9–12 months).

Postural stability is closely related to counterpoising for head and limb movements.

Counterpoising for movements of head, for lifting to the vertical (3 months), for looking everywhere and involved in 'hand regard' (4–6 months) and when visually reaching (6–7 months). The arms and hands are used together at first opposite child's abdomen (7–8 months) and then at shoulder level and later elevation above shoulder level (7–12 months). There are small weight shifts of trunk within the child's base (7–8 months) then larger weight shifts forward, backward and sideways while maintaining postural control. Sitting and turning the body increases from 7 to 12 months. This allows arm and leg actions and also recovery of balance when a child's body leans well out from buttocks in grasping a toy out of reach (Fig. 9.74). Weight shift elongates weight-bearing side with trunk muscles contracting on shorter side to avoid instability (normally 7–12 months). Postural stability with counterpoising is integrated with use of hands and during locomotion called 'bottom-shuffling' (scooting).

Righting (rising) reactions and actions. Head righting or head raising to the vertical position with trunk supported (3–4 months). *Head and trunk righting or rising* to the upright from a slumped sitting or leaning posture. This may be forward, backward or sideways (Fig. 9.73). Normally developed (4–12 months) depending upon the positions and support given to the child to re-erect.

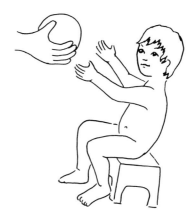

Figure 9.74 Counterpoising.

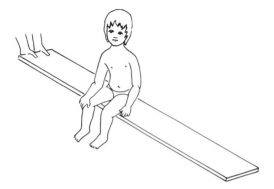

Figure 9.75   Tilt reaction.

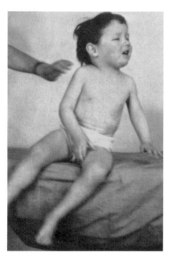

Figure 9.76   Saving reactions in the arms and legs.

Note: Rising to sitting from supine, see sections 'Supine development' and 'Prone development'. See discussion on rising from sitting to standing in the section 'Development of standing and walking'.

Tilt reactions (Fig. 9.75). These responses are activated as a child is tilted sideways, forwards or backwards with his bottom tilted off the horizontal. This tilt is much further than in weight shifts on a firm surface (9–12 months). Tilt responses are first with head followed by head and trunk adjustments.

Saving reactions (Fig. 9.76) and propping reactions in arms are protective responses if child tips or falls. Normally developed forward and downward (4–7 months), sideways (7–9 months) and backward (11–12 months). These are important for safety of upright sitting alone.

See *Stages in Sitting Development* in Figs 9.77–9.90.

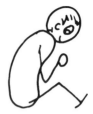

Figure 9.77   Sitting head uncontrolled, flexion in total child (*0–3 months*).

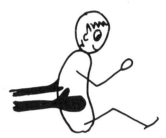

Figure 9.78   Decrease of flexion, vertical head control develops (*0–3 months*).

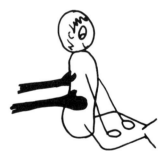

Figure 9.79   Sitting lean on hands, flattening of upper back develops, lumbar kyphosis still present (*4–6 months*).

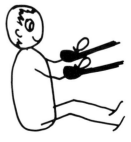

Figure 9.80   Sitting with less support, back straighter, legs straighter, turning out and apart (*4–6 months*).

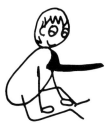

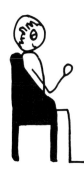

Figure 9.81 Sitting lean on hands, hips flexed–abducted–externally rotated. Less support and without support (*4–6 months*).

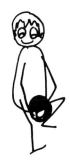

Figure 9.85 Sitting alone on the ground (*6–9 months*).

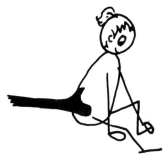

Figure 9.82 Sitting in baby chair with back and sides supporting or propped on a pillow support (*4–6 months*).

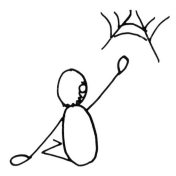

Figure 9.86 Sitting reach in all directions, hand support (*6–9 months*).

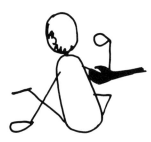

Figure 9.83 Sitting lean on hands and lift one hand to play, with feet or a toy (*6–9 months*).

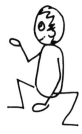

Figure 9.87 Sitting turn reach, no hand support (*9–12 months*).

Figure 9.84 Saving reactions and propping in arms (*6–9 months*). Tilt reactions begin.

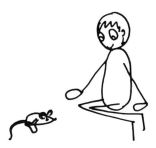

Figure 9.88 Sitting in various positions (*9–12 months*). Pivot in sitting.

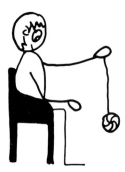

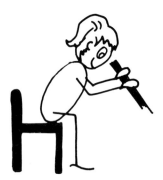

Figure 9.89   Sitting in a chair for daily tasks, no hand support. Sit alone on stool (*9–12 months*).

Figure 9.90   Rising out of sitting and getting into all sitting positions. Tilt reactions complete (9–12 months).

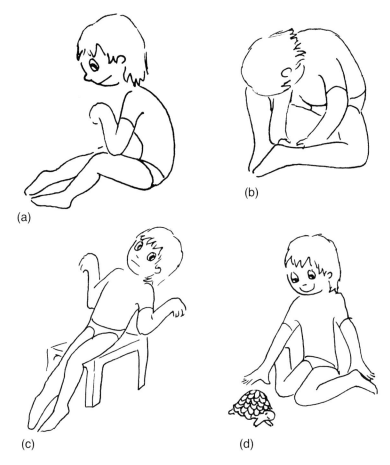

(a)

(b)

(c)

(d)

Figure 9.91   (a–d) Some abnormal postures in sitting.

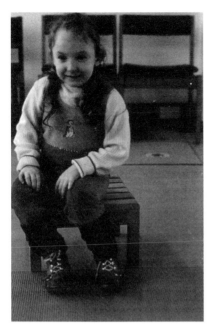

Figure 9.92 Sitting with 'windswept' legs to one side. A mild example which may be much more severe in other children.

Treatment and management at all developmental levels. Figs 9.94 to 9.107.

Aims

(1) *Absence of postural mechanisms.* Before postural mechanisms develop in normal early development, young able-bodied children have sitting postures which are also seen in older

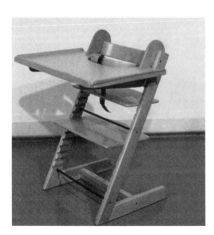

Figure 9.93 Tripp-Trapp chair for child with some balance.

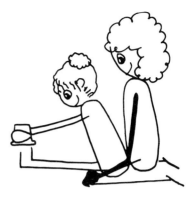

Figure 9.94 Support a child with your body when he is held on your lap or with you close behind him on a therapy roll, then gradually move away from the child's back. Give support at his waist level or at his hips and thighs. Shift the child laterally and then antero-posteriorly in preparation for movements.

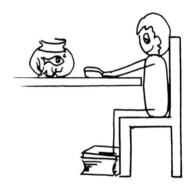

Figure 9.95 Sit with less lean against a table, feet supported and hands grasping a horizontal bar. Use eyes to follow interesting items. Later, child grasps bar with only one hand, using the other hand in play. Sit more upright leaning on hands on a table. Vary height of table.

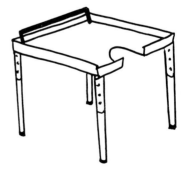

Figure 9.96 Cut-out table of adjustable height, with fixed grasp bar gives support. The cut-out offers support as a child learns to release grasps for support. One hand may grasp during movement with the other arm. Small vertical bars are also suggested for each hand to vary grasps.

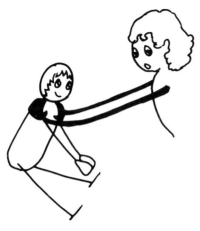

Figure 9.97 In floor or chair sitting positions, support is first given to the child's shoulders, then lowered to the hips and thighs (6–9-month level), sometimes to his feet only, and finally removed for sitting alone. Also train a child to sit on a downward incline of a floor wedge in long sitting to promote straighter back and legs. Knee gaiters may be used to assist knee extension. The correction of a round back is similar to that obtained by the forward seat incline in a special chair (Figs 9.109c and 9.110). A floor table may be needed for play and hand function.

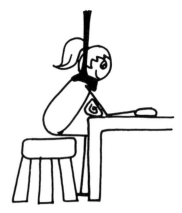

Figure 9.99 Use joint compression through shoulders with child leaning on forearms on a table. Encourage leaning on one arm and using the other for, say, eating, play, gesturing or pointing for communication. Place a roll of towels or small sponge wedge to keep forearms away from chest.

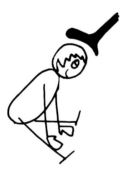

Figure 9.98 Gentle joint compression may be given through head, kept carefully held aligned with trunk. Joint compression can also be from 'bottom upwards' for a playful experience. Hold baby/child in careful vertical alignment and bounce him on his bottom on sponge rubber, trampoline, inflatable toy, beach ball or your lap. Check alignment of head with chin held in, with trunk and bottom.

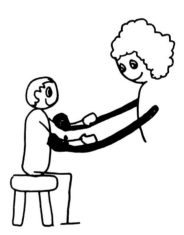

Figure 9.100 Train sitting with support given by an adult instead of by a table. Child leans on his forearms into adult's forearms. Joint compression may be given through child's forearms held directly below his shoulders. The child may hold the adult's shoulders whilst she supports the child's chest, subsequently his waist and finally his thighs, knees or just his feet on the ground. He may gradually not need to hold on.

children with cerebral palsy. *Aim* is to train postural stability. Fig. 9.93 is a chair to assist a young child who has some balance.

(2) *Spastic short muscles and overlengthened muscles* are seen in abnormal sitting postures such as in extended and adducted legs with flexed arms which have short muscles while the antag-

onists to these muscles are lengthened or overlengthened. The spastic synergies are also used to prevent falling. For example, the child holds on for balance with hunched tight shoulders, elbow flexors and excessively flexed wrist and hand grasp. A child fixes himself in sitting on

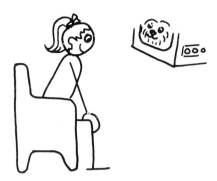

Figure 9.101 Visual and auditory stimuli at child's eye level for vertical head and trunk control in sitting. Upright posture is encouraged if given at child's eye level. Arm propping may be needed if stability is poor.

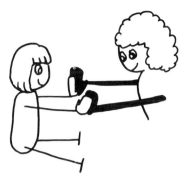

Figure 9.103 Child pushes his open hands against adult's hands with wrists in dorsiflexion. This brings him into a forward sitting position. Train active re-erecting to the upright and return to forward lean. The child may need to have assisted body support or holding of his arms. The child may have his arms on the back of a more able child and they rock forward and back.

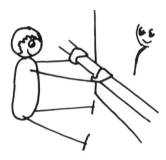

Figure 9.102 Child learns to sit with both hands grasping a pole, back of a chair, a table edge or adult's hands. Elbows are as straight and symmetrical as possible. The support may be grasped below shoulder level, at shoulder level or above shoulder level. Encourage a child to use one arm movement to reach a toy whilst the other arm is grasping a support. One arm is used for feeding, dressing and playing. Grasping with one hand and using the other to reach down, in front, at shoulder level and above shoulder level with maintenance of sitting develops.

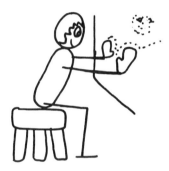

Figure 9.104 Child may also push against wall to make handprints on powdered or soaped mirror or push a large therapy ball or heavy toy on wheels to another child. From upright sitting, child reaches well forward to touch wall or toy with the other arm supported on seat or arm of chair and later without any arm support.

a chair by excessive knee flexion over the edge of the seat and pressing equinus feet against the legs of the chair. *Aim* is to maintain appropriate muscle lengths and correct abnormal limb positions while training postural control.

(3) *Children with dyskinesia and dystonia* also need to stabilise themselves with abnormal postures and control their involuntary movements with their muscle tension or dystonia. There are a variety of unusual postures, including flexing legs around chair legs. This aids balance and control of involuntary movements. Heel sitting on the floor and other positions may be useful as

they allow hand function which can be specially difficult for these children. *Aim* is to train postural control in a variety of postures that can be achieved by individuals and which can also be helpful for a child Figs 9.95–9.107.

(4) *Aim* is to assess and select correct chairs and tables with special adaptations for each child (adaptive equipment) irrespective of diagnostic type for comfort, communication, eating, drinking and hand function. Chairs, tables, pushchairs and wheelchairs which are too small or incorrect cause deformities and poor function.

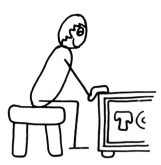

Figure 9.105   Child leans on hands on a seat or low box. If possible, his hands are flat with dorsiflexed wrists. Encourage a child to reach forward to a desired toy and then re-erect to an upright position. Hold the pelvis and tilt forward, sideways, obliquely and partial rotate for reaching in different directions. Cross the midline for added postural control. Tilt pelvis backward for leg lifting.

(5) *Aim* is to avoid prolonged sitting especially on a chair for more than 2 hours. Include *assisted or unassisted* rising to standing, supported standing, standing frames and strengthening of extensor hip and knees and arm muscles maintaining plantigrade feet on the ground.

(6) *Aims for all methods* depend on a child's age and size. Methods may be used for sitting on the floor and on the child's chair. Sitting on the floor is emphasised in babies and young children, whilst in older children at the same early developmental level, chair sitting is usually more appropriate.

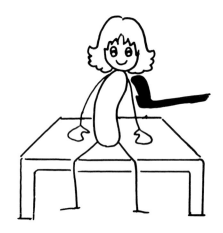

Figure 9.107   Give a child gentle quick and slow pushes expecting him to maintain balance. Push in all directions to train weight shifts within the base and later out of his sitting base without falling. At first a child supports on hands and then without support. Manual resistance may be given at the child's shoulder on the lateral, anterior or posterior aspects. This strengthens shoulder girdle, neck and trunk stabilisation muscles. Also give manual pushes or resistance with a child leaning on forearms (Fig. 9.99), on hands (Fig. 9.98) or grasping a support. For these actions suggest to a child to 'stay there' or 'keep sitting' according to his ability. *Note:* Give correct amount of resistance so that abnormal reactions are minimally provoked in limbs.

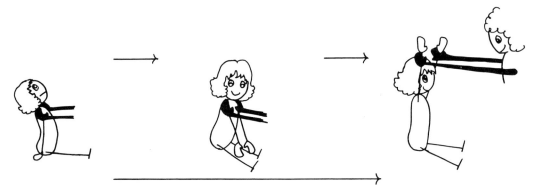

Figure 9.106   Stimulate head control, back straightening and arm elevation by bringing shoulders forward and then take the upper arms, turn them out and elevate them to hold a ball or touch adult's face. Later, if possible, a child raises arms for undressing. Make sure that the child's head is slightly forward for balance and tip head further down when top clothes are put on or taken off over the head.

Chairs and tables

Special chairs (adaptive seating) are selected according to the child's developmental level to:

(1) Train sitting.
(2) Correct abnormal postures.
(3) Provide stimulation in the upright position to develop a child's social, visual and hearing abilities.
(4) Develop hand function in the *upright* position of *supported* sitting (see the subsection 'Basic arm and hand patterns' below.)
(5) To enable better communication and speech as well as for oromotor function for eating and drinking, especially for swallowing.
(6) Meanwhile, training of sitting balance and correct posture without special chairs must continue and be associated with hand function and daily life activities as soon as possible.

Regular chairs and stools of different sizes are used:

(1) To increase development of sitting balance and independent good posture.
(2) To develop hand function together with sitting balance.
(3) To make standing up from sitting possible.
(4) To make pivoting in sitting and transfers possible.

Measurements. If chairs are not of the correct measurements for the child, they can obstruct the development of sitting, cause or increase abnormal postures and prevent hand function (Fig. 9.108). Only use an armrest if that support is needed. The backrest is at 100° to seat. Slight forward lean to a table is active for daily activities carried out by a child. Table should be up to the height of child's waist or higher if he lacks trunk control. There should be a *large* area of work space.

If the chair is *too high*, the child will find lack of foot support for his dangling feet disturbing to his poor sitting balance. Plantarflexed feet may become plantarflexion deformity. If the chair is *too wide*, the child may take more weight on one side as he slumps to that side. The lateral lean or slumping decreases balance and may lead to scoliosis. Place rolls of towel, sponge-covered blocks, sandbags or magazines to decrease a chair which is too wide. The seat could be made to fit his buttocks. If the chair seat is *too short*, the child may not be able

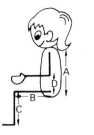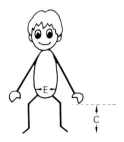

A	Height of backrest
B	Seat depth
C	Seat to floor
D	Armrest height
E	Seat width

Figure 9.108   The measurements for a chair. See modifications in text on evaluation of special chairs.

to balance without support to his thighs. His feet may twist or curl around the chair legs in his efforts to balance. Deformity of his feet and of flexed, adducted and internally rotated knees may be encouraged. If the chair seat is *too long*, he may slump backwards to the back support and increase hip extension–adduction–internal rotation, knee extension and plantarflexion or hip extension–adduction, semi-flexion of the knees and plantarflexion of his feet. Rounding of the back is inevitable. In all the above situations the child's hand function is made impossible or difficult. Concentration on schoolwork, social situations and communication is usually disturbed.

Evaluating a chair for a child

Most therapists use trial and error to assess which chair and table is most suitable for an individual child. Research continues among therapists and bioengineers to clarify when particular designs are indicated for specific problems. Stavness (2006) has reviewed research on chairs. Among different views on seat inclination, forward tilt or neutral was preferred rather than backward tilt. Carlberg and Hadders-Algra (2008), in their study of postural control and arm reaching, found that forward tilt of the seat was better for hemiplegia and the neutral position better for children with bilateral cerebral palsy. Controversy still exists between different workers. The studies of the following are among many others which can guide clinical therapists: Trefler *et al.* (1978); Nwaobi *et al.* (1983); Nwaobi

(1987); Mulcahy *et al.* (1988); Myhr and von Wendt (1990); Myhr *et al.* (1995). Controversy about seating may arise when clinicians are really comparing children at different stages of development of quiet sitting versus sitting for hand function, vision and communication or for balance training. An *assessment chair* with different elements which can be removed according to each child helps to make decisions as to which chair is suitable. Try this with a child in quiet sitting and during functions and where relevant during transport. Bardsley (1993) describes

an assessment chair which affects details of design which can be custom-made if this is financially feasible. Zacharkov's (1988) book is on seating. The GMFCS levels for special chairs are III-V.

Potential seat elements (Fig. 9.109a–d)

There is an increasing range of seating systems for children produced by different manufacturers as well as custom-made individual seating and the use

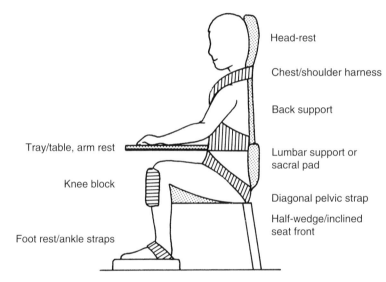

Head-rest

Chest/shoulder harness

Back support

Tray/table, arm rest

Lumbar support or sacral pad

Knee block

Diagonal pelvic strap

Half-wedge/inclined seat front

Foot rest/ankle straps

Figure 9.109   (a) First stages.

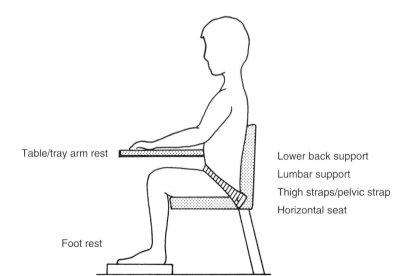

Table/tray arm rest

Lower back support
Lumbar support
Thigh straps/pelvic strap
Horizontal seat

Foot rest

Figure 9.109   (b) Second stages.

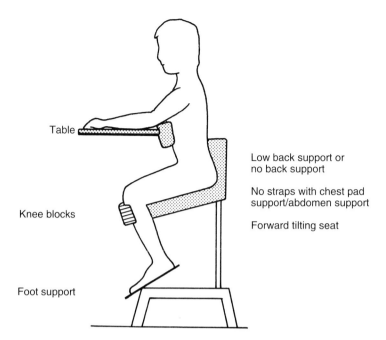

Table

Knee blocks

Foot support

Low back support or
no back support

No straps with chest pad
support/abdomen support

Forward tilting seat

Figure 9.109 (c) Third stages.

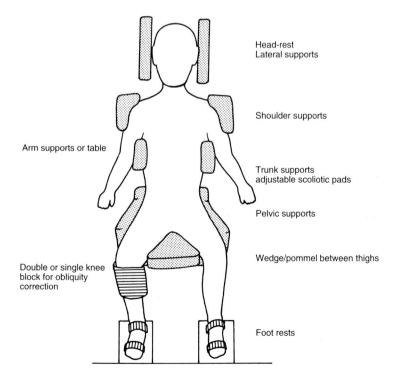

Head-rest
Lateral supports

Shoulder supports

Arm supports or table

Trunk supports
adjustable scoliotic pads

Pelvic supports

Wedge/pommel between thighs

Double or single knee
block for obliquity
correction

Foot rests

Figure 9.109 (d) First stages.

of orthotics for desirable sitting positions. For most mild and moderately involved children with physical disabilities, for babies and for children with motor delay, mass-produced regular chairs and tables are suitable. A few modifications with foot rests and foam pieces or firm cushions can be used to obtain the desirable posture in each child (see Fig. 9.93).

General considerations in selecting a chair/wheelchair

In a study by McDonald *et al.* (2003) there are suggestions on how to resolve disagreements between therapists and parents regarding seating for severe children.

(1) Parents and child find the chair aesthetically acceptable. Consider if chairs are culturally acceptable.
(2) The chair should be comfortable not only during quiet sitting but also when a child moves his head, body and arms. It should be comfortable and safe when the chair is moved from place to place.
(3) The chair needs to be portable from room to room or transportable for outings. It should not be too cumbersome for homes, classrooms or doorways. Storage needs consideration.
(4) A chair should enable a child to join his family, friends or classmates around a table, on the floor, in a sandpit or at picnics and camps.
(5) A chair does not substitute for therapy sessions and practice for a child's own development of postural control, changing positions or locomotion without a wheelchair.
(6) A child may need more than one chair: one for practising his emerging postural adjustments during looking, listening, reaching out and hand use in all directions, and another for safely supporting him during transport and when he is unsupervised and may fall. The additional support by a special chair maintains postural alignment and stability at times when a child concentrates on difficult communication, visual, hearing and self-care activities. He may have a floor seat and one for a regular table, or the floor seat can be strapped to a frame at table level with proximity to others at home or at school. An armchair for relaxation is also appreciated by many individuals. There are supports and abduction wedges included in those available on the market. Various adjustable chairs can serve more than one purpose.

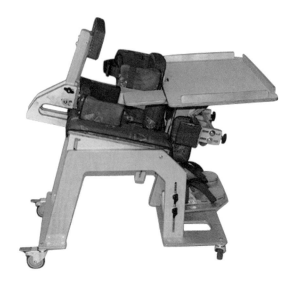

Figure 9.110 Tilted seat with chest support. Tilt is adjustable and back of child can be observed for symmetry and weight bearing on buttocks. A table can be attached. (Image supplied courtesy of Jenx, Sheffield.)

Specific considerations. See Figs 9.95, 9.109 and 9.110.

Pelvis, hips and thighs. The position of a child's pelvis is the keystone for better alignment of his head and trunk. It is positioned in association with hips, knees and foot rests. As in postural control training, a child is taught to sit well back in his chair and take weight equally on hips, thighs and feet. When his pelvis is smaller in girth than his trunk, a sacral pad supports his pelvis as his trunk is supported by the back of his chair. When his body and buttocks change in size, the sacral pad is removed so that protruding buttocks can be accommodated and a lumbar support is used. At the same time, assessment is made of the developmental stage of a child's pelvic tilt forwards and lumbar mobility. A lumbar support promotes the normal minimal lordosis with vertical pelvic alignment, when a child is at that stage. If not, discomfort and pressure marks are caused.

In order to hold a child's pelvic alignment when he cannot yet do so himself, use the following suggestions according to each child:

■ A diagonal strap across the front of his hips which ties below the level of his seat to keep hips back against the sacral pad or back of chair.

- A thigh strap for each leg nailed well back between a child's thighs and tying behind and below seat level. Use padding or rubber tubing on the straps to prevent chafing.
- Incline the front of the child's seat (half-wedge) so that his hips flex and his thighs receive support while his buttocks rest on a flat contoured seat. This prevents a child from sliding forward, sacral sitting or hip extensor stiffness. When extensor thrust or tension is severe, a roll of towel under the knees may help to overcome it by the increased hip flexion. The head and back may also flex as a result, and a firm back support with lumbar padding may correct this. If not, try flexing the child's hips with his chest supported in a forward leaning chair with table (Figs 9.109c and 9.110) or against a padded table edge as he stretches his arms forward to grasp bars or lean on forearms. McClenaghan *et al.* (1992) have studied backward inclination of the seat on postural stability and arm and hand function. See also Stavness (2006).
- Some therapists prevent extensor positions of the hips and sliding out of chairs by tilting the whole chair backwards with the hips flexed between 95 and 110°, as 90° creates forward sliding. This backward tilt has advantages in that it can be a relaxed position for those children who do not have a Moro response, head and trunk thrust in semi-lying or increased athetosis. Parents welcome this for rest in a wheelchair. Backward leaning also fixes the vertebrae in alignment in some cases of scoliosis and in severely involved children with excessive flexion which cannot be straightened otherwise. Most therapists prefer to avoid backward leaning chairs as a child can only see the top of a room, cannot explore visually or locate sounds below him or make face-to-face contact with other children on the floor or at eye level. Reaching and hand function is more difficult, and feeding development needs either a slight forward lean (about 20–25°) or an upright and slightly flexed head posture. This head posture prevents swallowing problems, and gagging. Backward leaning often gives a sensation of falling without the proprioception of the vertical posture essential for the development of postural stabilisation (Fig. 9.111a,b).
- Knee blocks which are padded hold the child's pelvis in position against a sacral pad or back support. They are also used in the forward-leaning chair or forward-tilted seat for back extension.
- Thigh supports with foot rests may have to be adjusted in relation to the hip flexion used. Take care to avoid pressure behind the knees. Thigh length discrepancies may require shortening of one side of the seat. Observe the position of the knees, and check whether pelvic obliquity is the cause of the apparent shortening when knees are not level with each other. Thighs may also straddle a bolster seat (Stewart & McQuilton 1987) in this special design which provides a wider base for head and trunk control (Fig. 9.112). Reid (1996) has used a saddle seat to improve postural control and arm function.
- Knee blocks are needed to correct pelvic obliquity in the presence of *windswept hips*. The trunk may also be laterally flexed in a scoliosis. It is not always clear whether the trunk posture is secondary to the legs and pelvis or vice versa. All need correction in sitting (in standing and lying) and so avoid a secondary hip dislocation on the adducted hip. A wedge-shaped pommel, thigh or diagonal straps suffice in mild cases of wind-sweeping legs. For more severe windsweeping the forward side, the least abducted thigh is pushed back to position the pelvis backwards on that side into a symmetrical sitting position. This is not possible if that hip is already dislocated. The other thigh is abducted as far as possible to achieve a symmetrical sitting position (Scrutton 1978). Some severe children benefit from bilateral thigh abduction splints alone or when attached to a trunk corset (support) (Fig. 9.113a,b). Trunk posture is then supported and may correct a scoliosis.
- If both hips are dislocated, the trunk and pelvis appear symmetrical, but there is not enough hip flexion for sitting. Prevention is essential and this is discussed more fully in section 'Hip dislocation' in Chapter 11.
- If the pelvis is tipped down on one side, then the thigh on that side is flexed on to a small wedge to position the pelvis up and level with the other side and maintain a straight spine.
- Lateral pelvis supports with pommels for a wider base also stabilise the pelvis in a symmetrical posture (Fig. 9.109d).

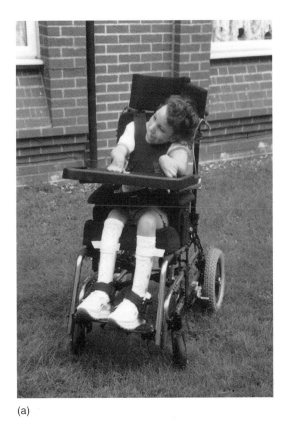

(a)

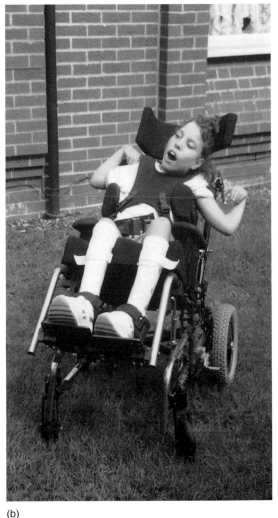

(b)

Figure 9.111   (a, b) Effect of backward tilt and upright position of a chair. Upright position with tray assists head control and arm function for daily activities, use of vision and communication.

Head and trunk. Once pelvis and hips are aligned, head and trunk are examined further. Add the following if necessary:

■   An H harness or shoulder straps to maintain the upright position. A V or crossed harness may be dangerous if a child often drops his head and catches his neck in the harness. Harnesses may be tied behind a child if he enjoys playing and opening the harness buckles.

■   Lateral chest supports with lateral pelvic supports hold some children in midline if they frequently tip to the side.

■   Shoulder supports together with pelvic supports or with trunk supports, or even all three supports can hold a child more upright.

■   Shoulder supports may be used to bring retracted shoulders forwards so that a severely involved child can reach the table or touch his hands and body.

■   The table needs to be adjusted so that kyphoses are corrected and both a child's arms can be lifted to correct lateral tipping or other asymmetries.

■   Hand grasps on correct tray/table heights also assist head and trunk alignment.

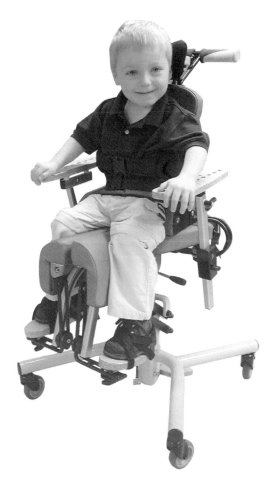

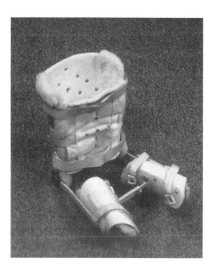

Figure 9.113   a

Figure 9.112   Image supplied courtesy of Jenx, Sheffield.

- Scoliosis pads are attached to some chairs. The pads need to be moulded to the child's ribs first on the convexity and also on the concavity side at the axilla and at both sides of the pelvis.
- Scolioses may not be corrected by seating on its own, and trunk orthoses are necessary. When wearing a corset or other orthosis, the child can be upright and the backward tilt of the chair may then be avoided. Sacral pads or other lateral padding need to be removed to give space for a spinal orthosis. Check that the orthosis does not rub against the child and therefore needing chair adjustments.
- Head control is often activated with adequate trunk and pelvic support with or without a trunk orthosis (see trunk-and-thigh orthosis in Fig. 9.113a,b). Stimulation to hold a child's head up in a chair is usually necessary.

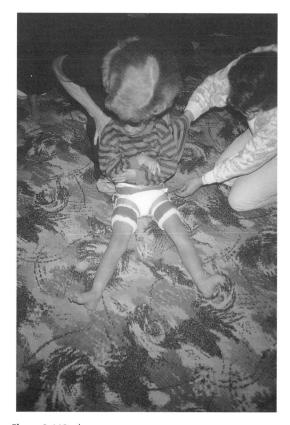

Figure 9.113   b

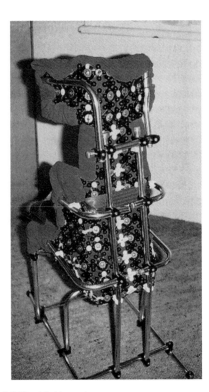

Figure 9.114   Matrix seat.

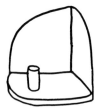

Figure 9.115

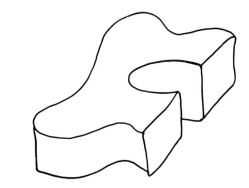

Figure 9.116

However, severely involved children may still benefit from a collar or chest and head support.

■ Sometimes severely involved children are placed in moulded seats, custom made to the shape of their own heads and bodies or to their bodies only (Bardsley 1993) (Fig. 9.114).

■ Lateral head supports remind children to keep their heads centred, but are unfortunately not always effective. A child often drops his head outside these head blocks. Improved designs are being developed by manufacturers.

Floor seats. Select the correct floor seat so that the young child can play with toys on the floor or join other children playing on the ground in playgroups, playgrounds or sandpits (Figs 9.115–9.117). Sitting on the ground is more acceptable in some cultures.

(1) A well-padded pommel for adducted legs. Two small pommels may be used close together and gradually moved apart as the child develops more abduction of legs for a wide base.

(2) Height of the back should be at shoulder level of the child if he tends to fall back or arch back when sitting. Occasionally the head may require

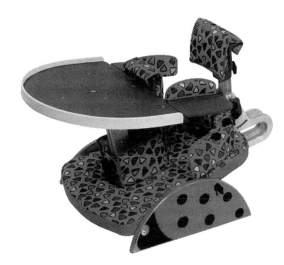

Figure 9.117   Floor seat with tilt down and forward. (Image supplied courtesy of Jenx, Sheffield.)

a padded back support. Curve the chair to prevent shoulders and back of the child arching into extension. See cylindrical chair (Fig. 9.116) which helps midline hand use.

(3) Height of the back and sides of the floor seat should be cut down to the child's waist level

as he acquires more head and trunk control. A square back may be used, as well as triangular and cylindrical ones.

(4) The width of the chair should be such that the child does not slide from side to side. Pad up the sides with sponge or newspapers so that this does not occur. A canvas or inflatable seat allows the child to sink into his own area of support. These seats must be stabilised and child supervised.

(5) Seat of chair is measured from child's hips to his knees.

(6) The floor seat may be placed on wheels for locomotion if the child requires this; it may be used in a toilet seat; it may be tied on to a sturdy adult chair next to the family table. A table can be fitted to it.

(7) The floor seat may have to be raised off the floor for those children who have a very rounded back. The height of the seat with foot support off the floor should be tested to see whether the child's back straightens. If this does not occur, it is important to give him a table which is high enough for his arms to be elevated to that point where his back straightens. A small firm pillow or back support may help to hold the back straight. Adjusting the position of the pommel or abduction wedge may help. If none of these

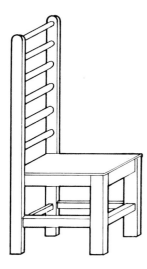

Figure 9.118 Slatted back based on a design by Petö Institute. Child can sit sideways and hook his arm through slats for balance; use slats to push chair for walking aid. Stabilise base by using a box as base or skis attached. A box base also prevents legs twisting under the seat.

methods corrects a severely rounded back, then a *floor seat should be used* with a tilted seat (Fig. 9.117).

(8) The seat is inclined down and forward to augment back straightening (Fig. 9.117).

Other equipment for sitting

(1) Chair swings, back and sides on toy trucks, rocking horse or pedal cars. Inflatable chairs, car seats, various special bath seats and also toilet seats practise supported sitting. There is more independence if a child can grasp a horizontal bar to sit.

(2) Toilet seats (Figs 9.120–9.124). See also Figs 10.1 and 10.2 in Chapter 10.

(3) Pushchairs and wheelchairs (Figs 9.109a–d, 9.111a).

(4) Additional suggestions for training sitting (Figs 9.118 and 9.119).

0–3-month normal developmental level

Common problems

Delay in lifting the head up from flexed or extended posture when the body is fully supported in a sitting position. Unsteady head holding in supported sitting. (Head lag in pull to sit, see section 'Supine development'.) There can be a total *absence of postural stabilisation*, resulting in a child falling backwards or leaning back as he slides out of the seat of his chair. When held at his pelvis, in sitting on the floor or on a chair, the child may drop head and trunk forward. Like an infant such children can sit in a reclining chair with supporting straps at this level of development (Fig. 9.91b).

Abnormal performance. An older severe child with totally absent postural stabilisation continues persistent backward lean against an inclined backrest, developing hip flexion tightness or fixed semiflexed hip deformity, as well as remaining unable to activate a floppy weak trunk. He may also use hip tightness to prevent falling backward or due to the prolonged sitting position. Some have infantile excessive extensor thrust. All these children cannot be flexed into the upright sitting position.

The head is held in an asymmetrical posture either laterally flexed, rotated or both. Arms, trunk and legs may be in infantile postures. The back is first

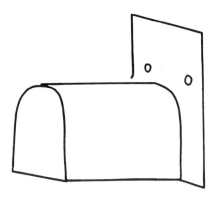

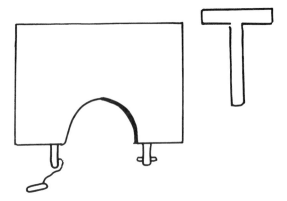

Figure 9.119   Legs are abducted over this roll chair (based on a design by Finnie). Knees must be just beneath the top of the roll, and the roll not too wide for the child. Check that the child does not slide down one side of the roll. Ordinary low table or fitted cut-out table is used. Leave 50 mm (2 in.) between the child's body and the cut-out edge for postural adjustments.

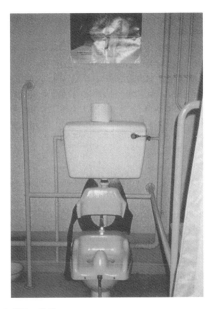

Figure 9.120   Toilet seat.

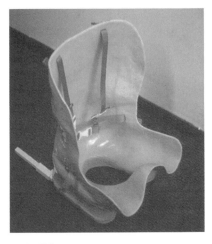

Figure 9.121   Toilet seat.

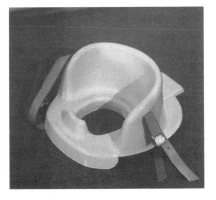

Figure 9.122   Toilet seat.

rounded, but unlike a normal neonate, the pelvis tilts backwards. Rounding of the back may become a kyphosis. Backward pelvic tilt may lead to short hamstrings on semi-extended hips and semi-flexed knees in this *sacral sitting* (Fig. 9.91a,b). Arms may flex and shoulders hunch tensely as a child avoids falling. An older child may use any grasp; he has to hold onto a support near his flexed arms. If sacral sitting with rounded back is excessive, the child attempts to hyperextend his neck to avoid falling forward and in order to look up. The abnormal postures are on the floor or on a stool.

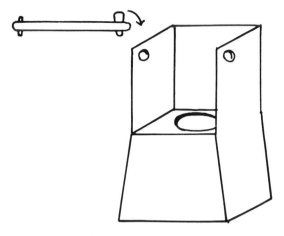

Figure 9.123   Watford potty chair. The bar is made from 1 in. (25 mm) dowelling. For a tall child the back height needs increasing and the 10 × 10 in. (250 mm) seat needs enlarging. Feet must be flat on the floor. Use foot stool or box for increase of flexion of hips and knees for a very extended child.

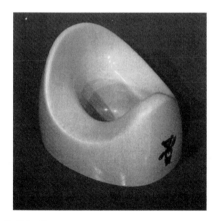

Figure 9.124   Potty.

Treatment suggestions and management

Severe children need fully supporting special chairs with head supports. Orthopaedic consultation for trunk orthosis and fixed deformity and physiotherapy to mobilise hips and strengthen trunk muscles in lying.

For less severe children, give support to the child's shoulders or under his axillae, holding him so that his total body is supported, so he can achieve vertical head control. Vertical head control may also be activated with his forearms onto a table as you hold his upper arms for support. This develops any of his shoulder girdle stabilisation, which activates head control. The child may need to lean forward against the rounded table edge for additional support.

Carry out any relevant methods suggested in Figs 9.94–9.105, but *giving support* to the child's shoulders and trunk and emphasising vertical head control. Correct asymmetry by holding both shoulders and facing child for communication. Train active head raise from a backward drop by bringing his shoulders or upper arms forward. Correct a forward drop by stimulating head lifting from the chest as you pull shoulder girdle backwards or lift upper arms. Raising the arms also extends rounded back and pelvic slumped posture. However, avoid child's fall or lean backwards by supporting his body during arm elevation.

Lifting of the head to the vertical prepares a child for eating and drinking and to avoid breathing problems due to the forward slump.

3–6-month normal developmental level

Common problems

Delay in supported sitting so that specially adapted chairs are needed from 6 months. Delay in looking up, down or around without disturbing balance. Delay of back straightening from the dorsal area to the whole back; delay of sitting propping on hands on the floor or on forearms on the table without some external support. Delay in re-erecting from lean to upright position (5–6-month level). (Delay in overcoming head lag in pull to sit, see section 'Supine development'.) An older child in floor sitting may still weight bear on buttocks thighs and also lateral legs and feet like a child at these early levels. Ring or tailor sitting with arms propped is used by an older child with minimal manual support.

Abnormal performance. The therapist can observe or anticipate additional individual abnormal postures, including the persistence of the abnormal postures from 0 to 3 months. Any abnormal posture may require manual support at this level. Postures are individually depending on severity:

(1) A child may lean forward and prop on his fists rather than hands for support. More weight may be taken on the less affected arm or hip, especially in hemiplegia. The arms are sometimes tensely extended and internally rotated

with poor shoulder stability. Head may be hyperextended with chin poking.

(2) When a child leans back against a chair, his head extends, his arms may be held up in abduction at his sides with shoulders hunched, neutral or retracted (Fig. 9.91c). With head extended a child may persist in earlier asymmetrical head and limb postures such as an asymmetrical tonic neck arm pattern. He may be able to centre the head and lift arms forwards at 45–90° in the air with elbows straight, shoulders hunched in an effort to counterbalance his backward fall or excessive extension. His feet may plantarflex to reach the ground for support or if the ground is near enough, his toes flex to 'hold on' and his feet may press into valgus for support (Fig. 9.91c). He is unstable.

(3) Some children have overcome their *extensor thrusts* or extensor positions by sitting in excessive flexion. They may even collapse forward with trunk floppiness once extensor stiffness has been overcome by them, by therapy or medication. With no postural stabilisation, the child has no sitting. Many children achieve a position somewhere between full flexion and extension. The falling backward or extensor thrust may remain *in the hips*, but trunk and arms flex and the head extends. The pelvis is tilted backward and knees bent as hamstrings are in a shortened position. If the child's knees are extended in long sitting on the floor, he may fall backward as the hamstrings do not allow this full extension. Less severe children can maintain long sitting with their pelvis tipped back, knees semi-flexed and weight on hips and heels (Fig. 9.91a). At this stage, support is usually needed either against a wall or leaning on one or both arms. In the next stage, this posture is maintained without support.

(4) A child sitting in the corner of sofa, the floor or on a chair which is too high may stiffly straighten, adduct and internally rotate his legs in sacral sitting with rounded back. On a child's chair he may find it easier if knees are flexed with feet in plantigrade position. The flexed knees decreases the pull of short hamstrings and so tips the pelvis forward to sit on his buttocks. Upright sitting begins to develop with trunk support. However, knee flexion deformities are particularly threatening, so avoid prolonged sitting on chairs. Some children have stiffness in

the trunk, often on one side only. Scoliosis together with torticollis may then be present. Rounded back or kyphosis is also present.

(5) If there is much instability, as in a child with dyskinesia or quadriplegia, he may strongly bend his knees over the edge of the chair, twisting his legs around the front legs of the chair or fixing them against the chair legs to avoid falling. Head and trunk may bend forward to avoid backward falls.

(6) Sitting on the floor with his bottom between his feet and his legs internally rotated and flexed is often seen in a child with cerebral palsy – *W sitting* (Fig. 9.91d). At this level he supports himself on arms. This is one way in which an unstable child can fix his pelvis and develop head and trunk control in preparation for hand function. Although this posture is seen in able-bodied children, it is not held for the many long periods which children with cerebral palsy persist in doing. Tightness of hip, knee and feet may then develop, if more variety of sitting positions and standing frames are not used.

(7) If a child at this developmental level tips forward from sitting and cannot yet save himself on his arms, this increases any fears of falling. Arm saving forward develops between 4- and 7-month normal developmental levels.

(8) A child may sit more on his better side or have stiffness in his trunk. Scoliosis with or without torticollis is present. Round backs may become unfixed or fixed kyphosis. Kyphoscoliosis may be present.

The abnormal postures above are compensations for lack of postural control and associated with short spastic muscles, if these are present. Prolonged sitting in any one posture causes deformity and disabling pelvic and flexion limb postures which interfere with standing and walking. The need for adequate arm propping and the presence of abnormal trunk postures interfere with use of hands.

Skin pressure points and tissue trauma are likely when a child cannot ask or is unable to change his abnormal prolonged sitting posture.

Treatment suggestions and management

Specially adapted chairs. Children aged 7–10 months in GMFCS levels III–V need such chairs for delayed sitting and to correct abnormal postures.

Hand function and communication can develop, but development of sitting itself involves training without the special chair.

Abnormal postures of head, trunk, arms, legs and feet are often corrected at the same time if the child sits on *both* his buttocks (ischial tuberosities), leans forward from his hips against a rounded table edge support, propping on his forearms or straight arms and grasping a fixed horizontal bar on the table. The table may need to be at his shoulder level and this support is lowered to waist level and finally removed near the end of the next levels (6–9 months). Make sure the child leans forward from the hips with back kept straight, chin in. Help him by pressing your hand on the small of his back, if he cannot manage alone. Feet should be supported on a firm surface. Legs need to be held apart for a wide base and turned outward if they adduct and internally rotate. When a child sits on a chair with the feet flat on the ground, improve stability by training him to push his feet downwards into the ground. Support him at hips, if necessary. Once this posture is achieved it is a functional position for feeding, communication and various hand functions.

Equinus and valgus deformities of feet. Minimise or correct them to obtain plantigrade feet which are extra supports for sitting balance. Use orthoses or special foot supports on a chair.

Hip and knee flexion deformity. Vary sitting positions. See below. Use standing frames and prone lying on wedges as well as sitting postures.

Scoliosis. Make sure the child sits equally on both his buttocks. Assist reaching overhead on the side of the concavity as you support sitting and later with less support. Sandbags or a roll of towels on his table under his forearm on the side of the concavity, or under the buttock on either the side of the concavity or convexity, should be tried to discover which props him into alignment.

Kyphosis is improved by height of table and training postural stabilisation in alignment with and later without support. Encourage or assist both arms reaching overhead in supported and much later in unsupported sitting. Check that any habitual head hyperextension, secondary to kyphosis, is corrected. Both the kyphosis and the head position can be corrected by motivating a child to reach forwards, just above the horizontal whilst keeping the chin in at the same time. Trunk orthoses or special supports in chairs are needed for many severe children with scoliosis or kyphosis.

Excessive hip, trunk and head extension is corrected within chair-sitting posture above, as well as having the child learn to sit on low chairs, sit in the corner of the sofa or room. Keep hip and knees flexed, feet flat to stabilise a child with dyskinesia or ataxia. Carry the child to a seat in full flexion, to counteract severe extension just before he is placed into his special chairs (see Figs 9.8–9.11).

Flexed knees. When knees are habitually in flexion, straighten knees on an inclined leg support which can be incorporated into a special supporting chair, particularly a floor seat, with trays for various hand activities (Fig. 9.117). Vary the angle of the incline according to the ability of a child to keep his pelvis level, without rounding his trunk. Also make sure that the pull of tight hamstrings is not causing rounding of the trunk. In less severe cases a small raise on to a platform for his floor seat is required. Use knee gaiters for flexed knees. Develop postural control with straight leg down the incline of a large floor wedge. At this level a child needs some support in these postures, but the control improves in the next levels.

Note: Side sitting should be avoided if there is a threatening hip dislocation in one hip or there is too much flexion in the child's hips and knees as well as the abnormal adduction and internal rotation. Feet need to be checked in case they are in abnormal postures in these sitting positions.

Leg adduction and internal rotation. Correct this position using supported sitting with legs apart and turned out on either side of large toys, a box of toys, bowl of sand or water, a small drum, straddling rolls, soft toys, the corner of the bed or chair and across your hip or thigh. Avoid having a child straddle anything of too great a diameter as he then increases hip internal rotation with such excessive abduction of his hips. Abduction splints may have to be worn during supported chair sitting for better hip posture. Sit behind a child on a roll supporting him with your body gradually remove this support, and hold waist or hips. An older child can practice pushing his knees apart himself using his hands or by having his hands on the floor or lower legs, pushing his legs apart with his forearms.

Sequence of training. Sitting on a child's chair may be achieved before sitting on the floor in children with dyskinetic (athetoid) or spastic type of cerebral palsy. *Involuntary movements* are decreased if a child pushes his own weight well onto his heels. Try tying ankles to regular chair with sides or in foot pieces with straps, if this does not stimulate involuntary movements in the rest of the child. Grasping and leaning well onto forearms often helps. Train head and upper trunk control supporting lower trunk and pelvis.

In all sitting postures a child develops postural control by first leaning forward, then he re-erects to the upright posture where more control is needed. A young child leaning forward in sitting on the floor with the legs flexed-abducted-externally rotated uses gravity to play with toys, his feet or pull off socks. Reaching down is initially more achievable than reaching up in supine against gravity.

In an individual, use a horizontal stick grasped by the child in both hands with straight elbows to correct either flexed arms, asymmetry, shoulder retraction or for a way of controlling involuntary arm movements (Cotton 1980; Tatlow 2005).

Additional suggestions are as follows:

- Tailor sitting or ring sitting, with lower trunk supported, corrects inwardly rotated, adducted and extended legs. This may be used for ball play provided that the child does not have excessive knee and hip flexion tightness and round back. Support head and trunk in floor seat and tray to correct back rounding and poor arm reaching out due to delay in development of postural control. Ring sit for symmetry.
- Carry out any relevant methods in Figs 9.94–9.107, but give adequate support at this stage so that a child can develop stabilisation of head on upper trunk. With further training of sitting, support may be lowered to the child's waist. Hold child's shoulders or body with him slightly forward for vertical head control. Sitting with a 20° forward lean is a functional posture for daily activities such as for feeding and hand function at a table. For communication, encourage head hold in the midline with eye-to-eye contact (Fig. 9.97).
- Tip a young child whilst carrying him on your hip. Encourage him to actively come up to the vertical. Holding a young child in upright suspension against your chest, tilt him playfully from side to side to songs. Give him time to readjust his head or head with upper trunk to the vertical, gradually move him away from the support of your chest during the song to see if he still manages to adjust himself. He may

not be ready for tilting on a therapy roll but might enjoy being in a special chair seat for a swing. Moving through space gives both visual and proprioceptive experience.

6–9-month normal developmental level

Common problems

Delay in acquiring independent or even momentary sitting alone, as a child still needs to use one or both hands for support. He cannot then use his hands for other functions. Some children at these levels may achieve sitting alone but cannot yet use the arms and hands or they fall over. This is due to a delay in the postural adjustment or counterpoising of the body for use of limbs. A child may be delayed in sitting lean on one hand and using the other. He may manage to grasp a bar attached to a table and begin to use the other hand first on a table surface and later above it to waist level. Individuals vary in their achievements at these levels.

Special chairs with tables are still needed to support a child's body due to delay in achievement of sitting alone and/or when using hands.

There is also delay in re-erecting to the upright from backward, forward or side-leaning positions.

Abnormal performance

(1) See abnormal postures in sitting above, which are now carried out *without* support to the child.
(2) Abnormalities of arm reach are associated with abnormal postures (Fig. 9.91a–c).
(3) A child may not have saving responses if tipped sideways and forwards.

Treatment suggestions and management

Sitting on a thick cushion, or inflatable seat on the floor, may give a child more stable sitting with firstly support at the lower trunk and then at the pelvis and finally without support. This is useful for play or when sitting alone has been achieved.

Various methods of giving and reducing support. At this level, carry out the sitting postures from (1) to (5) given above in levels 3–6 months but with gradual removal of support from waist to pelvis to

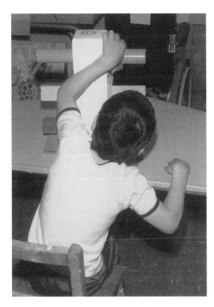

Figure 9.125 Absence of counterpoising the arm. This may lead to a scoliosis. The table is too high. The object is too high for child.

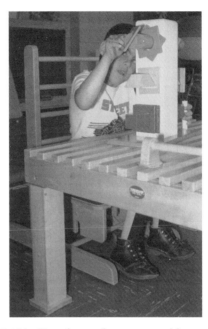

Figure 9.126 Use of grasp for support and lower table to assist until counterpoising develops for arm elevation.

independent sitting. Methods for removing support are given in Figs 9.94–9.107.

Additional suggestions for sitting development are:

- See supine development for methods to develop rise to sitting.
- Upright sitting, with hands propped at sides, and trunk turn to look behind are developed. However, this cannot yet be combined with reaching to side and behind him or he will fall.
- Use methods for sitting with the child using *one leg or arm movement*, such as stretching a limb up in the air to receive clothing, a shoe or sock, kick a ball or place foot on a foot stool or even the seat of his chair. He now has adequate pelvic and trunk control for these activities. Sitting balance is best maintained without any back support, but *with* the child's own hand support (Figs 9.125–9.128). These positions may be used in daily activities such as dressing, brushing hair and washing with one hand grasp, propped or his leaning onto a table. Later do this without support.

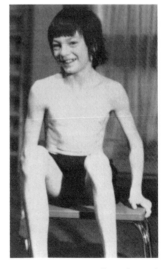

Figure 9.127 Leaning on more affected arm during counterpoising improves stability of that arm as the more skilful arm is used. However, develop arm movements of the more affected arm so that counterpoising is activated on each side.

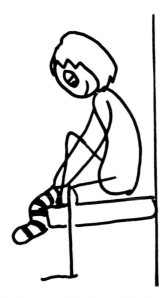

Figure 9.128   Counterpoising during daily living activity.

9–12-month normal development level

Common problems

Delay in acquiring sitting steadily (for about 10 minutes) without support on the floor and on a normal chair; sitting and playing without loss of balance; sitting, turning and reaching out or up without falling; changing from one sitting position to another or to lying; to crawling or sit change to standing. Delays in transfer from wheelchair to bed or chair to chair. Delays in sequences of any change of position, from and to reassume sitting. Delay in positive tilt reactions sideways, forward and backward, in saving reactions of the arms in all directions including backward. If these reactions are absent, sitting is insecure on any moving surface. A Moro reaction or startle occurs instead of backward tilt reactions. Delay of sit and pivot, of sit, reach across, to side and above a child's head. Bottom shuffle is delayed in children who will use this locomotion.

Abnormal performance as described in abnormal postures in sitting, but carried out *without* support. Stiff, jerky, unsteady or slow patterns may exist when rising to sitting and changing positions. Unusual patterns of rising devised by a child are acceptable if no other patterns are possible (Figs 9.70 and 9.71).

Treatment suggestions and management

Use methods in Figs 9.94–9.107, but encourage increased variety of arm patterns in play and daily tasks, and without supporting a child. Encourage his reaching overhead, across his body and behind his body. Use both arms simultaneously. Specific arm patterns correct abnormal trunk postures, for example the child's arm elevation corrects his kyphoscoliosis; arm abduction and external rotation and trunk turn with reaching behind a child correct round backs. You may need to hold his thighs for initial support and a child may use one arm support or grasp while using the other in particular activities (see section "Development of Hand Function', Figs 9.190–9.199).

Changing postures into and out of sitting position or rising reactions.

(1) Rise into sitting from supine or prone (see sections 'Prone development' and 'Supine development').
(2) Rise from sitting to standing up from a chair or the floor (see section 'Development of standing and walking').
(3) Sitting on the floor with legs in front of the child, change to prone. The child either places his hands in front of him, between his legs or to one side and goes down to lying, or he places one or both his hands to one side of him and moves into side sitting (Fig. 9.129). Help a child learn to change from floor sitting to prone kneeling (crawling position) and back again to sitting.
(4) Train the child to get on and off low wide stools of different heights (Fig. 9.130) and then chairs (Fig. 9.131). He often needs to reach out and grasp chair arms or backs, and to lean on the seat, the back of the chair or the table nearby.
(5) Train the child to get in and out of his wheelchair, in and out of a motor car, toy pedal car, tricycle and other apparatus. Teach transfers from bed to chair using the child's own arm support and from chair to standing holding on and later without support. Strengthen weight bearing on arms for transfers.
(6) The therapist either moves his leg (or legs) and child pivots his body, or moves his arms, allowing child to pivot his body. Move one of the child's hands on a table to allow him to move

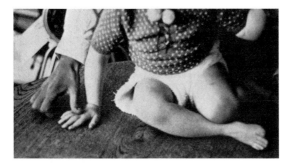

Figure 9.129 Changing from sitting to side sitting and back again. Change from side sitting to four-point postures or to lying.

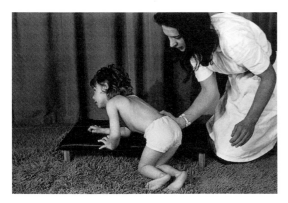

Figure 9.130

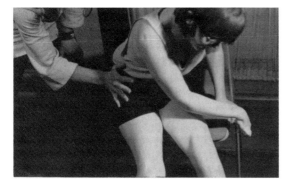

Figure 9.131 Getting on and off chairs of various heights and widths.

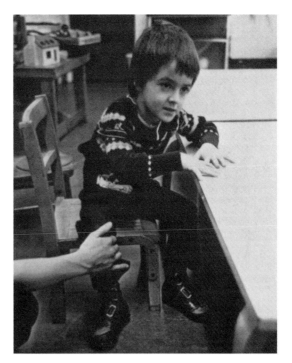

Figure 9.132 Pivoting on a chair.

the other arm in the pivot. Try pivot training on each side, so a child can get in and out of seats. Sitting on a stool/box and completely swivelling himself around on a stool/box is a useful motor ability for independence and for transfers (Fig. 9.132). Pivoting needs to incorporate the child's active leg abduction, arm action and postural control as he moves one leg or arm for the pivot.

Enabling a child to achieve a variety of postural changes can simultaneously involve correction of unfixed deformities such as separation of adducted legs, use of trunk strengthening, improved arm support and extension of bent elbows. Open hands and bent elbows are corrected by active reaching out and grasping supports or leaning on lower tables. Body rotative patterns are used and these together with other aspects appear to reduce hypertonus, lengthen and strengthen muscle groups.

It is easier for a child to go down to lying from sitting first before having to learn how to lift himself up against gravity, to sitting from lying *if* rotation is used. It is not so when straight patterns are used for lying down as a collapse into lying may happen. Slow control of lying down demands more muscle control.

■   Practise as many different sitting positions as possible: side sitting (Fig. 9.129); sitting with one foot flat on the ground, the other bent or straight; sitting with both knees bent and feet flat on the ground (crook sitting); sitting in various types of chairs of the correct size and in adult chairs if the child is correctly placed and has adequate balance. Sitting with his legs dangling and no foot support is an advanced posture. Therefore, avoid training sitting on a plinth with feet dangling in early stages.

Remember: Some children stabilise better on one side of their hips or trunk and prefer to sit sideways onto one buttock. This is obvious in children with hemiplegia but also in asymmetry in other types of cerebral palsies. There are also *windswept* legs to one side (Fig. 9.92). Scolioses and pelvic obliquity may result from persistent asymmetrical weight bearing in sitting. If a child can only use one hand or one visual field, this also increases asymmetry in postural stabilisation and counterpoising. Avoid side sitting to only one side in these children as windswept legs become associated with dislocation of the internally rotated hip. See special chairs for correction of pelvis trunk and windswept hips.

■   Augment sitting with manual resistance given laterally, with one hand in front and the other behind to resist rotation and your hands on anterior and on the posterior aspects of child's body (Fig. 9.107). ('Stay there' or 'Don't let me push you over'.)

■   Postural adjustment during weight shift as well as tilt reactions and saving reactions in the limbs are all stimulated by slow and by quick pushes (Fig. 9.133). Develop tilt responses and a sense of security in sitting by use of rocking chairs, rocking horses, swings, see-saws, vestibular rocking board, rocker boat or inflatable toys. Play 'see-saw' games on parent's lap or body. Pony riding and horse riding also stimulate tilt responses (Fig. 9.134) and a variety of postural adjustments within a child's base.

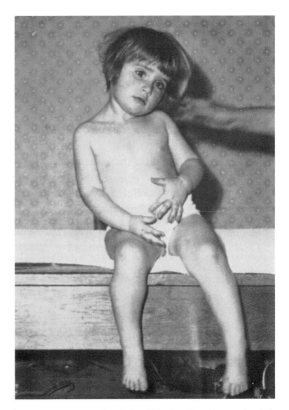

Figure 9.133   Lateral weight shift stimulated by push off the vertical. A more vigorous push of a child's pelvis/hips well off the horizontal plane stimulates the tilt reaction. If the child falls, saving responses in limbs are activated.

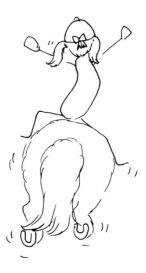

Figure 9.134

■ Use of incorrect size and type of chairs, tables, pushchairs or wheelchairs and of repeated placement of a child in only one or more poor sitting positions.

Development of standing and walking

The following main features should be developed according to an individual's developmental stages:

Antigravity support or weight bearing in an infant is on semi-supinated or forefeet when held supported under shoulders. Legs may stiffen with co-contraction. No head control with head forward. Pelvic tilt backward with hips flexed, knees slightly flexed with legs on a small base. Normally present at birth and temporarily absent (3–4 months) in some babies. On tipping the child forward, automatic stepping is produced and stops around 2–3 months.

Postural stability of head and trunk (Fig. 9.135). Supported weight bearing under axillae is modified when upright head and trunk control develop. At first, head stabilises on the trunk and then trunk on pelvis in supported standing (4–6 months). There is a widening of the standing base, with increased weight bearing, hip and knee flexion, posterior pelvic tilt and legs increasing abduction and external rotation with pronated feet (5–7 months). Support is still given by the adult while the child takes support onto a table, first on his forearms, then on his hands (7–8 months). The child first leans against a table/couch as he stands without adult help, but grasping or leaning on his hands (7–9 months) and then moving away from the trunk support (8–10 months). He gradually releases his one hand support and then both hands to stand alone (10–12 months and more steadily 15–18 months). Arms are held up in 'high guard' abduction–extension for stable scapulae to maintain head and trunk stability for standing and walking alone. High guard decreases and base narrows with feet as apart as shoulders and pelvis or slightly further apart for increased postural control. Legs are straighter, feet are plantigrade, with pelvis in neutral position, and with the head and trunk upright. The postural alignment has changed from head being anterior to hips to the head being in line with hips.

Postural stability of the pelvic girdle in the vertical is first in posterior tilt (0–6 months), then neutral (7–10 months) and then anteriorly tilted between 9 and 12 months in standing holding on and then alone. Also pelvic stability in upright kneeling supported, but only in kneeling unsupported at 15 months.

Postural stability is closely related to counterpoising of head and limbs.

Counterpoising in the standing position holding on and removing one hand (Fig. 9.136), holding on lifting an arm overhead, holding on, trunk turn and also bend down to reach a toy with one hand. He also holds on lifting one foot (10–12 months). Later a child lightly touches a bar without holding on

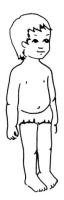

Figure 9.135   Postural stability, head on trunk on pelvis and whole of child in standing.

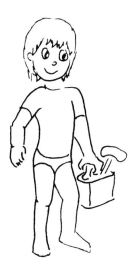

Figure 9.136   Counterpoising a weight or movement of the arm.

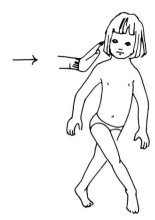

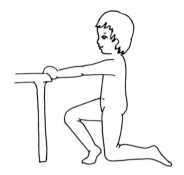

Figure 9.138 Rising to standing.

Figure 9.137 Saving from falling with a protective step.

or manages alone to carry out these counterpoising actions (12–18 months). The postural control and counterpoising become more varied in the second and third year of life, until he stands on one foot, not holding on, (2$\frac{1}{2}$–3 years). Standing on one foot is a most important counterpoising action. The child can then take weight on one leg for long enough to allow the other to step sideways in cruising or later to swing through and step forward or backward with and without hands supported. The child prepares for one foot balance by weight shift within the base holding on (7–9 months) and with less hand support increasing amount of weight shifts outside the standing base (9–12 months) for cruising holding on.

Control of antero-posterior weight shift of the child's centre of gravity to initiate walking (propulsion) and to stop (retropulsion) first with both of his hands held, then with only one hand held and then alone using a number of the postural controls outlined. Later he steps in a diagonal direction and in turning (12–24 months).

Control of lateral sway from one foot to the other. This is developed further in cruising with lateral stepping as well as when walking with each hand held laterally by adults. At first the child steps forward and laterally when held by adults or holding onto the sides of some walkers (12 months). Lateral sway is very obvious in toddlers and becomes modified with development.

Rising reactions and actions (Fig. 9.138) from lying (prone and supine) to standing, from squatting or from sitting to standing and from kneeling to standing (7–10 months). Support using hands pre-

cedes rising without support. Around 7–8 months a child may pull to stand but be unable to return to the ground, calling for help to do so. He finally learns to drop to sitting on his bottom without much concern. Other rising abilities have already been discussed in the sections on prone, supine and sitting development (see also Fig. 9.179).

Tilt reactions in standing are antero-posterior and lateral and later diagonal. They are acquired after standing and walking alone. Tilt reactions are not essential for walking. However, children without tilt reactions will be unsure especially in the dark and on rough ground.

Perturbations of a child in standing. Nashner *et al.* (1983) have shown in their studies that the sequence of muscle activation in a cerebral palsied child differs from that of an able-bodied child. Nevertheless, such a child with cerebral palsy does not fall over. Nashner *et al.* (1983) have also demonstrated slower timing on the spastic side compared to the normal side in childhood hemiplegia.

Saving from falling (Fig. 9.137). If pushed from behind the child will first bend forward adjusting pelvis backward in response to a slight push, but if push is more vigorous the child takes a protective step forward to save himself from falling (staggering). Responses are present in all directions. Later small lateral hopping may be used. A child also flings out his arms in protective (saving) reactions. Normally these develop at 12–24 months of age. They are important as the child will have less fear of falling if he can protect himself, and may then become willing to walk.

Typical toddler's gaits described under section 'Abnormal gaits' below have normal components due to lack of development of postural mechanisms in the early developmental levels of children without cerebral palsy. As older children with cerebral palsy have not yet developed specific postural mechanisms, they too show a number of these characteristics of gait.

See *Stages in the development of standing and walking* in Figs 9.139–9.150.

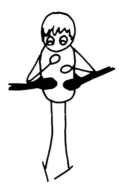

Figure 9.139 Weight bearing on legs (supporting reaction) (*0–3 months*). Body held.

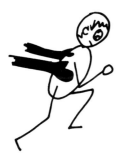

Figure 9.140 Automatic stepping if infant is tilted forward, body held. (*0–3 months*).

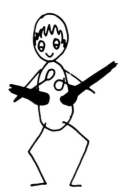

Figure 9.141 Sinking or astasia (*3–6 months*). Head control.

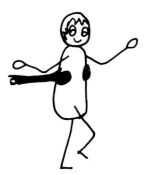

Figure 9.142 Trunk supported standing and bouncing in standing (*5–7 months*).

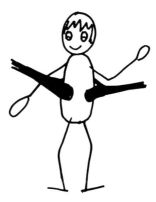

Figure 9.143 Supported standing (*5–7 months*). Weight bearing of legs.

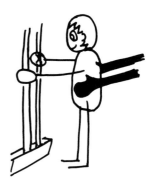

Figure 9.144 Stand holding on to support with pelvic support (*7–9 months*).

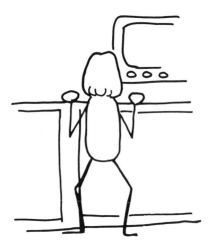

Figure 9.145 Stand holding on to furniture (*7–9 months*). Begin weight shift.

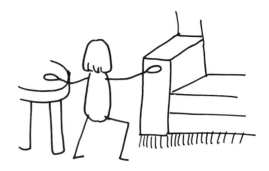

Figure 9.148 Cruising (lateral stepping) (*9–12 months*).

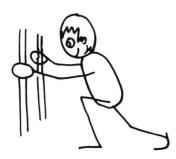

Figure 9.146 Pull up to standing from various positions (*9–12 months*).

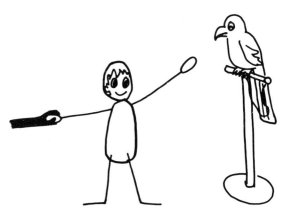

Figure 9.149 Stand supported, reach in all directions (*9–12 months*). Weight shift.

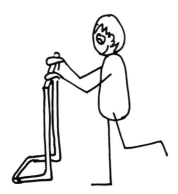

Figure 9.147 Standing holding and lift one leg off the ground or one arm released (*11 months*).

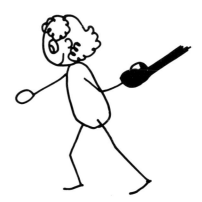

Figure 9.150 Stand alone and walk with two hands, then one and then no hand support (*12–18 months*).

Prognosis for walking

Montgomery (1998) reviewed seven studies identifying predictors of walking (ambulation). Walking was acquired between 3 and 9 years and was unlikely afterwards. Sitting by 2 years and crawling by $2^1/_2$ years were strong predictors, but some children who only sat by 4 years did eventually achieve walking. Children with *obligatory* primitive reflexes at 2 years were most unlikely to walk. Scrutton and Baird (1997) found that children not rising to sit and sitting alone by 2 years were less likely to walk by 5 years. Molnar and Gordon (1976) emphasised that failure to achieve sitting by 2 years does not exclude the potential for walking, though they found sitting at 2 years important. The majority of children who eventually walked sat by 4 years. Bottos and Gericke (2003) in their review documented that children who lack independent sitting at 3 years are unlikely to walk independently.

Clinicians need to avoid being dogmatic that if a child does not sit by 2–3 years, that child will not walk. Other studies have different views:

Wood and Rosenbaum (2000) carried out a historical study of children using the Gross Motor Function Classification System (GMFCS) (Palisano *et al.* 1997). They followed changes in the GMFCS level from age 1–2 years to age 6–12 years. The data (their table IV) show that only about 40% of 78 children stayed in the same level, with about 20% improving and about 40% getting worse. Two children went up three levels and one child dropped three levels. So the figures show that although the GMFCS levels of a *group* of children do not change much as they get older, the level of an *individual* child may change dramatically. This study is used as a prognosis for walking. The Ontario Motor Growth Curves (Rosenbaum *et al.* 2002) have been discussed under section 'Functional measures' in Chapter 8 and are used by some clinicians as a prognosis for walking.

Wu *et al.* (2004) determined the probabilities of walking at ages up to 14 years by using records for a total of 5366 children who could not walk (with or without aid) at age of $2–3^1/_2$ years. They found that children who do not roll by age of $2–3^1/_2$ years (GMFCS Level V) have about a 10% probability of walking (with or without aid) by age of 14 years. Those who can roll but not sit by age of $2–3^1/_2$ years (Level IV) have about a 40% probability of walking (with or without aid) by age of 14 years, and these

children include about 10% who walk well alone. Those who can sit but not walk by age of $2–3^1/_2$ years (Levels II and III) have about an 80% probability of walking (with or without aid) by age of 14 years.

Prognosis for walking to adolescence and adulthood

Beckung *et al.* (2007) comment that children had the greatest achievement of walking at 9–10 years on the basis of the Gross Motor Function Measure but that after this age there was great variability on maintenance of walking.

Details of studies after childhood are presented in the section 'Studies of function' in Chapter 7 on older people.

Treatment and management at all developmental levels

Aims

(1) *Develop postural mechanisms.* Emphasise stability and counterpoising with weight shift and postural alignment in functional standing *first, and also* in phases of gait for a child learning to walk or already walking alone with an abnormal gait. A number of abnormal gaits involve compensation for poor postural control in standing.
(2) *Correct abnormal postures and movements as much as possible in the context of standing and stepping.* See Chapter 11 for further details on deformities and gait.
(3) *Assess and select appropriate* designs and sizes of standing equipment, orthoses and walking aids according to the individual.
(4) *Bone density problems need early use of appropriate standing and walking frames.* Bone density is due to delayed or less weight bearing, nutrition and some medications for epilepsy.

The physiotherapist needs to take particular care with selection of techniques according to abilities of others involved in management of the individual. Some parents or carers are highly motivated to teach standing and walking and need to learn that they train at a child's individual pace.

Note: Weight bearing and stepping are not walking. Children who are able to bear weight and step needing trunk support for balance are really at the 6-month normal developmental level. These children are frequently the ones who need support on chest and lower trunk in walking frames. Some children, mainly with dyskinesia will use a walker on wheels to run headlong, but are unable to stand alone, having not yet developed the postural stability of head, trunk and pelvis of later developmental levels. If children with ataxia use wheel-walkers, they stagger in all directions. The training of standing and walking in such children should concentrate on their next levels of development which build up trunk and pelvic control.

0–3-month normal developmental level

Common problems

Delay in taking weight on feet, when fully supported under shoulders. Poor head control, round back with pelvic posterior tilt and semi-flexed hips and knees. Reflex stepping (primary walking) if tipped forward until 2 or 3 months. In some normal babies there is a temporary loss of weight bearing (3–4 months) which may perhaps be due to increasing weight of a baby on legs that are too weak to support him (Thelen *et al.* 1989). Sole contact may also include grasping reflex of the foot on the ground, which is normal until 9 months.
   Abnormal performance.

(1) There may be an excessive antigravity posture onto toes with stiff straight knees in a 'pillar of support' with legs adducted or crossed (scissoring).
(2) When fully supported, there may be various abnormal stepping reactions as each sole of the foot contacts the ground. There is an *athetoid dance*, when each leg jerkily withdrawing outwards with each foot everting. Some athetoid individuals on sole contact 'conflict between grasp and withdrawal reflexes' (Twitchell 1961). One leg may exhibit a *pawing* repetitive involuntary motion.
(3) Excessive infantile *crossed extension response* apparently like the jerky high-stepping pattern seen in older children as the other leg rigidly extends as its sole contacts the ground. This is similar to automatic stepping above but more obligatory.

(4) Withdrawal reflex of both feet on contact with the ground, as opposed to alternate leg withdrawals.

Treatment suggestions and management

From 0–6-month developmental levels. See below.

3–5-month normal developmental level

This is the level at which some normal babies may not take weight in standing but sag (abasia) and infantile primary stepping is no longer present (astasia). Children with cerebral palsy also sink down without weight bearing for a period. The children may be at this developmental level which is due to weakness and absent postural stabilisation. Later this is augmented by short hypertonic flexor muscles.

Treatment suggestions and management at 0–6-month developmental levels

Increase weight bearing on both feet. Develop weight bearing on plantigrade feet with a fully supported child, which counteracts delay as well as the various abnormal reactions to foot contact with the floor. Manual extension of a child's legs assists his weight bearing. Trunk support or trunk and pelvic support is needed at this stage. Encourage head and upper trunk control which may have been achieved in sitting development between 3- and 5-month levels.
   Use the following methods with *full* support at this level in children aged 12 months and over:

(1) Use of knee gaiters with pelvic supports, knee splints or long leg orthoses.
(2) Periods of weight bearing in prone standing frames with tables at upper chest level (Fig. 9.155d–e).
(3) Joint compression through hips and pelvis or through knees, giving full trunk support.
(4) Desensitise soles of feet by weight bearing on feet with heels pressed down in sitting, squatting and then in standing. Use shoes and various floor surfaces, sponge or a trampoline, etc. to find which the child can tolerate. Inclined *prone stander* allows partial pressure of child's weight on his feet (Fig. 9.155d). This develops toleration of a firm surface on the soles.

(5) Prone standers are used to correct postures of trunk, pelvis and legs. Select support and correct positioning elements for each child. Miedaner (1990) suggests 20–30° incline for an appropriate posture. See discussion on standing frames below.

Prone standers or inclined frames do not train standing itself, but correct postures and desensitise soles of feet. Upright positions are needed to train standing (later stages).

6–9-month normal developmental level

Common problems

Delay in weight bearing with flexible knees, if supported, in active *bounce* when held in standing, and in alternate stepping (not automatic high stepping), if held. Delay in achieving upright pelvis and straighter trunk. (Figs 9.142–9.145). *Abnormal postures* are likely to be seen from this level on, that is from the 6–12-month normal developmental level.

Abnormal postures in standing (see Figs 9.151–9.154)

These may be due to:

Absence of postural stability. The child may be able to maintain equilibrium, even inadequately, by attempting an abnormal posture to compensate for this absence (Figs 9.151–9.154). He may show the following symptoms:

(1) *Sinking* into hip flexion, knee flexion and dorsiflexion.
(2) Adduction–internal rotation of the legs.
(3) Lordosis may compensate for hip flexion.
(4) Round back and head flexion or head thrown back and chin-poking may be present.
(5) Feet in valgus or in overdorsiflexion. If overdorsiflexion is limited by tightness of ankle or plantar flexors, the child may stand on his toes.
(6) *Children with dyskinesia* compensate for tendency to fall or for their precarious backward lean, with head flexion, chin poking or head stiffly rotated to one side, hip extension, knees semi-flexed or hyperextended, valgus feet. The arms are initially held stiffly extended backward or in an asymmetrical pattern like the

ATNR when the child is supported from the back. When standing alone, arms are brought forward and up in the air or clasping hands as additional counterbalance for their body extension behind their feet.

These postures, to maintain equilibrium under difficult biomechanical circumstances, are also seen in normal people on slippery surfaces or when first attempting ice skating or skiing. Some of these biomechanical compensations are also seen in young able-bodied children before the development of adequate postural stability and postural adjustment for early weight shift.

If a child also has spasticity or rigidity with short stiff muscles, he may use that to prop himself up into the abnormal postures above.

If the child has *good* upper limbs or at least a grasp in poor upper limbs, he will use them for support. Such children *stand and walk on their hands* with walking aids (Fig. 9.153). They bear so much weight on their hands that fatigue of the good arms is common.

Fear of falling is naturally appropriate when postural control is so inadequate. Fears exacerbate all these abnormal postures.

Asymmetrical postural fixation (stabilisation) and counterpoising. The child will take weight on the better side, and the leg with poor postural stability will flex, adduct and internally rotate at the hip, flex at the knee and remain propped on the forefoot, or have no weight bearing (Fig. 9.154). An athetoid child may have one leg *pawing* the ground with an involuntary motion.

Scoliosis may compensate for the body weight being distributed to one side only. This asymmetry may or may not also have been seen in other weight-bearing positions such as sitting, kneeling or four-foot kneeling. Sometimes, it is the postural stabilisation mechanism of the pelvis in only standing which fails, but which may be able to cope at lower levels of development, such as sitting and supported upright kneeling which provides wider and lower bases than standing on only two feet.

The unaffected side in hemiplegia obviously takes all or most of the child's weight. The hemiplegic leg is usually rotated back from the pelvis. It may be abducted or adducted, internally rotated, knee flexed, straight or hyperextended, and foot flat or in equinus, toes may claw the ground. If the young

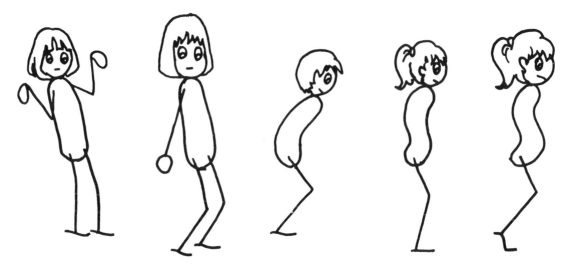

Figure 9.151 Falling or extending backwards is compensated by hip and knee flexion and adduction, lordosis, valgus, overdorsiflexed feet or plantarflexion.

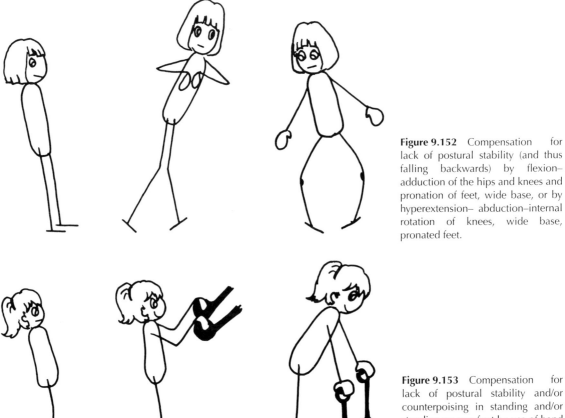

Figure 9.152 Compensation for lack of postural stability (and thus falling backwards) by flexion–adduction of the hips and knees and pronation of feet, wide base, or by hyperextension– abduction–internal rotation of knees, wide base, pronated feet.

Figure 9.153 Compensation for lack of postural stability and/or counterpoising in standing and/or standing on one foot by use of hand grasp or *walk on hands* for support. Children increase spasticity in their arms if they flex and grasp.

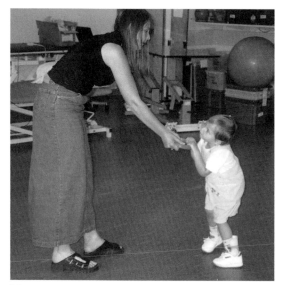

(a)

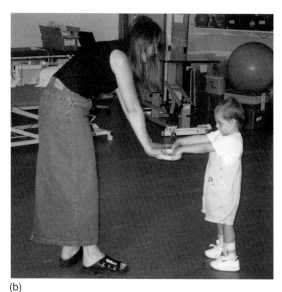

(b)

Figure 9.154 (a) Standing with flexion and asymmetry, and poor postural control. (b) Correction with arms symmetrical elbows extended and both hands either grasping in front, below and in front, or at each side. Equal weight on each leg, head and trunk in midline, facing mother for motivation.

child's weight is taken on the hemiplegic leg and the good leg is lifted, he may collapse or sink into flexion. Lack of counterpoise of one arm may lead to the child leaning abnormally to one side or on to the other hand for support. This creates asymmet-

rical postures. Presence of tilt reactions to *one* side only may be associated with scoliosis (Levitt 1984, p. 115).

Absence of protective saving reactions of arms or legs may delay standing and walking in some children because of a justified fear of falling. This absence of saving will create crouching postures as seen in normal people who fear falling. In addition, absent tilt reactions also make them even more unsure and they will increase those abnormal postures which compensate for lack of postural stability and counterpoising. Normal postural mechanisms seen at this level are:

(1) Parachute or saving reactions in the arms on falling forward or sideways (see section 'Development of sitting', Figs 9.76 and 9.133).
(2) Propping reactions in the arms to *break* the fall (see sitting in Fig. 9.84).
(3) Tilt reactions in sitting which may make standing more secure if not directly related to its acquisition.
(4) Presence of toe clenching in supported standing until about 9-month level.

Persistence and use of primitive reflexes. Unwitting constant stimulation of reflex stepping, excessive positive supporting reaction (Bobath & Bobath 1984) and repeated withdrawal reflexes *in some* cases may increase abnormal leg postures. Repeated stimulation of one pattern of movement particularly on one side may increase tension into abnormal posture. However, a child occasionally uses the ATNR to step alone. The increased co-contraction on the standing leg on the side of the face turn is used for stability as the other leg flexes to step. This is observed in a child with dyskinesia which also serves to control involuntary motion or the 'athetoid dance'.

Growth of legs. Growth increases existing deformities as muscles do not grow as fast as bones. Unequal growth of legs may be causing abnormal postures during standing; for example, weight bearing on the longer side leads to an equinus on the shorter leg in order to reach the ground. Weight bearing onto the shorter side leads to the hip flexing or both hip and knee flexing on the longer side to tend to equalise the balance. Scoliosis to one side may occur to compensate for leg length. This is mostly observed in hemiplegia.

Asymmetrical distribution of spasticity may be present and add to the abnormal asymmetry in postural control of weight bearing in standing (see below).

Use of spasticity for compensation. If there is no postural stability and counterpoising mechanisms and the child has a spastic type of cerebral palsy, he will *use his spasticity* to *fix* him against gravity in the upright position. Thus, if a child is *standing on spasm*, he will collapse to the ground if his spasticity is removed by physiotherapy, drugs or surgery for spastic muscle groups. He may be left with straight legs but completely lose his independent standing or even his previous ability of stumbling around. Spastic legs are also weak.

Biomechanics and spasticity.

(1) The spastic muscle groups, particularly those that flex one joint and extend another, such as hamstrings, rectus femoris and gastrocnemius act on bony and joint levers. Abnormal limb alignments result, which may not be corrected, especially with weight bearing. In time they become established producing bony torsion and joint subluxation. The muscle actions are then even more ineffective. Bony torsion or joint subluxation reduces the muscles ability to generate an effective moment (Graham 2004). Stiff soft tissues including muscles, bony and joint abnormalities impair the biomechanics of gait (Gage 1991).

(2) One joint deformity with short spastic muscles and weakness has an effect on the whole limb. There can also be an effect on the whole body in the biomechanics and so a child can be able to maintain a fairly upright posture. Thus, one spastic muscle group with its weakness or with the weak antagonists should never be considered alone in treatment, with or without orthopaedic surgery.

Examples of abnormal postures of the whole leg or body to maintain a fairly upright posture are the following:

- Hip flexion may be dictated by equinus in order not to extend and fall back.
- Hip flexion may be dictated by greater knee flexion.
- Knee flexion may be dictated by too much hip flexion to avoid falling forward.
- Valgus flexed knees may be dictated by hip flexion–adduction–internal rotation.
- Hip extension may occur by short hamstrings flexing the knees and tilting the

pelvis backwards. A long kyphosis or a flat back may then be associated.

- Knee flexion or knee hyperextension may compensate for short, tight plantar flexors or equinus.
- Excessive dorsiflexion may be secondary to excessive hip and knee flexion. Equinus may instead result if spastic plantar flexors cannot remain stretched by the mechanical overdorsiflexion.
- Lordosis and kypho-lordosis compensate for hip flexion.

Clearly, abnormal postures are not only due to the biomechanics of spasticity but also due to inadequate postural mechanisms controlling balance (Figs 9.151–9.153).

(3) The important clue is the presence or absence of the postural mechanisms of postural stabilisation and counterpoising (postural adjustments). In some children, the posture may have normal alignment in quiet postures up against gravity without movement. When voluntary movement is used, these children cannot balance due to lack of counterpoising and compensate with abnormal postures. In more severe conditions these biomechanical compensations for poor postural control (balance) can even take place during both quiet postures and postural adjustments. Therefore, abnormal body alignments are seen during quiet postures against gravity as well as during hand, arm or leg motion. Body alignment in locomotion is also abnormal when poor postural control affects crawling, knee-stepping and walking.

(4) Abnormal postures in standing and walking can themselves further disturb balance as they continue to be used in standing during growth.

The child's abnormal posture may be different when he has to maintain his balance on his own. Thus abnormal postures are:

Well-supported standing.
These components are similar to those of a normal infant held supported under the axillae (0–2 months).

- Hip extension or semi-flexion, adduction with legs together or crossing (scissoring), internal rotation.
- Knee extension.
- Plantigrade feet or on toes.

Later, child in unsupported standing or if child holds on for balancing alone.

- Hip flexion, adduction–internal rotation with feet apart, wider than pelvis or beneath hips.
- Knee flexion or hyperextension, closely adducted (valgus) or in midline.
- Feet in equino-varus, varus (supination), valgus (pronation), or sometimes, heel may be down and forefoot everted.
- Toes may clench and evert.
- Lordosis, kyphosis, flattening of lumbar area or kypho-lordosis may be present.
- Excessive pelvic tilt backwards is associated with flat back, pelvic tilt forwards with lordosis. This has similar components to a normal child of around 7–12 months. Typically, the pelvis normally develops from posterior tilt to neutral then anterior tilt, hip–knee flexion to extension, on toes or pronated feet to plantigrade feet and clenched toes relax. The wide base changes to narrower bases, flat lumbar area to lordosis.

Arm and head postures

These are similar to the abnormal postures seen in sitting development. However, if the hands are grasped by an adult or the child holds on for support, he may use an abnormal pattern in arms and hands. The child with the spastic type of cerebral palsy usually increases flexion–adduction in shoulder, shoulder hunching, flexion-pronation in elbow, palmar flexion with or without ulnar deviation in hands, adduction of thumbs. Increase in flexion in the arms in quadriplegia often seems to be associated with flexion in the legs and abnormal postures of the whole child (crouch posture).

Treatment suggestions and management at developmental levels of 6–12 months with support (see Fig. 9.155a–g)

Standing equipment (frames)

Individual children may use standing frames between 6- and 12-month developmental levels. However, severe children (GMFCS levels III–V) who are not at 6–12-month developmental levels need

full supporting standers around age 12 months for threatening deformities especially of the hip. Hip dislocation is discussed in Chapter 11.

Aims for the use of standing equipment are the following:

(1) Opportunity to experience a standing posture and develop weight bearing and head control.
(2) Reduce deformities of trunk, pelvis and limbs using maintained stretch and improved alignment.
(3) Improve joint ranges.
(4) Promote hip integrity and minimise threatening hip subluxation.
(5) Encourage visual, proprioceptive and perceptual experiences in a different position.
(6) Enable communication with peers and family in play or social activities at tables in school or home.
(7) Develop hand function in an upright well-supported posture. Supporting arms are partly or fully freed for actions, gestures and eating and drinking in standing position. However, there are children with limited understanding of how to use their arm support or grasp to stand, but need standing experience not only for reasons given in this list but also for arousal of their limited attention.
(8) Contribute to prevention of bone density problems.
(9) Offer physiological benefits for bladder, bowel, circulation and respiration by position change.

Research is needed for each of the aims which are based on clinical views. There are studies for specific aims for hips (Phelps 1959), muscle stretch (Tremblay *et al.* 1990) and bone density (Stuberg 1992; Wilmshurst *et al.* 1996; Caulton *et al.* 2004). Studies exist but there may either be few subjects, non-blinded assessors and other difficulties in order to give more evidence for the use of standing frames.

Choice of standing equipment

The following aspects need to be considered:

Typical posture achieved.
Comfort.
Child/adolescent and parent view of aesthetics or acceptability.
Space in the home, school or playgroup.

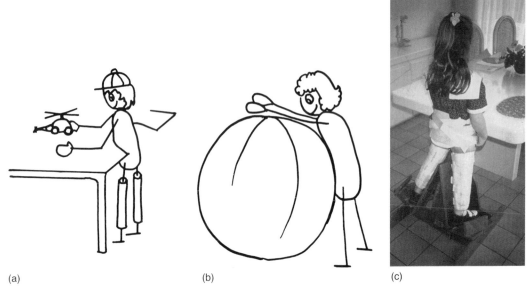

(a) (b) (c)

Figure 9.155 (a–c) Child's arms symmetrical, head and trunk central, weight equal on each foot. Keep child's weight forward onto his feet. Trunk is supported by a roll, a large ball, table, high couch or the body of the therapist behind him. Also use a high couch, ordinary table with padded, rounded edge or cut-out table. Later remove the trunk support and use his hand grasp on support, or lean only on forearms, lean on hands on low table (9–12-month level). Legs are apart and externally rotated, hips flexed or extended, knees straight, feet flat on the ground. Use orthosis or abduction splint, knee splint, foot supports according to the child's difficulties. Later remove knee splints. Rhythmically shift the knees into semi-flexion to avoid rigid infantile stance and if the knees also hyperextend. Later shift weight from foot to foot. (d) Prone stander. Height and angle are adjusted so that pelvis is aligned *without* hyperextension of back or head. Lateral adjustment of pelvic band with derotation and adjustment of knee blocks obtain symmetrical weight bearing. Incorporate foot block if legs are of different lengths. Table is adjusted for hand function and for head control with chin in. Table may be angled or horizontal. Time in any stander needs supervision so that excessive use does not increase hypertonus or fatigue (30–60 minutes). (With acknowledgement to James Leckey Design, Dunmurry, Northern Ireland.) (e) Standing frame, supporting chest, hips, knees and feet. (f) Joint compression through hips, later through knees. Child may stand on floor, but trampoline, sponge rubber, inflatable mattress may be used if posture is kept corrected, and *bouncing is restricted*. The trunk may be supported by his own grasp or holding your shoulders (9–12-month level) or if his trunk requires more support (6–9-month level), lean child against table, roll, couch, large stuffed stable toy or large ball. Head and body alignment must be well over straight legs and feet on the ground. Avoid hyperextension of knees and any abnormal postures. (g) Stander used for mobility before walking with aids is established. Upright position enhances socialisation. (With acknowledgement for photo, Dynamic Stander by Rifton Equipment).

Manoeuvrability and manual handling.

Adjustability of trunk, pelvic tilts, asymmetry pads and straps. Further adjustments may be needed for hips, knees, feet as well as for any presence of different leg lengths.

Adjustability needs to be easy for carers, classroom assistants and parents.

Daniels *et al.* (2004) report on details of different types of standing frames available in the United Kingdom.

Training methods for development of independent control of standing include:

1. Equal distribution of weight on each foot and begin weight shift equally on each.

2. Correction of abnormal postures.

3. Building up of the child's stability by decreasing support.

4. Consideration of severe delay in standing and walking alone.

5. Continuation of development of active head, trunk and pelvic postural stability and essential weight shift needed to counterpoise each limb in standing.

6. Continuation of the practice of upright postures, in sitting and chest-supported kneeling.

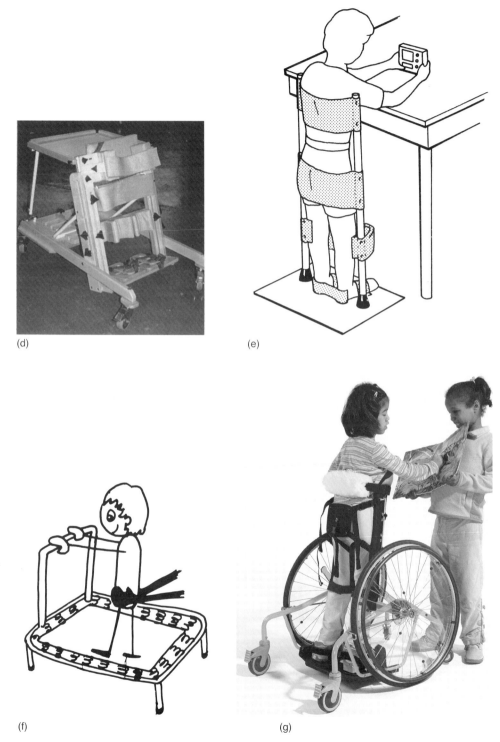

(d)

(e)

(f)

(g)

Figure 9.155   (Continued)

Make standing training interesting with, say, songs, standing at tables of toys, sand and water play tables, as well as watching television. Remember to smile approval with positive comment for child's own efforts to control aspects in his standing. After all, standing on only two feet is more challenging for children than earlier postures, but the rewards soon become obvious to them in psychological and social benefits.

(1) *Equal distribution of weight bearing on each foot. Supported and later unsupported standing according to developmental level.*

 (a) Check this by having child standing on two weighing scales and help him correct this as you read the equal weight borne on each scale. Also use biofeedback (Winstein et al. 1989), for example biofeedback with force plates and visual display for training an older person (Hartveld & Hegarty 1996).

 (b) Head and trunk in midline is first supported and then unsupported if possible.

 (c) Teach weight shift onto one leg to free the other leg for a step. First show this weight shift onto the less involved leg. Then, teach weight shift on to the side that bears less weight, with and later without support. Assist the child with manual support to waist and pelvis. He may move himself onto one leg as he places the other on a footprint or picture on the floor. If possible, ask the child to weight shift against your hand placed firmly against his lateral hip, increasing manual resistance according to child's strength. Carry this out initially with support to child's chest or having him lean on his forearms, on hands or grasping a support with elbows straight. Practice weight shift from side to side for stepping, using a rhythm. A more able child may hold hands and move together with him as you give the less able child support.

 (d) Use a mirror for both you and the child to see that he is in correct alignment with his weight on both feet. A white stripe on the mirror gives added visual cue for his midline vertical alignment.

 (e) Use a wide base and bring both feet together for standing, and then stand with one foot in front of the other to maintain postural control. Do this with and without support.

 (f) Correct any deformities, especially of the feet, such as equinus, so there are two plantigrade feet for equal weight bearing. Equinus may be developmental delay or secondary to other deformities, see below.

 (g) Check length of legs in case of growth asymmetries and raise shoe if there is more than half-inch (12.5 mm) difference. This avoids the child needing to take more weight on either the short or the longer leg.

 (h) Remember to keep the child's weight forward over both feet and help him avoid any twist or lean backwards. Try *not to have a child lean back* against the wall or against an adult. Avoid a child's arching back in prone and upright standing frames. This aggravates the tendency to fall or extend backwards when developing standing ability.

 (i) Practise standing him in a corner with a stable chair in front of him to help him overcome fears of falling. He then also actively and equally sways laterally from wall to wall and antero-posteriorly towards the chair and to midline, posteriorly to wall and back to midline.

 (j) Whenever possible face a child. He uses your presence as motivation to stand in correct postural alignment with gravity and initiate weight shifts forward (to greet you/touch you in a game).

 (k) Stand on different surfaces, for example carpet, sponge rubber, rough ground with (and later without) support.

(2) *Correct abnormal postures or deformities.*

 See correction of abnormal postures in sitting and use similar methods for kyphosis, scoliosis, hip adduction and internal rotation, feet deformities. See subsection 'Standing equipment (frames)' (Fig. 9.155c–e,g).

 (a) Place the child's legs apart in line with the pelvis in standing, hips and knees straight, head, trunk, pelvis upright. Hips flex when a child plays with toys at a table and when initial standing alone begins as the child maintains balance over the feet. The straight knees will slightly flex and vary with extension for control of posture. Keep feet flat on the ground. If legs are in internal rotation, turn child's thighs and feet to face outwards. Stand him like this straddling in abduction over a roll, inflatable toy, sponge rubber or large stuffed toy. You can hold him like this when you are seated on the floor and the child's legs are abducted over your thigh or legs. If necessary, hold the child's knees and thighs facing apart and outward (in external rotation), to overcome excessive adduction–internal rotation. The toy he straddles needs to avoid valgus knees by keeping both his *knees and feet* apart. Press his heels to the ground by pushing down through his knees to his heels (joint compression/approximation). Sway child laterally and also forwards and backwards to a slow rhythm.

(b) Equal weight distribution and weight forward over feet will correct many abnormal postures. Symmetrical postures and head in midline are trained and progress made to asymmetrical control during limb actions. Motivate and facilitate child's arm reach behind at shoulder level or overhead to touch something that interests him. This activates muscles to decrease a rounded back or bent hips and knees (Figs 9.164 and 9.165).

(c) Splints and orthoses reinforce training of active correction. If abnormal positions cannot be actively corrected by the child *in every joint*, at the same time, use splints or orthoses for one joint whilst the others are actively corrected by a child. For example, correct abnormal adduction with an abduction splint, whilst a child actively stretches his knees and keep his heels down with his weight taken towards the external surface of his feet. Another possibility is to correct bent knees with the knee gaiters/splints, whilst the child actively corrects the position of hips and feet. Yet another possibility is to correct the feet in below-knee orthoses or in plaster casts whilst the child actively corrects hips and knees, head and trunk.

(3) *Building up a child's own stability by a decrease of support given to him.*

Carry out methods with trunk or shoulders supported by your hands and by selected standing frames in which supports can be decreased. As child progresses, decrease support of a child to the waist and pelvis and even just knees and feet. Well-fitting shoes or orthoses provide stability as a child actively controls standing posture.

(4) *Consideration of severe delay of standing and walking.*

Abnormal weight bearing, without the trunk and pelvic control of 6–12-month developmental levels, is seen in severe cases of much older individuals as well as in young children (GMFCS Levels IV and V). Excessive antigravity reaction of hip adduction (scissoring)–internal rotation, hip and knee extension, toe standing occurs when the child is held in standing. This cannot be manually corrected. A child may try control by using excessive demands on hands for supports and not be able to use them for other hand skills in standing. There may also be an increase in deformity due to overuse of specific muscles in the upper limbs and trunk.

Train such an individual with methods of below 6-month levels given above and have treatment concentrate on lengthening short muscles, practising rising, arm support in prone, supine and sitting. Practise upright trunk control with activities in sitting. Improve limb and trunk postures and partial weight bearing in an inclined *prone stander* with control of feet, knees, hips and pelvis with an abduction wedge. A child can then be placed at eye level with his peers and family who are standing. This incline is adjusted to 20–30° for correct weight bearing (Miedaner 1990). A *supine stander* instead of a prone stander is more helpful for children and older people with very poor head control and deformities, particularly of the spine. The standers need to be easily raised mechanically or electronically for manual handling by carers.

Use a well-supported upright standing frame as soon as a child can tolerate this without excessive increase in tension, involuntary movements or spasticity. This may be seen in head, arms, hands or trunk, as well as the withdrawal of legs due to oversensitive soles. Check whether this *overflow* can be slowly corrected with assistance during play and other activities which appeal to a child. Treatment suggestions for standing are followed if and when the child becomes more able and ready to respond to them (see subsection 'Prognosis for walking' above).

Meanwhile it is most important to plan other forms of mobility such as standing frames on large wheels ('dynamic standers', Fig. 9.155g) if upper limbs are able to manage this, electric wheelchairs or play vehicles with special switches. Special switches are available and experts need to be consulted for ages 2–4 years and over.

(5) *Continuation of training of head, trunk and pelvic stability and counterpoising in all vertical postures as well as standing.*

Children within all levels of severity need training of the postural mechanisms. Development of these postural mechanisms does seem to decrease excessive hypertonus and in dyskinesia minimise involuntary movements and in hypotonia activate weak postural muscles, during weight bearing in standing. Train this control mainly in upright postures, in sitting, knee walking (sideways, forwards, backwards), half-kneeling and upright kneeling. *Do not use upright kneeling* if the child has hip or knee flexion tightness or lordosis.

9–12-month normal developmental level

Common problems

Delay in standing, holding on and able to shift weight forward and back and laterally preparing for limb movement. Standing may be stable but become unsteady if releasing one hand from support, reaching with one hand and turning to look behind him without reach. Delay in holding on and standing on one leg, stepping sideways or cruising. Inability to stand alone momentarily, step two-handed support, one-handed support. Delay in rising from prone or supine to standing with help given in the transitional positions of sitting, squatting, kneeling on all fours, upright kneeling or half-kneeling. Later, there is lack of holding on and pulling himself to standing from these postures. Delay in standing first with base wider than pelvis followed by a narrower base in line with hips. Delay in pelvic tilt forward with normal lordosis. Weight shift forward/back, later-

ally is delayed when standing alone using hands to hold on for balance and later with no support.

Abnormal performance See above section 'Abnormal postures in standing' and the treatment suggestions which follow it.

A measure of standing abilities, sit to stand and reach are given in the Berg Balance Scale (Kembhavi *et al.* 2002). For example:

Standing alone progresses from 30 seconds after many tries, alone for 30 seconds, then 2 minutes with supervision and 2 minutes alone and safely. There is also progress for standing with eyes closed, and progress in standing with feet together and standing on one leg. These are not given in developmental levels, but do have standing abilities and sit-to-stand which are recommended in this section on standing.

Liao *et al.* (1997) in their research show that standing balance does not automatically lead to walking, though dynamic balance significantly correlated with walking performance. They, therefore, recommend that rhythmic weight-shift training is much needed to improve walking performance. Walking itself very much needs to be trained in walking activities. Balance function and walking have various parameters and they suggest that it is not clear which aspects of standing balance correlates with which aspects of walking and this prompted their research. This book recognises that standing postural control is an important prerequisite for walking but other aspects are also needed such as leg and trunk strength, muscular organisation, minimal deformities, space perception, adequate vision (visual flow) and energy for endurance as well as confidence and motivation. Family and therapist's encouragement support a child's motivation. Treadmill walking does not provide visual flow, space perception, though fitness is promoted. Treadmill walking is discussed in section 'Adjuncts to therapy' in Chapter 3.

Shumway-Cook *et al.* (2003), in a study of standing balance in six children (four with spastic diplegia and two with hemiplegia), demonstrated a significant improvement in their ability to recover stability following training. Woollacott *et al.* (2005) explored possible neural mechanisms that contribute to improvements in balance control on a movable platform. Both these studies were on reactive balance control. More evidence is given in Shumway-Cook and Woollacott (2001).

Abnormal gaits

Typical toddler's gait

This is well described at around 12 months by Aubert (2008) before gait changes rapidly to mature elements at 3 years and less dramatic changes until 7–10 years. The characteristics of early gaits are normal when the postural mechanisms are not yet fully developed. Similar gait patterns and biomechanics are present in older children with cerebral palsy as their postural mechanisms are delayed.

Gait patterns include the following:

- Wide base or use of walking aids to widen base. Feet pronated with legs in very wide base.
- Weight shift more excessive to each side ('waddle'), single leg stance is limited.
- Pelvic mobility is absent.
- More steps taken per minute (cadence), low velocity, short uneven steps and stride.
- Pronated feet, sometimes with flexed toes and more double-leg stance used for stability.
- Dependent on supports each side or in front before toddler gait is fully independent.
- Appears to 'run' as more postural control is needed for slow walk. Unable to stop easily.
- Unable to walk backwards or to turn a corner.
- Hip and knee flexion with abduction–external rotation in wide base on weight bearing.
- Excessive hip and knee flexion with some abduction–external rotation during swing.
- Hyperextension of knee when stepping slowly. Flat foot contact with floor for stance.
- Inadequate balance and arms persistently held up in air (high guard), even after standing is achieved (Fig. 9.168). Arms gradually become low guard and swing is a later achievement.

The problems in standing will affect gait, therefore walking alone should not be 'pushed' if standing is absent or very abnormal. Fears of falling may increase abnormal gait patterns in such cases. Appropriate well-supporting walkers are used until the standing postural control and postural alignment become more reliable for walking alone. There are children who use speed as momentum in 'running headlong' or 'hasty walks' though they cannot stand alone.

Additional abnormal features to the toddler features of gait for therapy:

(1) Excessive hip and trunk sway more to one side in the pelvic waddle.
(2) Excessive hip and trunk sway antero-posteriorly with jerky gait.
(3) Asymmetry of weight bearing and unequal steps.
(4) Abnormal postures of head, trunk, pelvis, knees and feet (Figs 9.164–9.169).
(5) Abnormal stepping patterns in spastic diplegia and quadriplegia, for example *toe walking*; *crouch gait* (overflexed hip–knee and dorsiflexed feet) and *jump gait* with equinus on foot contact and hip–knee extension during stance among other variations.
(6) A dyskinetic *running gait*; *drunken gait* in ataxia or dyskinesia (athetosis); *high stepping gait* and *scissoring gait* in either spastic or dyskinetic type of cerebral palsy.
(7) Overactive arms to maintain balance, *tightrope walking* patterns, persistent abnormal arm postures with lack of reciprocal arm swing. There may be excessive involuntary arm motion seen in dyskinesia.

Delay or abnormal walking patterns may be due to:

Poor or absent stability and counterpoising or asymmetrical ability to counterpoise.

(1) The child may *waddle* from side to side without counterpoising each leg; that is, he 'falls' from foot to foot as he cannot maintain posture for any length of time on one side. There may be excessive trunk sway from side to side. The pelvis and trunk may rotate forward on the side of the swing-through (stepping) leg instead of counterpoising on to the weight-bearing leg in an upright position. The child may have a better postural mechanism on one side, most obviously seen in hemiplegia or asymmetrical tetraplegia, diplegia or triplegia ('asymmetrical ability'). A limp and more weight bearing on to the more able side are characteristic of the gait.
(2) Children mainly with dyskinesia may *run headlong* as they cannot bear weight long enough on each side for a step. Children with dyskinesia or ataxia stumble about and were thought to be drunk by some members of the public. There are also children and especially adolescents and

adults with dyskinesia who stabilise themselves in stepping to avoid prevailing extension or lean backwards behind their feet. The compensation used is the following:

■ Head bent down or chin juts forwards, arms held down and forwards, hands may clasp or thumb held. To control involuntary arm movements which disrupt balance, these arm postures are also used.

■ Hips remain extended with knees flexed, feet plantigrade and toe-clutching the floor.

■ Stepping may be in flexion (*high stepping*) with rigid extension or knee hyperextension during stance, as compensation for balance.

(3) Children with cognitive or perceptual impairment as well as other individuals with cerebral palsy may not wish to walk, show fear of walking and hang on to adults excessively and on to their walking aids. Cognition and perception are relevant to walking in other situations such as when instructions need to be understood and that walking through doors needs to be accurate.

(4) In any of the types of cerebral palsies there may be excessive arm flinging movements or emphasis of the saving reactions in the arms or arms reminiscent of tightrope walking, coming into play to help the child balance on each unstable leg. 'Sinking' patterns of standing and compensation for falling back are seen as in standing (see Figs 9.151–9.153) and walking (Figs 9.164, 9.166–9.168).

Absence of antero-posterior shift. This makes it impossible for the child to *start* walking. A walking aid on wheels may start him off. Stopping is also difficult if this mechanism is not operating. He may also *mark time* and then stop, as he is unable to stop or reverse the antero-posterior shift. Some young children only stop by a collapse onto their bottoms as seen in able-bodied toddlers. This is not socially useful and more painful for large adolescents.

Absence of lateral sway. This is obvious in the children with dyskinesia (athetosis) who run headlong and in other children pushing wheel-walkers. This compensates for inadequate postural stabilisation. Develop lateral sway and weight shift with training of standing on one foot (counterpoising), and emphasise cruising sideways and any activities which promote lateral weight shift from leg to leg.

Lack of tilt reactions in prone, supine, sitting, upright kneel and standing rarely delays walking. This training in walking should not be delayed if these reactions are not yet acquired. Martin (1967) found that labyrinthectomised adults could walk although tilt reactions were not possible without their labyrinths. Similar observations have been noted in children who walk but have absent or poor tilt reactions. Nevertheless, tilt reactions should be included in the programme as it makes the child more steady in changes of terrain and in the dark. As Dr. J. Foley puts it, 'you cannot walk across a ploughed field at night if you do not have tilt reactions' (personal communication).

Saving or protective reaction (arms and legs). These must be trained to prevent the danger of the child falling on his face, and giving him confidence to walk. *Remember* that the protective step in falling is not the same as a voluntary step which the child takes as he is being trained to walk. Foley observed the presence of voluntary stepping without the presence of protective stepping and vice versa (personal communication). Therapy must, therefore, train both of those stepping movements. Excessive saving reactions in arms or legs may occur to compensate for the absence of the other mechanisms. It is most noticeable in ataxic children and athetoid children. The *drunken walk* may be excessive staggering reactions in the legs. Children with dyskinesia cannot *stand still* but take little protective steps. A wide base is used for better balance by children with ataxia and by those who have motor delay without cerebral palsy.

Forssberg (1985) and Leonard *et al.* (1988, 1991), among others, have contributed studies on abnormal gait patterns and compared them to the gaits of normal children. Gage (2009) and Miller (2007) provide detailed normal and abnormal gait analysis and orthopaedic procedures in cerebral palsy.

Abnormal gaits in the spastic type

All the problems above are included with the addition of the pull of short or stiff spastic muscles and associated weakness. There may be various abnormal postures which are associated with each other, as described in the discussion of abnormal postures in the section on standing. There is lack of selective motor control which may also contribute to aspects of gait. For example, dorsiflexion cannot be isolated from knee flexion to obtain initial heel contact with extended knee, positioning for mid-stance with knee extension and during the phases of swing through of the stepping leg (see the right leg gait analysis in Fig. 8.3; see also section on 'Deformities and gait' in Chapter 11).

In Chapter 11, the section 'Deformities and gait' describes abnormal gaits in spastic hemiplegia, diplegia and tetraplegia (quadriplegia) in relation to orthopaedic procedures and physiotherapy.

Automatic reactions expected at 9–12-month developmental level are the postural adjustments of dorsiflexion, hip flexion and beginning of protective forward step (Fig. 9.137). There are also the saving reactions developing in the arms if falling backwards as well as propping on hands to break the fall (see beginning of 'Development of standing and walking').

Treatment suggestions and management at 9–12-month developmental levels

Continue methods from 6–12-month developmental levels but with less to no support.

Aims and methods at 9–12-month developmental levels for all conditions include:

(1) Further improvement of stability.
(2) Training *appropriate* lateral sway (weight shifts) and antero-posterior sway and lead this to stepping and to cruising along furniture or parallel bars.
(3) Standing and counterpoising single leg positions and motions of greater variety.
(4) Correction of abnormal postures as much as possible.
(5) Older children and adolescents need to be kept fit during walking as there is *an energy demand* on a person managing to walk with poor balance, weakness and/or deformities.

Deformities. Those who have potential ability for walking may need stable orthoses on their feet and therapy for plantigrade feet for stability in standing and walking and for improvement of abnormal gaits. Mild flexion deformities of hip and knees allow standing and transfers, but feet that are very deformed and painful in the older child are a major hindrance (Graham 2004).

Many individuals with different abilities use standing frames or knee gaiters to assist passive and active control of hips, pelvis and trunk. Botulinum toxin A (BTX A) for spasticity together with physiotherapy is discussed in Chapter 11.

Select the activities below according to each child.

(1) *Improve stability* with the following techniques: the child stands, holding on or alone. At this level, support pelvis, thighs or knees according to individual ability. To overcome any fears, let a child tell a therapist when she should 'let go' so that he can balance with less or no support.

At 9–11 months his own hand grasp is spontaneously used for support, but if absent, place the child's hands on to horizontal or later vertical bars for maintained grasp. Increase the grasps by gently pressing down on the wrists.

At 9–12-month development level a child is more able to stabilise against manual resistance. Start with child's hands resting on your shoulder or place a child in a corner of a room on a non-slip floor. Apply manual pressure at his hips or shoulders, pushing him off balance; he must actively maintain his upright standing – 'Don't let me push you over', 'Stay there'. Do this laterally and also antero-posteriorly (Fig. 9.156). Do this with rotation – 'Don't let me

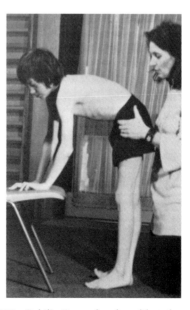

Figure 9.156 Stabilisation on hands and feet, then more upright. Lateral sway, antero-posterior weight shift.

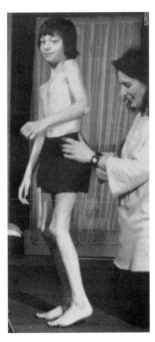

Figure 9.157 Activate an individual's own lateral sway against manual resistance and 'pushes' for postural adjustment. Active sway by person/child is the next stage.

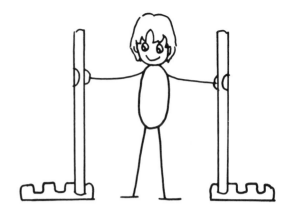

Figure 9.158 Lateral sway practised with lateral grasp for trunk and hips extension. Use externally rotated arms.

turn you'. Another way of using manual resistance is to ask the child to push against your hands placed in positions on his hips or shoulders or on one hip and one shoulder – 'Push against my hands'. Resistance should not be *so great* that the child twists his limbs into abnormal positions or increases involuntary movements, or even falls over.

Once standing is present, practise standing with blindfold or eyes closed and with a veil or in light subdued by sunglasses worn by child. Also have a standing child balance on different surfaces such as sponge rubber, on an inflatable mattress and on rough ground. Do this with and without use of vision.

(2) *Stand and sway* or weight shifts (Figs 9.156–9.158). Continue methods of weight shift at 6–9 months above and establish standing against manual resistance 'Don't let me push you', 'Stay there' (Fig. 9.182). Have his body lean laterally against your body at his side or move him laterally holding his pelvis, so he releases the other leg for a step. Move the child forward for a step for walking or lat-

erally for cruising. Decrease your guidance as he gains control. Once he has managed sway sideways and to sway forwards, he shifts his weight against your hand on his hip, shoulder or both hip and shoulder as you offer manual resistance described above. Manually resist the forward and backward sway which is used for step and stop. Assist maintaining of postural alignment of head and trunk upright with slight truncal curve towards the leg with less weight bearing during sway.

Train lateral sway with legs apart then closer together, for a more challenging base for balance.

Check that feet are plantigrade using the articulated orthoses which allow antero-posterior sway.

Encourage a child's active sway in a corner of the room to allay fears of falling. A child may practise sway between two stable chairs or parallel bars and in a static walker. The child's grasp should be in front or at the sides and at waist or shoulder level. Lateral grasp on poles is preferable to parallel bars as it improves upright, symmetrical weight bearing and trains supinated grasp (Figs 9.159 and 9.160). *All these actions can be done to rhythm and song.* The lateral sways can become steps included in a simple dance routine together with another child as partner.

(3) *Standing and counterpoising limb or trunk movements* (Fig. 9.161). The child stands holding on with both hands and then with one hand

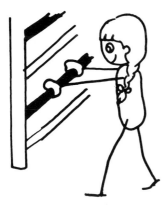

Figure 9.159　Antero-posterior sway in preparation for step.

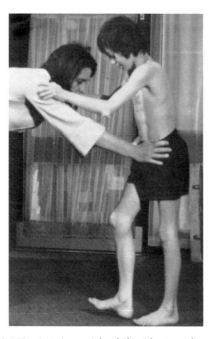

Figure 9.160　Anterior weight shift with step taken against therapist's manual resistance. Note activation of dorsiflexion.

whilst lifting one leg to different heights on the bar or in the air. He could lift one of his legs up in front, to the side and backward, on to bars, box, a step, a small beach-ball, onto your hand, or you put his sock or shoe on or off.

Arm patterns for function are shown to a child in the context of reaching for an object or daily care activity whilst holding on with one hand and later when the child is able to stand alone. Use objects that interest a child to encourage reaching out in all directions. Arm patterns should also be used in the following ways. With the child standing holding a support with one hand or leaning on one hand, correctly facilitate the other arm into elevation–abduction–external rotation without and against resistance. Encourage assisted or active reaching for a toy overhead. A child could also stand and balance while 'walking' his hands up the wall, sliding them up the wall, up a soapy mirror or in other play activities devised by you. It depends on the task, the postural control and the strength of a child as to which way the arm elevation is developed.

A child progresses to stand and reach behind him for toys offered, to touch a wall, as well as to stand and bend down to fetch an object on the floor or low box. He could also move hands down or up each wall bar to fetch a toy hung on either the bottom bar or on a high bar. At first, support a child at his chest or pelvis. This activity also helps to stretch hamstrings and stretch elbows to reach toy. Help him re-erect to standing if this is needed. Later increase demands with tasks such as stand and pick up a cup of water or a heavy object and place it back on a table or on stools of different heights. Assist the grasp, as mentioned above.

When a child stands either grasping a support with one hand as the other moves, it may be necessary to maintain alignment of his legs during normal asymmetry of the trunk in postural adjustment. Therefore, hold his weight-bearing legs straight or in external rotation. Hold one leg and both arms straight while he moves the other leg with normal asymmetrical postural adjustment (counterpoising) of the trunk. The weight-bearing leg is straight in Figs 9.161–9.163. Facilitate the movements against manual resistance shown in Figs 9.162 and 9.163 given correctly, which preferably needs to *be shown clinically*. Heavy objects may be pushed, pulled or lifted by a child who can manage this. It is possible to use desirable arm or leg patterns instead of the habitual patterns which relate to deformities.

A child is shown leg patterns and weight bearing in his phases of walking in parallel bars or in a stationary walker. Leg patterns that may be used are flexion–adduction–external rotation (stepping pattern) from and to

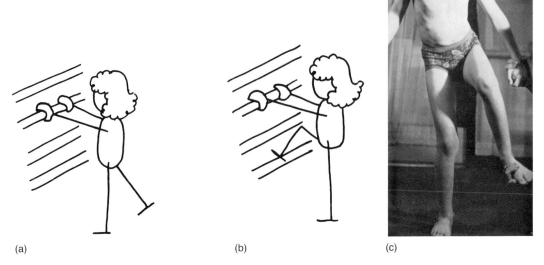

(a)   (b)   (c)

Figure 9.161   (a–c) Counterpoising exercises for walking and climbing stairs as well as for putting on and off socks, shoes and trousers, and for washing and play activities.

extension–abduction–internal rotation (push-off pattern), the knee extended and foot dorsiflexed in *stepping*. Hold toes and forefoot in dorsiflexion in *push off* and to prevent extensor thrust.

Note: Use leg and arm patterns *without* giving resistance if excessive overflow of spasticity cannot be controlled and if methods are not easily nor skilfully carried out.

(4) *Correction of abnormal postures.* The arm and leg patterns (synergies) are not the only ways tasks are managed but selected to activate counterpoising and to correct abnormal positions of arms and legs. In addition, rotation of the pelvis and trunk with the arm or leg movements appears to decrease hypertonus and improve postures (see the subsection 'Basic arm and hand patterns for all levels of development').

(5) *A functional assessment of strength* in both active and passive ranges can take place in the context of standing and preparation for stepping. A child or older person who can cooperate is placed in supported standing on one leg, on a block or on the ground. The other leg to be tested is not weight bearing. The ranges of movement of hip extension and flexion, knee extension and flexion and foot dorsiflexion needed for the walking pattern are tested. This will not be the full range needed

as approximately a range of 0–25° or 35° is usual. Muscle actions of plantarflexion and hip extension for push off (pre-swing), hip and knee extension for stance, and hip flexion, knee extension and dorsiflexion for initial contact (heel contact) are also tested in this functional position. Training of these elements or components of standing and stepping can follow and so impairments of strength and ranges are treated within a function.

(6) *Correction of some common abnormal postures in standing and walking.* These are from approximately the 9-month developmental level (supported) to over 12-month developmental level (unsupported) until adolescence and adulthood (see Figs 9.164–9.170).

■ Flexion and *sinking* posture (Figs 9.164 and 9.167).

■ Asymmetrical posture (Fig. 9.165).

■ Internal rotation of legs (Fig. 9.166).

■ Hip extension, knee flexion, plantarflexion, arm flexion and there may also be arm abduction–extension in the air, elbow flexion, wrist palmar-flexion (arms in *high guard*) (Figs 9.167 and 9.168) or held down.

■ Hyperextended knees and lordosis (Figs 9.169 and 9.170).

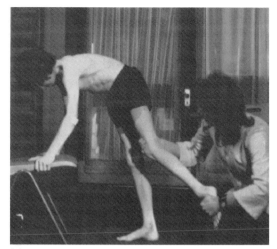

(a)

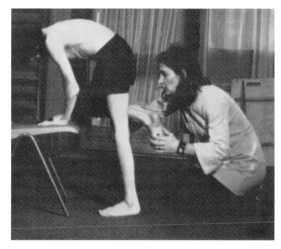

Figure 9.163 From this hip–knee flexion–abduction–internal rotation pattern facilitate *stance* of extension–adduction–external rotation in his right leg.

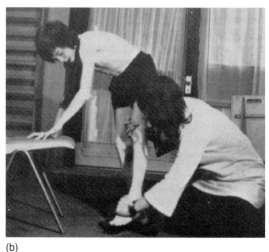

(b)

Figure 9.162 Correction of stepping pattern, that is facilitation of leg flexion–external rotation, knee extension with dorsiflexion. *Push off* pattern (a). *Heel strike* pattern (b). Progress to use within stepping while pushing chair/ladder or in parallel bars.

■ See posture and gait in dyskinesia below. Correction may not be indicated in these adolescents and adults if biomechanical compensation is effective for these people.

Additional suggestions for training walking and gaits other than ideas shown in the figures:

Correction of a waddling gait or running headlong must include training of lateral sway and this is also developed in cruising around furniture. The

9–12-month level of development includes the important development of cruising. Counterpoising activities involving standing on one leg often improves waddle gait as well as other abnormal gaits. *Asymmetrical gaits need increased weight shifts* to more affected side and rhythmic weight shift from side to side and lateral cruising in each direction. Place a more desirable toy on the side which bears less weight for cruising or when reaching out at play in standing at a table.

Crouch gait. Postural stability and counterpoising activities improve this gait if it is due to delayed development of balance. Damiano *et al.* (1995a) in their research studies showed that strengthening quadriceps in children with mild-to-moderate cerebral palsy improved crouch standing and walking. Both postural training and strengthening are recommended.

Toe walking may be present in able-bodied toddlers. Hips and knees are straight and flexible. I have also observed this in toddlers with severe visual impairment without any cerebral palsy. Rising onto toes may be a response to avoid a fall as in a postural adjustment of initial rise on toes before leg protective reactions. In cerebral palsy, persistent toe walking needs modification of the elongated plantar flexors by strengthening the dorsiflexors, stretching any shortness of plantar flexors and training for poor postural control.

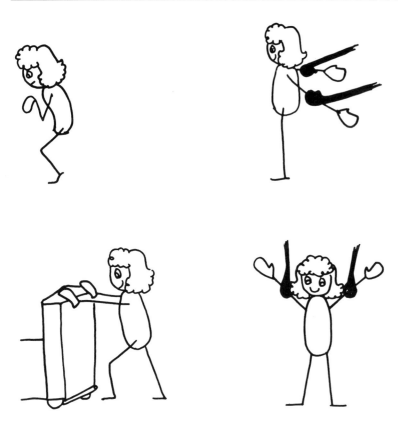

Figure 9.164 Correction of a flexed child whose limbs may also adduct and internally rotate, in standing or in walking. *Keep child's weight forward as in these exercises, there is a tendency to lean too far backwards.* Arms are extended and externally rotated. This corrects head, trunk and legs. Hold child's shoulders, elbows or wrists. Encourage weight shift from side to side by tipping child from your hold on his arms. Stand and walk by pushing walker at shoulder level. Open hands overcomes too much flexion. Keep elbows straight, elbow splints (gaiters) may be needed. Knee splints to maintain extension of knees and/or to get heels down, if required. Calipers or back-slabs for knees may be needed in older children. Slow walk and a long lunge forward when stepping and pushing truck helps to stretch tight heel cords and tight knee flexors.

Cruising or stepping sideways. The child holds horizontal bars and takes a step sideways. At first, there is hip flexion for postural control. Emphasise hip extension with abduction in lateral step in both supporting leg and stepping leg, as soon as is possible. At first, give support and then expect him to keep his pelvis and/or trunk upright so that he takes weight through the standing leg with plantigrade foot. Improve this activity by joint compression through the standing hip or knee whilst manual resistance is given to the abduction of the stepping leg. Some children respond to resistance of the abducting leg which automatically increases stabilisation by their own weight through the standing leg. Others may require you to correct any abnormal positions of hip, knee and foot by holding the thigh and knee extended and externally rotated, shifting the child's weight onto the outside of the foot. Observe that a child's pelvis is symmetrical and in vertical alignment (neutral). Manually correct any retraction on one side and tip the pelvis forward into neutral.

Walk holding two hands or one hand. To prepare for the *walk holding two hands* below use the technique for weight shift sideways given above for cruising. This developmental level of walking (normally about 12–13 months) is the level at which children are functioning when they walk with walking aids of many different types. The walkers stimulate locomotor actions of initiation of stepping and lateral sway, used at age 2-6 years and over.

Examples are as follows:

(a) Walk holding parallel bars or parallel ropes. If the child has not yet achieved grasp and release, a felt cuff or moving hand grip which slides along the bar may be used.

(b) Walk with a walking frame grasping in front or at the sides. Progress from using walkers (Figs 9.171a,b–9.173a–c) to having the child grasp a horizontal stick which is held at each end in your hands. He may hold a small stick in each hand which you grasp at each side of him. Decrease these hand supports further by having

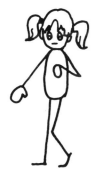

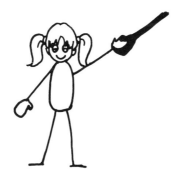

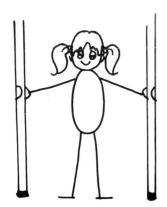

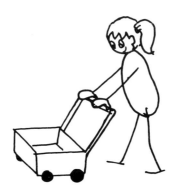

Figure 9.165 Activities to increase weight bearing onto more affected side or on to hemiplegic side. Hold arm in position to counteract arm flexion–adduction–internal rotation. Bring arm forward if shoulder re- tracts. Symmetrical grasp, or *both* hands open and pushing truck. Use elbow splints to maintain elbow ex- tension. Weight distributed equally on feet. Shift weight to more affected side. Child tries to grasp with his arms apart and turned out or with his arms abducted in mid-position but not with shoulders turned inward.

him grasp rubber rings lightly held in each of your hands.

(c) Both of you hold on to a large ball (netball size) simultaneously as you step backwards. Always ensure that the child's weight is well forward over his base.

(d) Walk holding someone's hands on either side or in front of him.

(e) Walk pushing a weighted doll's pram, another child in his wheelchair, a kitchen chair, with studs for sliding, a chair on wooden skis or with set of runners, or a metal walker on four points which slide.

(f) Walking using crutches, elbow crutches, tripods, quadripods or sticks.

(g) Walking using vertical poles at either side with thick rubber bases (Fig. 9.165).

(h) Walk with both hands grasping for hemiplegia. Walk with the ladder-back aid (Peto aid) which improves extension as a child pushes the aid with wrist extended grasp (Fig. 9.173c) (Cotton 1980).

(i) Weight crutches, quadripods or have weights on ankles for children with dyskinesia.

(j) Orthoses provide stability as well as correction of feet.

When selecting and using walking aids consider the following:

Grasping a support at the side of the child tends to train lateral sway for walking. However, if the support involves elbow flexion, this may be con- traindicated as the grasp-elbow flexion and hunch- ing of the shoulders increases spastic stiffness in in- dividuals and may also overflow into the legs. The child's grasps need to be low down and slightly in front with straight elbows (Figs 9.171–9.173). Use elbow gaiters to assist extension. You may instead support at both the elbows or hands holding arms straight (Figs 9.167 and 9.168) as you bring his weight within and slightly in front of his base.

Grasping the hands support in front helps to train the anterior weight shift needed to start walking. Once again avoid shoulder hunching and excessive arm flexion, so use of elbow gaiters to assist in re- minding child to keep elbows as straight as possi- ble is advisable. A posterior walker may be more effective if a child already has an anterior weight

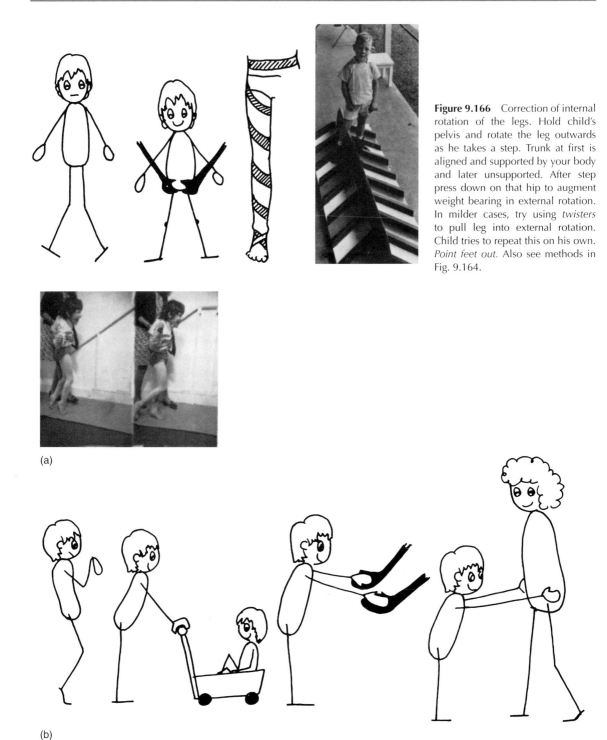

Figure 9.166   Correction of internal rotation of the legs. Hold child's pelvis and rotate the leg outwards as he takes a step. Trunk at first is aligned and supported by your body and later unsupported. After step press down on that hip to augment weight bearing in external rotation. In milder cases, try using *twisters* to pull leg into external rotation. Child tries to repeat this on his own. *Point feet out.* Also see methods in Fig. 9.164.

(a)

(b)

Figure 9.167   (a) Hip extension, knee flexion, plantarflexion. (b) Correction of hip extension, knee flexion, arm flexion, plantarflexion (toe walk). For arm abduction–extension in the air, elbow flexion, wrist palmar flexion.

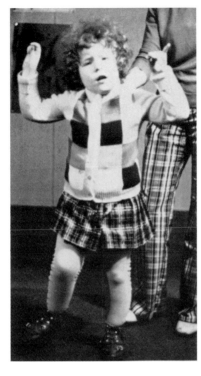

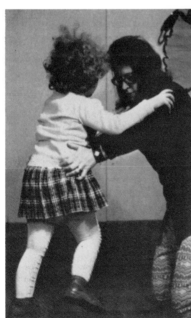

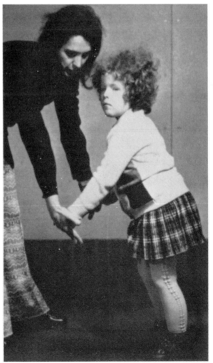

Figure 9.168 Methods to gain confidence and correction of hip extension, knee flexion, arm flexion, plantarflexion (toe walk). For arm abduction–extension in the air, elbow flexion, wrist palmar flexion or 'high guard' arm posture.

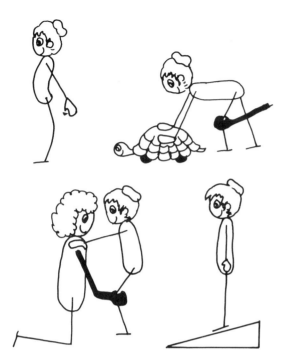

Figure 9.169   Correction of hyperextended knees and lordosis. Check tightness of plantar flexors and stability of pelvic girdle.

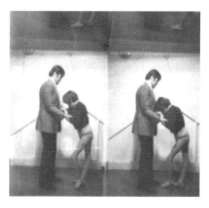

Figure 9.170   Hyperextended knees.

shift and is ready to step with hip–trunk extension (Fig. 9.173a,b). Although Logan *et al.* (1990) prefer posterior walkers, this is an individual assessment which does not apply to all children. Normally early walking uses hip–knee flexion (similar to a mild crouch gait in cerebral palsy) to maintain balance. It may also be helpful to press a child's wrists down to improve his grasp. Try having him lean forward

and down onto open hands or forward onto his grasps. This is most effective in training the active initiation of stepping and continuation of stepping. In Fig. 9.168, note the open hands of the therapist allowing the child to press down and forward to actively initiate stepping.

Inadequate hand use for walking aids. Some involuntary movements, tremors or poor grasp ability with weakness interfere with a child's maintenance of grasp. Children with severe intellectual disabilities or perceptual problems may not manage to use walking aids as well as concentrate on balance and stepping. Hold these children's hands on to the bars directly or by pressing through their wrists as they grasp. Use particularly stable walking frames, weighted trolleys or doll's prams. The ladder-back walker or a chair on padded wooden skis is often helpful. Avoid walkers with castors or wheels, which run too quickly for a child. Later, walkers or crutches/sticks with weighted bases may be managed by some children.

Do not use baby walkers or walkers with a body ring and canvas sling or seat with castors. These mass-produced walkers are not safe for any baby as they tip over easily and lead to other accidents. The wheels on all four corners create undesirable postures and prevent a child from taking weight within his own base and keeping his feet plantigrade. Development of independent and better patterns of walking is prevented as standing, and weight shift by the child himself is disrupted by the wheels. The child will, therefore, sit into the canvas or hang on to the rim of the walker and clutch it with tense bent arms and may stiffen and walk on toes. However, older children do use walking aids which suspend a child from an overhead bar in a parachute design between the legs. Weight bearing is taken through both plantigrade feet, and as some of the suspension lifts the child's weight off his feet, there is less hypertonus and better weight shift. This partial weight bearing is also used in treadmill walking.

Children who run headlong are most likely to hang on the rims of any wheel walker and run dragging their feet. Their walkers should be weighted or a brake applied to the back wheels or, perhaps, remove all wheels. Remind these children to walk more slowly, and in a stationary walker practise standing still with feet together or as little apart as they can manage.

Grasping someone's hand or a quadruped/tripod aid with one hand by a child is usually a progression

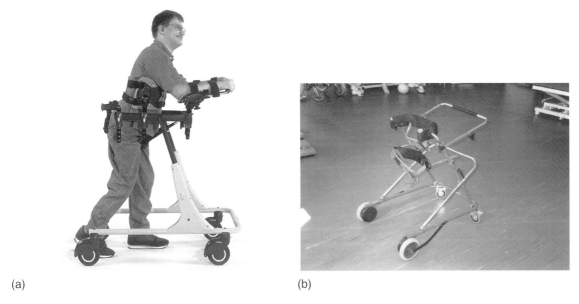

(a)   (b)

Figure 9.171   (a) Walker for a person needing chest support. It can be adjusted forward or upright. Forearm supports assist symmetrical shoulder stability and grasp. (Acknowledgement to Rifton for Rifton Pacer Gait Trainer.) (b) The Orlau Walker for a person needing chest support and symmetrical elbow extension with grasp. A similar walker is the Arrow Walker (Pony).

from walking holding on with two hands. However, if the child takes weight abnormally through one side more than the other or if there are asymmetrical postures, then *two* aids need to be used until he walks alone. Some children progress to grasping a quadruped stick in the centre and in front of them, instead of using two aids. Some children manage aids if they are weighted with small sand bags.

A *child 'walking on his hands' and 'hanging on his armpits'* in walking aids so that he hardly takes weight on his feet needs to be discouraged from doing so. If not, he will step in this way for years and his independent walking will not have any opportunity of developing. Give extra training in all aspects of head, trunk and pelvic stability in both standing and sitting development for these children. Try training their walking restricting holding onto aids but onto more unstable supports such as holding a ball, rings or sticks that you also hold. Use ropes instead of bars in the parallel bars.

Abnormal postures of the head, trunk and legs need to be corrected as much as possible (Figs 9.154, 9.174e, 9.164–9.173). There are regularly new designs of walkers available on the market. If correction is not possible with a particular walking aid, then explore a better one and, if possible, train walking without walking frames. In most cases train the earlier levels in the development of standing or walking more thoroughly. It is important to find suitable tricycles or wheelchairs for mobility until control of abnormal posture improves. Orthopaedic surgery or procedures and muscle relaxant drugs are indicated in individuals. Some people may not be able to walk due to severe deformities and multiple impairments. They require suitable mobility aids if walking is considered unlikely.

Note: Pushing a trolley with handles which are too low or sticks and other walking aids which are too low may increase head and back rounding.

Walking aid giving too much aid. Reassess walking aids regularly to monitor the child's own ability to weight bear, step, control head, trunk and pelvis, and grasp. Select or omit walkers according to each individual and so too much aid is avoided. However, for longer distances, poor weather conditions or unfamiliar environments, more aid may be indicated.

Other forms of mobility should always be available for people who need them, for social and exploratory reasons, to counter fatigue, for experience of space and speed, and especially for a sense of their own control of moving from place to place. For these reasons, mobility aids such as wheelchairs,

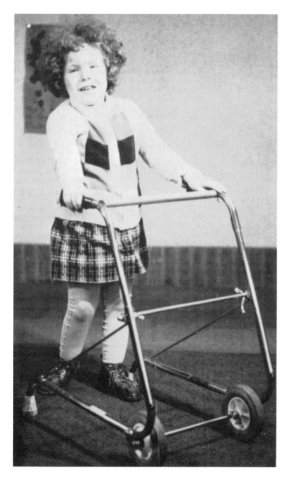

Figure 9.172   Rollator.

play things, standing frames on large wheels and well-supporting special tricycles are also necessary for children who have not yet learned to walk with or without walking aids.

Lower limb orthoses for standing and walking

Lower limb orthoses are used for standing and walking depending on assessment of joint ranges, muscle action and biomechanics. They are used for support, alignment, prolonged stretch of hypertonic muscles and as part of the whole functional programme. A physiotherapist works closely with an orthotist and/or an orthopaedic surgeon. Gait anal-

yses are used in research and clinical work for the most effective designs for individuals (Morris & Dias 2007). However, the following orthoses are commonly used with clinical assessments when gait analyses are not available:

(1) Hip abduction with trunk brace for correction of hip deformities and pelvic and trunk deformities in lying, sitting and standing positioning equipment and/or standing, walking and sitting hip (SWASH) orthosis (Fig. 9.174e).

(2) Knee gaiters or splints correct and support knees in standing and weight shift and so trunk and hip control and some foot adjustments can be practised. This can also be managed in stationary walkers or a standing frame when supports/straps are removed for training and for periods of the day (Fig. 9.155c) (see Appendix 2).

(3) Ankle–foot orthoses are of a number of designs and can also correct the hip and knee. These consist of the following designs used within shoes, trainers or boots.

■ Solid ankle–foot orthosis (AFO) (Fig. 9.174a) of moulded thermoplastic material. It is often set at 2–3° dorsiflexion to counteract the plantarflexion deformity. The range of motion in the ankle with knee straight should be neutral. If not in neutral, then other parts of the foot, especially at the subtalar joint, will compensate and become hypermobile. In addition, the plantarflexion can persist and may become a contracture. There will be rubbing by the orthosis which will alert the therapist that the fit is incorrect. Inhibitive plaster casts for such ankle limitation or surgery will need to be used before the AFO is recommended. The stability in standing is enhanced, but gait patterns remain in a rigid pattern. AFOs may impede crawling, half-kneeling rise to standing, sit-to-stand and use of large stairs.

■ Hinged ankle–foot orthoses (HAFO) (Fig. 9.174b). The hinge at the ankle allows some dorsiflexion, so an individual can use correct biomechanics in rising from sitting, from squatting or from half-kneeling to standing. Weight-shift forward is better and improves the gait. An HAFO in a hemiplegic condition may allow more

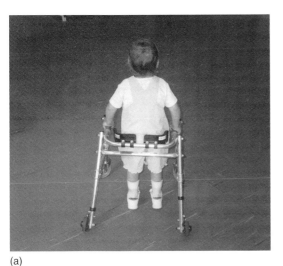

(a)

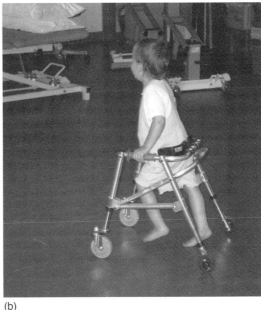

(b)

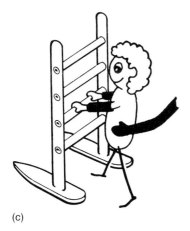

(c)

Figure 9.173   Walkers to promote extension.

symmetry. Orthotists may adjust a hinge to allow minimal plantar and dorsiflexion. The solid AFO sometimes leads to weakening of push off by plantar flexors in gait.

■ Dynamic foot orthosis (DAFO). This is a moulded orthosis for calcaneous, mid-tarsal joint and toe flexors inhibiting hypertonus. Longitudinal and trans-

verse metaphalangeal arches are corrected. DAFO can be small above the malleoli when ankle control is needed with minimal tibial forward travel. The DAFO can be incorporated with a tibial component. A plantar stop is usually included (Hylton 1989).

■ Ground reaction (Floor reaction). Ankle overdorsiflexion may increase a crouch hip–knee flexion posture or not overcome hyperextended knees. Range of motion test of ankle and knee needs plantigrade at the ankle with a straight knee, preferably assessed in standing. The orthosis is moulded to the front or sides of the lower leg to limit ankle dorsiflexion. A knee element or knee piece is necessary to increase knee extension. As the heel touches the ground, there is an associated reaction of knee extension, which also improves hip extension. A posterior walker is best used for extension (Fig. 9.174c).

Hyperextended knees decrease if they are compensations for plantar flexor tightness. However, increasing the set of an AFO to 5–7° into dorsiflexion increases the knee flexion and so midline of the knee is promoted. A hyperextended knee needs assessment to confirm that it is not due to the quadriceps or hamstring weakness, short spastic quadriceps, anterior pelvic tilt with weak hip extension pushes knees into hyperextension. Poor pelvic stability may increase hyperextension for balance.

In older children knee–ankle–foot orthoses may be helpful in cases other than short stiff plantar flexors. Overstretching of knees may lead to pull on posterior joints, creating pain in later years.

■ Night-splint AFO can either be a solid AFO, bivalved plasters or a hinged AFO with adjustable straps to grade the amount of dorsiflexion over time. This prolonged stretch is used for spastic plantar flexors during sleep. However, positioning lying equipment for postural management includes such correction during rest or sleep (see Polak *et al.* 2008).

■ Inserts or foot orthoses. These correct heel position in footwear. However, the forefoot often also needs correction, so the heel-cup is extended to include correction of longitudinal and transverse arches. The sides of the inserts may be raised for extra support, the forefoot moulded or sponge and leather inserts included. The flat foot of early walking is seen in able-bodied children under the age of 3–4 years and may be present in delayed walkers with cerebral palsy. Discussion with orthopaedic surgeons is advisable as orthoses can prevent the activation of small muscles during weight shift, which corrects flat feet during standing and walking.

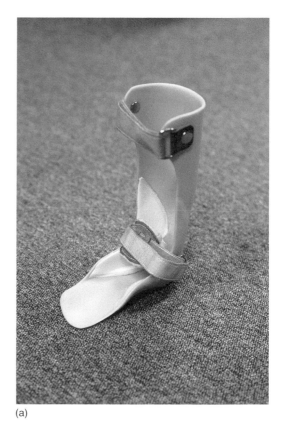

(a)

Figure 9.174   (a) Solid ankle–foot orthosis for dorsiflexion and moulding foot. (b) Hinged ankle–foot orthosis allowing dorsiflexion for gait, stairs, half-kneeling and sit-to-stand. Minimal plantarflexion for push off in gait. (c) Ground-reaction ankle–foot orthosis limits excessive dorsiflexion. Knee element maintains knee extension. (d) Ground-reaction ankle–foot orthosis with stiffening at ankle and with extended sole to correct flexion of toes. Front can be moulded to the lower leg in severe crouch-walk. (e) The SWASH orthosis, with variable hip abduction, dynamically corrects adduction and/or hip dysplasia. May need trunk support. Image is from Camp Scandinavia.

Shoes or special trainers should be checked for correct fit and support for all children whether worn with or without orthoses. Slow range of motion and stretch are useful before orthoses or shoes are applied.

Research studies showing the value of AFO continue (Butler *et al.* 1992; Radtka *et al.* 1997; White *et al.* 2002). See critical reviews by Morris (2002) and Figueiredo *et al.* (2008). Different materials are being developed as well as modifications of designs based on studies and experience, and the important reports by parents, children and older individuals.

Check comfort, pressure points and ease of application. Parents' and individuals' understanding of the purposes of orthoses is an important consideration for cooperation. Studies have shown prevention and correction of deformity, reduced plantar flexor hypertonicity, greater stability, improved gait and less energy expenditure in walking.

Botulinum toxin, baclofen and other drugs as well as orthopaedic surgical procedures aim to correct abnormal hypertonic postures. Physiotherapy precedes and follows these procedures with the methods above (see Chapter 11).

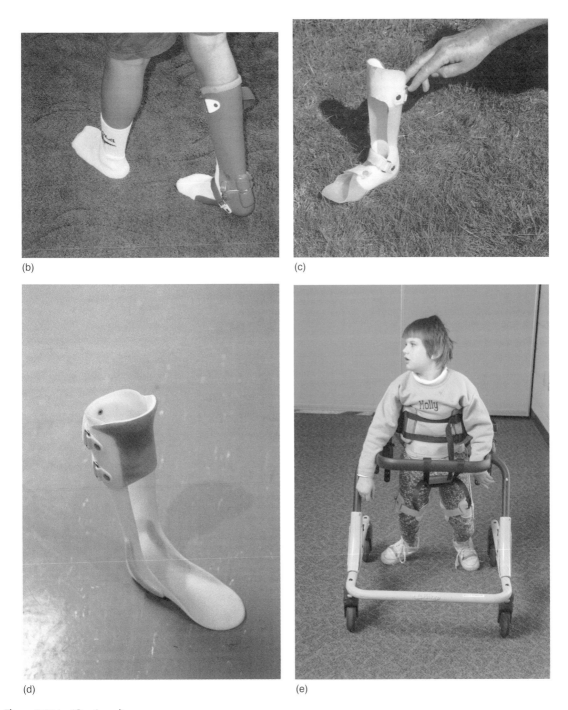

(b)

(c)

(d)

(e)

Figure 9.174   (Continued)

Treatment suggestions for rising to standing (0–12 months)

Mobility in bed and transfers

All the rising abilities trained are valuable for a child's independence in turning in bed and getting out of bed. Training includes the use of hand grasps with elbow extension for pushing blankets down and for support as well as the hand propping used in developing this independence (see section 'Hand Function' below).

Prone to standing. At earlier developmental levels the child has learned to roll over and get on to his hands and knees or rise from prone on to hands and knees (0–6 months). Train him to rise to half-kneeling and then to standing (6–12 months) (see section 'Prone development' (Fig. 9.179)). Some individuals may rise onto hands and feet to standing. Avoid the pattern pulling up to standing by dragging legs into extension and onto toes. However, this is a pattern seen in able-bodied toddlers, but it persists in cerebral palsy. It can be corrected using a roll and during bed mobility exercises when lying prone, dropping legs over the edge of the bed and rising to standing (Fig. 9.175). Pushing on straight arms tends to press heels down with straight legs.

Supine to standing. Rising from supine to sitting into squatting on both or one foot and pulling up to standing may be preferred by a child, rather than using the half-roll pattern. Help him to develop this by taking both his hands when he is sitting on the ground. Stabilise his foot with your foot and wait for him to pull himself forward over his feet and then extend his legs. From crook sitting or squatting, assist rising if child actively can stretch his legs. Use a hoist on his trunk if he is tall or heavy. The full rising can be carried out from supine to squatting and up to standing by holding the child's hands and feet flat on the table. Hemiplegic or asymmetrical children can be encouraged to take weight on the more affected side as they squat and rise (see section 'Supine development'; see also Fig. 9.177). Rising from the ground using squatting is a necessary skill in cultures where people use floor activities in daily life.

Sitting to standing. Rising from sitting on a chair (Fig. 9.176) or from squatting to standing (Fig. 9.177) can be carried out in a variety of ways.

Face a child on his chair with both of you grasping the same stick. Assist the child to push the stick towards you to bring his weight forward as he stands up. Use manual resistance applied on the top of the child's thighs. The child's thighs are carefully kept apart and in external rotation by the therapist who is either behind or in front of the child. If the therapist sits on the ground in front of the child, she has the advantage of making sure that his weight comes well forward over his feet. He may learn to bring his own weight forward over his feet if he is also told to reach forward and down to the floor and *raise his bottom* off the chair. In some children, resistance may be given at the lumbar area to augment this movement. Rising from the floor and from a chair to standing can be taught by careful verbal instruction. For example, rising from a chair involves 'Put your feet flat on the ground, bring your nose over your toes, lift your bottom and now stand up'.

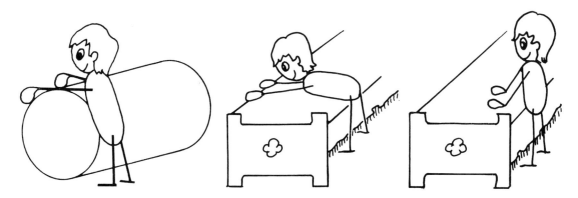

Figure 9.175   Assume standing from prone lying across a roll, large ball or bed. Check that heels are on the ground, knees and hips straight and, if necessary, turned outward.

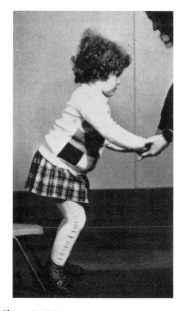

Figure 9.176

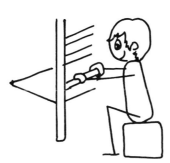

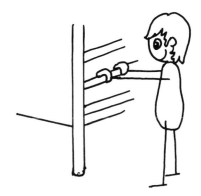

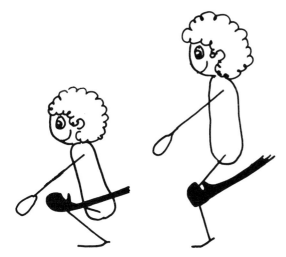

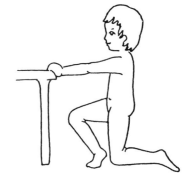

Figure 9.178

Figure 9.177

Teaching a child to bring his weight forward or *nose over his toes* is important or he will not become independent in rising. He will tend to use an extensor thrust or get up abnormally by pushing on his feet, leaning backwards and grasping your hands, being totally dependent on you in order to rise to his feet. Develop squat on a stable potty or from sitting on a toilet chair to practice the correct use of this rising action daily. Legs are exercised, grasp

may be practised on a bar and independence is promoted. Sit to stand is an important motor function for many daily activities in school or in the community.

Teach getting up to standing from kneeling (Fig. 9.178), holding crutches or other walking aids. Other rising problems have to be solved. Rising from bed to sit/stand must be included. Figure 9.179 gives various sequences for rising reactions. A child, parent and therapist work together to choose which sequences suit their daily lives.

Supine lying to squatting and then to standing is only learned by people functioning at the 3–5 year developmental levels, which involves a straight

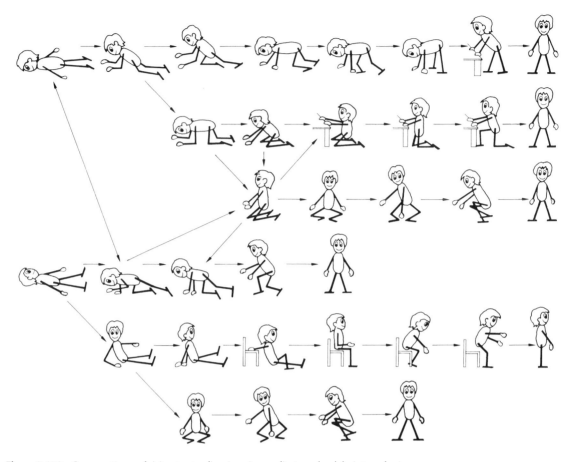

Figure 9.179   Some patterns of rising to standing (see Appendix 1 – wheelchair transfers).

lying-to-stand pattern with no/minimal rotation, with a child often using hand support on the floor. *Slow rising and hold* prepares for attainment of maintained squatting, perhaps at play, in the next stage. Individuals use a momentum to rise from different postures, as postural stability in each transient position is not necessary for independence. It is the training of slow controlled rising sequences which augment stability in the transient postures and establish safety.

Transfers. The rising experiences above are used in transfers, but specific training of transfers is needed. Transfers use arms and hands as supports when a child moves himself from chair to bed and vice versa, or a person needs to give support. Transfer from a chair without arms to a chair with arms and progress to seats without arms using less and less of a child's own arm propping for support. In Fig. 9.132, a child is being taught to pivot on a chair

for transfers, and pivot in standing is also a way for a person to transfer from, say, bed to stand, to chair.

Transfers are achieved or established in the next stages of development. They are important for carers as well as allowing the child to feel that he is participating in changing his position. Hoists or turntables may still be needed for more severe cases.

Stand and stoop to floor now without giving child support. Use wall bars to move hands down from bar to bar and move up bars. Child rises or re-erect to standing from stoop to floor. Make this activity more meaningful by inviting the child to pick up clothes, socks or soft, hard, large and small toys. Hold child in standing with legs apart as he stoops to push a ball between his legs to another child. He rises to standing and plays throwing a ball over head to another child. At first, a child may tend to topple forward in reaching for an object and be unable to reach the floor. Start with objects on a low box and progress to the floor. Use assistance and then gradually remove this with his achievements. This is motivating as a child clearly sees his own achievements over time and would enjoy this as a 'goal'.

Such activities provide both counterpoising and rising elements, as well as perceptual experiences with hand function.

12–24-month normal developmental level

Common problems

Delay in walking alone, improvement in walking pattern, for example narrower base, arms coming down from being held up in abduction high guard to medium guard and later arm swing. The steps need to be more rhythmical, equal and smoother. Delay in stable standing alone and during play in

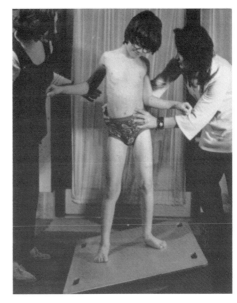

Figure 9.181 Tilt reaction sideways.

standing. Delay in rising to standing completely independently, starting and stopping walking with and without sticks, stair ascent and descent, use of inclines and walk on rough ground is not achieved or not improving until second year (and still further in third year). Delay in walking, carrying an object with both hands, as well as a cup or a heavy object. Delay in standing, picking up an object from the floor.

Abnormal performance. See the section 'Abnormal gaits' above, for a variety of motor patterns.

Reflex reactions. The following are expected at this level:

(1) Saving from falling by staggering (protective) reactions in lower limbs, forward, sideways, backward, crossing over and hopping.
(2) In standing, tip child backward which results in dorsiflexion of feet (Fig. 9.182), then trunk flex forward and, when child is pushed more vigorously, a protective step results. When child is pushed forward, this results in back extension, with or without a rise onto toes. A lateral push results in trunk incurving towards the upright, inversion of the foot opposite to the push and pronation of the other foot (Fig. 9.181). If the tip (push) is slight, only feet respond symmetrically. A tilt board is also used to activate these reactions.

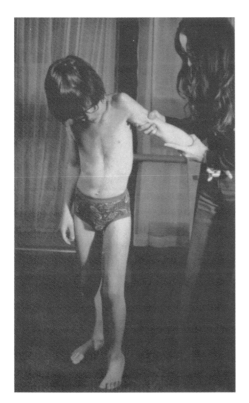

Figure 9.180

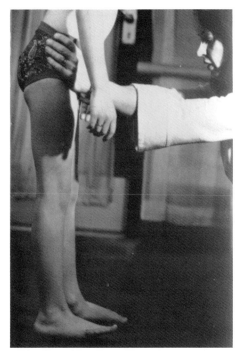

Figure 9.182 Tilt reaction backwards using hip flexion with dorsiflexion. Slight push activates dorsiflexion only.

(3) Rotate child in standing, feet apart, results in one foot inversion on the backwardly rotated side and the other foot in pronation.

(4) Arm-saving reactions become more established in all directions.

Treatment suggestions and management

Standing. Practice lifting heavier objects or toys, maintaining standing balance. Stand and stoop to pick up toy from different table heights and floor. Stand, stoop and re-erect; stand, kick and throw balls.

Gait. See Figs 9.164–9.168. Continue improvement of gait. Child becomes able to self-correct gait and control balance.

Other techniques. See 9–12-month level without walking aids. *Stair climbing* is also dependent on standing on one leg long enough for the other to deal with the step. This should be trained on and off a low box, progressed to higher boxes as well as staircases, pavements, and wall-bars or stable ladders. These activities also trains perception of height or space. Use of banisters, two hands, one hand and

independent stair climbing is achieved by 3–4 years developmental levels (see Tables 9.1 and 9.2).

At first a child uses an exaggerated foot lift, but by 3 years there is an economical foot lift to stair.

Train walking and stop, walk and turn, walk between and around objects, walk on different terrains. *Develop walking up and down inclines.* Walk backwards. Run holding child's hand. Teach child to push and pull large toys.

Train a person to pivot (turn) in standing by assisted trunk turn while he moves his legs in steps to turn. Once achieved, pivoting is usually valuable for transfers and turning in small spaces.

Train protective and staggering reactions. First push the child's anterior pelvis slightly backwards for dorsiflexion with or without hip flexion (Fig. 9.182). A more forceful push results in a protective backward step. Also hold hips and sharply rotate child to provoke a protective step. Hold a child's upper arm and push and pull him in all directions to stimulate staggering or hopping reactions (Fig. 9.180). One foot may be held instead and the child pushed forward and a protective step provoked.

Tilt reactions (Fig. 9.181). Tilt the child back, sideways or support him at his hips. Tip (push) slightly at shoulder/trunk. Use a rocker board.

■ In order to stimulate tilt response, tip child well off the horizontal to develop a safe postural control. A child also tries to sway himself forwards and backwards using an active postural adjustment to maintain balance. Later try this laterally with supervision.

    Perturbations on a moving surface can be developed on a train, tram or in moving floors at the airport.

■ To provoke reaction in his feet on a rocker board. See also discussion on the treatment of valgus feet in Chapter 11.

More advanced counterpoising on one foot is shown using a scooter (Fig. 9.183a) and when stepping over benches or toys of different heights (Fig. 9.183b) as well as in activities such as climbing and kicking balls (see Tables 9.1–9.3). Standing and throwing balls, sandbags and other activities devised by you. All these activities improve postural control and balance as well as keep a child fit and increase strength.

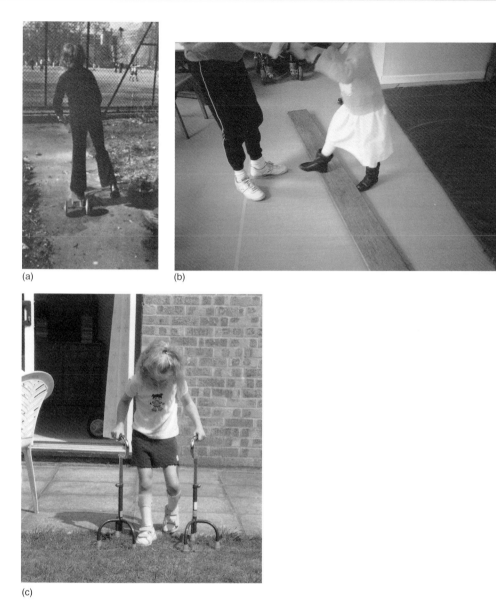

(a)   (b)

(c)

Figure 9.183   (a) Counterpoising on one foot. (b) Variety of benches for stepping over, walking along and sitting activities. (c) Negotiating different surfaces when walking with tripods and ground reaction ankle–foot orthoses.

2–7-year levels (see Tables 9.1–9.3)

Train tricycling (Fig. 9.184), hop, skip and jump, and the variety of activities at the different developmental levels described in Tables 9.1 and 9.2. Functional strength training can be motivating in groups such as circuit training classes (Blundell *et al.* 2003).

Development of hand function

The development of hand function not only depends on the motor control of the shoulder girdle, arms and hands but also on visual, perceptual, perceptual-motor and cognitive development.

The *main motor aspects* of hand function involve the type of grasp, the pattern of reach, the pattern

Table 9.1 Motor developmental stages, 2–7 years.

2 years
Climbs onto furniture
Pulls wheeled toy by string
Ascends and descends stairs holding on, two feet per stair
Gait pattern changes from wide base, short, flat footsteps to narrower base, more heel–toe action established by 3 years
Arms held in abduction during gait come down to relaxed flexion at child's sides
Legs change from external rotation to facing forward
Walk, run and stop alone
Avoids obstacles while running or walking, steers wheeled toys
Throws ball without good direction and excessive effort
Arms held out when asked to catch a ball
Walk backwards, sideways, between obstacles
Walks into a ball to attempt kick

2.5 years
Jumps two feet together
Ascends stairs, holding on, alternate feet
Descends holding on, two feet per stair, ascends two feet, no hold
Steers tricycle while 'walking' his feet on ground
Stands and kicks ball with one foot
Stands on tiptoe by imitation

3 years
Ascends stairs, no holding on alternate feet
Descends stairs usually two feet per stair, no holding on
Jumps from bottom stair or pavement
Climbing furniture, apparatus well
Runs and turns, runs and pushes large toys
Walks on tiptoes, on heels, heel–toe action in walk up inclines, uneven ground
Balances on one foot alone, momentarily, enough to walk on line unsteadily
Pedals tricycles and pedal cars
Imitates movements, e.g. wiggles thumb, asymmetrical arm position unless very complicated

4 years
Throws and catches ball with more control, less effort, more direction and does not need to place arms out to catch
Bounces ball, picks up ball or object with bend from waist
Walks on wide balance beam, near ground, walks heel to toe on line steadily
Stands on one foot 3–5 seconds alone
Hops on right or left foot increasing distance
Imitates finger plays including fine pincer actions
Gait pattern now with arm swing, as adult: stops suddenly; turns on the spot

5 years
Climbs trees, ladders, apparatus
Expert at sliding, swings, 'stunts'
Dances, hops and skips to rhythms
Throws and catches ball in various directions, smaller balls
Kicks ball on the run
Counts fingers by pointing

6 years
Wrestles, tumbles
Roller skates
Jumps rope, begins skip with rope
Stands on one foot with eyes closed
Bounces and catches balls

7 years
Walks on narrow and high balance bars
Throws ball about 30 feet
Begins team sports

Source: Based on Cratty (1970), Gesell (1971), Sheridan (1975).
Note: Movement development shows improvement in speed, precision and decrease of effort or extraneous movements, and increase of endurance. Perception of space, timing and rhythm become integrated with many of the motor skills; see physical education literature for further details and for patterns of performance.

Table 9.2 Character sketch of developmental stages, 1–7 years.

Item	Stage 1	Stage by age (years)	Stage 2	Stage by age (years)	Stage 3	Stage by age (years)	Stage 4	Stage by age (years)	Stage 5	Stage by age (years)
Gait in walking	Early toddler	1.6	Late toddler	1.9	Young child heel strike	2.3	Adult. Heel toe push off	6.0		
Upstairs	Creeps on hands and feet	1	Walks two feet/step + hand. Exaggerated foot lift	1.9	Walks two feet/step + hand. Economical foot lift	2.3	Walks one foot/step and hand	3.0	Walks one foot/step. No hands	4.0
Downstairs	Sitting bumps or creeps backwards	1.3	Walks two feet/step+ hands (giving much support)	2.0	Walks two feet/step + hand	3.0	Walks one foot/step and hand	4.0	Walk s one foot/step. No hands	4.6
Tiptoes	Balances momentarily but lowers heels to floor before walking	2.0	Walks on toes but with much ↑↓ movement of heels which touch floor often	2.6	Walks well on toes with no ↑↓ movement of heels	3.6	Runs well on toes	4.6		
On heels	Toes raised when standing but lowered to floor before walking	2.0	Walks with toes raised and whole forefoot off floor only for some steps	2.6	Able to walk on heels with forefoot only occasionally sinking	3.0	Walks well on heels	3.6		
One foot balance	Tries but unable (may *cheat* by holding on to something)	2.0	Momentarily succeeds 0–2 seconds	3.0	3–9 seconds	4.0	10–12 seconds	5.0	12–16 seconds	6.0
Hopping	Unable – may jump up and down 2 feet together	2.0	1–4 hops	3.6	5–8 hops	4.0	9–12 hops	5.0	Over 12	6.0

Note: Ages given are in years and months. With acknowledgements to Dr P.M. Sonksen from her thesis (1978) for MD entitled: The neurodevelopmental and paediatric findings associated with significant disabilities of language development, University of London.

Table 9.3   Developmental stages of the kick, 1–8 years.

Stage I: boys <1–2.6 years/girls <1–3 years
The child walks, runs or *straddle-toddles* towards the ball, and then walks into it, displacing the ball rather than actually kicking it. Some children who are standing near the ball or have come to a stop near it, lift up one foot and then step on to the ball. Children at this stage sometimes overbalance and fall.

Stage II: boys 1.6–>7 years/girls 2.6–>7 years
From a standing position the child propels the ball forward by flexing the leg at the hip and maintaining his balance on the other leg. If the child has run to the ball, he will stop just in front of it, adjust himself and/or the ball and then kick the ball.

Stage III: boys 1.6–>7 years/girls 2.6–>7 years
The child can now run towards the ball and kick it whilst running, propelling it forward with some force and good direction. He anticipates the kicking position and brings the supporting leg at the side of the ball before swinging the kicking leg forward. The latter leg is not kept fully extended throughout the kick, but is kept slightly flexed during the swing and then fully extended for the actual kick.

Stage IV: boys 4–>7 years/girls 5.6–>7 years
The child and the ball are moving towards each other, and the running child can now kick the oncoming ball with good direction and force. He can anticipate the slight modification of the ball's position moving towards him as he brings himself to the kicking stance, and he hits the ball end on, suddenly reversing its trajectory towards the examiner.

Source: After P.M. Sonksen.

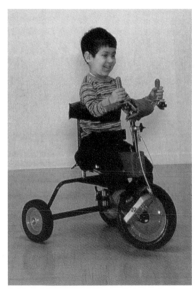

Figure 9.184   An adapted tricycle for handgrips, trunk support, knee extension, flexion and dorsiflexion. (Acknowledgement to Rifton for Tricycle.)

of reach-and-grasp and the pattern of release. These aspects may develop independently of the gross motor activities. Such development of upper limb function depends on well-supported lying, sitting and standing postures, so a child can concentrate on fine motor development.

However, although hand function can develop if a child is well positioned and appropriately supported by equipment, this is limited for the child's whole development. All arm and hand actions activate the anticipatory postural adjustments, so it is unwise to omit stages of unsupported trunks in a hand function programme. Assess child's level of postural control in prone, supine, sitting and standing development to plan activities for interaction of postural control with upper limb function.

As postural control can be at different motor levels to hand function, therapy and management is planned to accommodate this discrepancy using appropriate support. It is essential to develop fine motor ability in its specific developmental levels as:

(1) Use of hands is helpful for perceptual development, cognitive development and for communication with and without augmentative and alternative communication aids, including computers. The use of gestures and development of as much self-care as possible are essential. All these activities provide emotional

satisfaction and socialisation of the child (see Chapter 10).

(2) Use of hands is particularly important for a child with motor disabilities so that he can use them for support on open hands or grasp in order to support himself to sit, stand, walk or pull himself into any position.

(3) Hands can be used to help establish shoulder girdle stability which is fundamental to many of the fine and gross motor skills. This is distal to proximal control and different to the proximal to distal traditional sequence used in the past. Observation of able-bodied babies reveals hand use in breastfeeding, thumb sucking and hand placing when the dorsum of the baby's hand is touched against a table/toy. Children with dyskinesia first benefit using maintained hand grasp to stabilise shoulder and trunk. Depending on a task, both proximal to distal and vice versa in upper limb function is used in therapy. The principle of proximal-to-distal development does not apply in upper limb function in cerebral palsy.

(4) Abnormal patterns may not only be due to spasticity, athetosis or ataxia, but include arm and hand patterns seen in able-bodied children at an early age of development and not at the chronological age of the individual with cerebral palsy. These are outlined below and there may be much variation between individuals.

(5) Hand function development may not be in agreement with developmental levels of gross motor function (see Chapter 1) (Eliasson *et al.* 2006).

Aims

Upper limbs and the postural mechanisms.
(1) Establish head control (stability and movement) for hand/eye coordination.

(2) Establish postural stability and weight shift of head, shoulder girdle, trunk and pelvis in many gross motor activities in prone, supine, sitting, standing and stepping, which are also necessary for hand function. This allows arm and hand function in postures other than in lying.

(3) Develop particular stabilisation of the whole body, shoulder girdle stabilisation on arm/forearm support and wrist stabilisation with fine motor activity. Non-slip surfaces,

stable furniture and stabilising of objects by child or therapist need to accompany training. For example, body, shoulder and wrist need to stabilise for pouring liquids onto a stable container.

(4) Decrease manual or other supports in developmental stages, especially in sitting, standing and upright kneeling, so anticipatory postural control (counterpoising) is associated with arm and hand function. If not, essential anticipatory postural adjustment for daily function remains dormant (Fig. 9.185). There is more support when a child concentrates on new or difficult skills. The supports or straps in chairs and standing equipment are increased at such times. Some therapists use two chairs, one for learning postural control (balance) with hand function and the other with more support for hand function in feeding, finer skills, communication aids and switches and for speech therapy.

(5) Develop rising reactions. Hands and arms are used to help in the change of various postures or the assumption of posture in gross motor development. A child also needs to assume a position in which he will carry out his chosen task in various environments.

(6) Develop saving reactions in the arms. The upper limbs are thrown into various patterns involving active contractions of the muscles in synergies (patterns) to save and prop the child as he falls off balance. Although the hands and arms participate in *automatic* saving and propping reactions as well as in various rising reactions, these will rarely be enough to contribute to *voluntary* movements. Voluntary movements of reach, grasp and release have to be specially trained in fine motor activities and may find a variety of synergies necessary.

(7) Some of the arm synergies trained for gross motor function are also used in voluntary reach (Fig. 9.186). However, these patterns need to be practised in the context in which they are used in daily tasks. There is then integration with sensation, perception and understanding. If the task is chosen by a child, or special interest is shown by the child, then emotional satisfaction, motivation and social needs are satisfied.

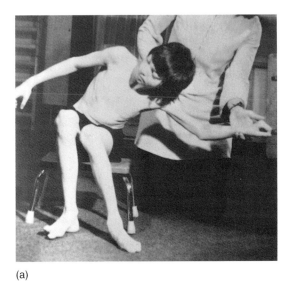
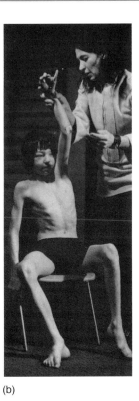

(a)   (b)

Figure 9.185   Training reach (strength, synergy and postural control). (a) Absence of counterpoising in the trunk leads to child falling over the arm during its movement. *Note* attempts to counterpoise with the better arm or by grasp or arm support by child is used initially and progressed to trunk adjustment without arm support or grasp. (b) The trunk is counterpoising the arm movement. Patterns of arm movements should be trained together with counterpoising, in all positions. *Note* the height of the chair controls the position of the legs. A lower chair should be used to prevent any extensor activity in legs, to stabilise the child or to diminish athetosis.

Upper limbs and abnormal motor behaviour.

(1) Treat abnormal postures of the whole child including the abnormal postures of the arms and hands (Figs 9.187–9.189). Improving posture of the whole child often positively improves the arms. Conversely, correcting postures and arm patterns improve the rest of the child (Fig. 9.190). Deformities are minimised by specific arm actions avoiding secondary deformity. The aim is to minimise deformities and prevent secondary impairments in hands which may block further function. However, in severe children or adolescents some abnormal hand postures have been used effectively for function. For example, palmar flexion to open a tightly flexed hand and grasping with marked wrist dorsiflexion.

(2) Consider how to decrease involuntary movements in the hands or whole arm which disrupt hand function. These involuntary movements may stem from the whole body. There may be involuntary motion in another part, for example the 'kicking about' of legs or sudden extension of legs hitting tables, which disturb the use of the hands.

(3) Counteract any abnormal asymmetries. For example, only one side is used; fisting of one hand is greater. Various visual problems affect one side and reaching across to the opposite side. There are desirable asymmetries when a child stabilises on one arm whilst using the other more able or dominant arm.

(4) Develop the ability to rotate trunk and shoulder girdle to reach across the midline. This

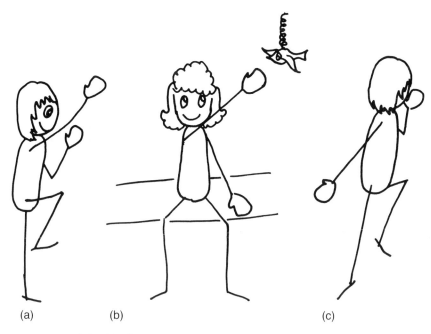

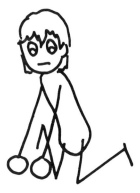

(a)   (b)   (c)

Figure 9.186   (a) Arm pattern of shoulder flexion–adduction–external rotation trained within training of rolling. (b) To reach a toy in lying or sitting. (c) Arm pattern of shoulder extension–adduction–internal rotation within rolling prone to supine, or within creeping pattern in prone, may be used in reaching back and behind child as, say, in putting on a coat.

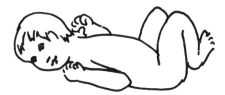

Figure 9.187   Shoulders protracted or retracted with arms flexed–adducted and hands clenched in a predominantly flexed child similar to the newborn. Inability to reach out or can only reach near his body. Problems of release occur if hands flex or clench excessively. Asymmetry may exist with visual input only available from hand on one side.

Figure 9.188   Arms flexed–adducted and internally rotated with elbows flexed and pronated, wrists flexed or mid-position and hands clenched or open. Shoulder flexion–adduction–internal rotation may also occur with elbow extension-pronation. Shoulder flexion–adduction may also occur with elbow supination and flexion in children with dyskinesia who *fold their arms in* towards their bodies.

first develops in supine and much later, between 2 and 3 years, in sitting and standing.

Basic arm and hand patterns for all levels of development

Although one should not be dogmatic about the pattern in which a child uses his arms and hands to achieve his goal, it is important to select corrective patterns below in treatment because:

(a) Abnormal patterns can be inefficient. However, some are efficient because they are easier for cerebral palsied children, but they offer a limited repertoire. These grasps are not suitable for

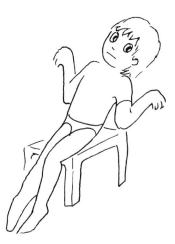

Figure 9.189 Arms held up in the air in abduction–external rotation, elbow flexion and supination with palms facing toward the child. Elbows may also be flexed and pronated with palms facing outward. Hand may be hanging down or clenched; this is also called the *bird-wing position* and is seen in supine, sitting and standing positions. This may alternate with an asymmetrical tonic neck reaction or other asymmetry. There is inability to reach forward, bring hands together and develop *hand regard* and bring hands down for support.

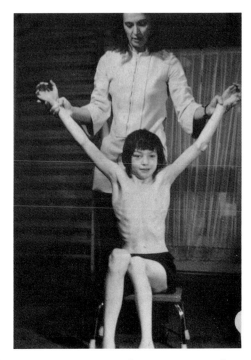

Figure 9.190 Correction of asymmetry of arms, flexion–adduction–internal rotation and other abnormal postures of the arms also corrects abnormal postures of head and trunk (kyphosis, kyphoscoliosis) and vice versa. *Note* child tries to maintain postural fixation in vertical alignment and not fall backward against the therapist. Use arm elevation for dressing, ball play and other activities.

more developmentally advanced tasks and for different situations. The repetition of cerebral palsy grasps tends to create deformities which often make control more difficult.

(b) The child with poor hand use has much less sensory experience or perhaps loss of sensation. He may have no idea on how to move and needs training in basic neuromuscular patterns. He may later modify these patterns within his individual development and discover what he finds as the most effective hand use through experience and learning. Visual impairments or other perceptual difficulties result in the choice of atypical or very clumsy hand function.

There are atypical grasps I have observed in various able-bodied receptionists and bank clerks which are efficient for writing. There is an adapted tripod grasp, finger–thumb and lower fingers 4-point grasp and pen held between index and long fingers and pressure of thumb beneath them.

Constraint-induced movement therapy

This is a treatment for hemiplegia based on the view that the affected arm and hand are restricted because of lack of experience and practice (Taub *et al.* 2004; Gordon *et al.* 2005; Charles *et al.* 2006). Therapy involves restriction of the unimpaired limb so the child has to use the affected arm to carry out tasks and so enhance perceptual-motor function and motor learning with that arm and hand. Therapists following DeLuca *et al.* (2003) have modified the plaster of Paris restraint on the uninvolved upper limb. A thermoplastic paddle splint restricts the hand and wrist within a puppet, so bilateral propping and assisting support by the uninvolved side can take place. The splint is contained within a puppet. This is for 2 hours every day for 4 weeks while engaging the child in interesting one or two-handed tasks. Others have used an arm sling, ski-glove or mitten on the uninvolved hand. In the past, therapists have regularly offered toys and other items on the side of the hemiplegia with their fairly unobtrusive holding of the uninvolved arm. Although the initial research was with a plaster on the uninvolved limb in order to gain intensive motor function in the involved arm, this approach is now more child friendly. However, therapy needs to be intensive with significant commitment of the family and carers. Care is taken not to frustrate a child with difficult tasks, and the family advises when it is best to trial this technique. The theory which has been proved is clearly that active function and practice improves motor control.

Charles and Gordon (2005) have carried out a critical review of constraint-induced movement therapy, and Steenbergen and Gordon (2006) have reviewed evidence that lack of arm function may be due to impairments in movement planning which are improved by bilateral hand function. The less involved hand activates motor planning in the hemiplegic side.

0–3-month normal developmental level

Common problems

Delay in eye focusing, visual fixation, visual following of an object. Clenched hands; thumb still held in palm. Opening begins and continues into next stage.

Abnormal performance. See abnormal patterns of arms and hand in supine, prone, sitting and standing above. If a child has hypersensitive palms, this can be associated with lack of experience in using the hands.

Reflex reactions. Grasp reflex, Moro reaction, tonic neck reaction, flexor or extensor spasms.

Treatment suggestions and management

Eye focus and following (hearing and vision)

(1) First offer visual interest in the midline and help the child keep his head in midline. You may need to hold both his shoulders forward, occasionally backward to allow him to keep his head upright (see sitting development, vertical head control; prone development, head control).

(2) At first, place your face or toys close to the child's eyes at about 8 in. (20 cm) from him.

Then gradually move further away with encouragement to follow you.

(3) Eye-to-eye contact is of first importance before interest in objects. This is best done at the child's eye level whether he is in side lying, supine, prone, supported sitting or supported standing.

(4) Associate vision, hearing and head control with face-to-face singing, talking. Vary tones of voice. Encourage a smile and general communication as he attends, follows and looks for your *voice*.

(5) Help him to look at and follow your face and then at shiny, moving, colourful noise-making mobiles, toys, fishes in a tank, marble runs, a torch light. Use coloured ribbons, Christmas decorations, shiny bottle lids and also objects which do not make any sounds. Following a visual lure on its own is more difficult for some children.

(6) Use red, yellow or primary colours and black and white pictures.

(7) Use jingling noises and not high-pitched or sudden loud noises as the child may still have a startle reflex.

(8) Hang tinkling bells, jingling beads or mobiles in the window or doorway, so they make a sound as the wind blows. Guide any visually directed early arm reaching with full body support of child (von Hofsten 1992).

(9) Put him in different positions, but start with well-supported upright sitting as well as lying on his back, side or stomach to carry out active looking and listening activities.

Use of vision is fundamental for hand function. There is therefore delayed development in children with visual impairment.

3–5-month normal developmental level

Common problems

Delay in hand regard, visual exploration; bringing hands together and to mouth, touching self. Delay in active grasp of an object placed in his hand, and delay in grasp and shake a toy. There is delay in early clumsy, random reaching for objects. Grasp is normally on the ulnar side of a hand, and this palmar grasp uses fingers but not thumb at this level. The clutching of child's hands on clothes on himself

Table 9.4   Development of hand function and eye–hand coordination (assessment guide).

0–3 months
Eye-to-eye contact (parallel eyes)
Fixes eyes on light; eyes follow object to midline (1 month), to past midline (2 months), over 180° (3 months), eyes down, then up hands opening from closed posture

Reflex reactions: Tactile grasp; stretch grasp; blink; doll's eye reflex. Moro, ATNR, reflex hand flare open

3–5 months
Grasps with his eyes when interested in object
Hand regard or studies his hands, brings hands together in midline, clutches and unclutches hands
Visual exploration of environment, visual tracking targeting and visual directed reach begins, swipes at objects when lying.
Clumsy reaching, bilateral; corralling an object; early hand shaping to object
Clutches clothes; touches body, mouth, face
Grasps object placed in hand; abducted thumb
Reflex reactions: Moro, ATNR disappearing, absence of grasp reflex

5–7 months
Reaching successfully in all directions, depending on trunk balance often trunk stable
Bilateral reach, unilateral reach; anticipatory excessive MP/finger extension
Grasps feet in supine and sitting – bilateral then unilateral; thumb pressed into opposition
Maintains grasp (grip) on stationary object
Ulnar grasp changing to palmar grasp; wrist flexed becomes straight
Mirror movements of grasp in the other hand
Moves head to see things, eyes converge and focus on pellet at 10 feet; smaller pellets seen by 9 months (Sheridan 1977); rakes pellet with flexing–adducting thumb, raking actions of all fingers. Thumb out of palm.

Continues to mouth everything, hand to mouth movement with object
Reflex reactions: Saving and propping downward, forward and beginning laterally; posteriorly later (12 months)

7–9 months
Transfers object from hand to hand
Unilateral reach and grasp; wrist extends trunk weight shift sitting alone
Radial grasp, beginning use of fingertips with opposed thumb
Holds one block while given another
Offers cube, but cannot release it; drops objects
Releases cube by pressing it against a hard surface
Bangs two objects together; compares them. Use sticks to bang all over a large surface
Pats, bangs, strokes, clutches, rakes, scratches – pats mother's face, pats image of face in mirror; thumb abducted or opposed

9–12 months
Protrudes index finger, pokes objects with finger, other fingers flexing
Grasps between fingers and thumb, then one finger and thumb (crude to fine pincer grasp)
Pick up and place in and out of large containers, then smaller containers; places lids
Reach and grasp possible in all directions, with supination and improved control of shoulder, arm; appropriate anticipatory grasp
Release with gross opening of hand, then more precise until places small objects in jar, peg in hole, for appropriate anticipatory release
Looks for fallen toy (permanence of objects); casts toys
Reflex reactions: Saving and propping backwards behind child; lateral and oblique

Table 9.4   (*Continued*)

12–18 months
Casting of toys stopping; mouthing stopping
Watches small toy moved across room up to 12 feet
Builds tower of two cubes; places pellet into bottle
Pushes and pulls large toys
Drinks alone from cup, often spills
18 months–2 years
Delicate pincer grasp and release
Takes off shoes, socks, vest, hat
Turns pages of book
Strings large beads, later smaller beads (29–36 months)
Scribbles with pencil; whole hand grasp, supinated
Feeds self clumsily
Hand preference more obvious

2 years
Pencil grasp, pronated fingers, wrist deviates
Throws ball inaccurately
Unwraps sweet
Screws and unscrews lids, toys
Imitates vertical line; scribbles and dots

3 years
Takes off all clothes, puts on most clothes
Feeds self completely, using fork
Copies line, circle; static tripod pencil grasp
Draws a man simply
Cuts with scissors
Washes alone

4 years
Draws simple house, more detailed man
Brushes teeth, dresses alone except for buttons and laces
Constructive building, including three steps with cubes
Matches and names four colours
Copies cross; static tripod grasp modified

5 years
Copies square, triangle, letters; dynamic tripod pencil grasp
Matches 12 colours
Drawing and copying improved
Uses knife and fork
Dresses and undresses completely

Note: Assessment measures of detailed hand function interwoven with conceptual, perceptual and ADL development are carried out by occupational therapists and psychologists. (See also the section 'Physical ability assessment guide' in Appendix 1, and sections on developmental stages of feeding, speech and language, dressing, play and perception in Chapter 10.)

or mother may be delayed. Hands are fully opened by this developmental level.

Abnormal performance. Asymmetrical bringing of hands to midline; beginning of reach or a grasp is mainly, or only, on one side. Child is touching with semi-flexed or closed hand. Sensory experience is therefore limited.

Abnormal patterns in reaching becoming more obvious in the next level. Imprecise clumsy reach is normal at this level. Abnormal grasps also becoming more obvious at the next level. The early ulnar or lateral grasp is not abnormal at this level.

Treatment suggestions and management

Hand regard and bringing hands to midline and early reach to a visual stimulus:

(1) Place the child in side lying or lying equipment, or in well-supported sitting, with shoulders brought forward and both arms placed in front of child's eyes. Have a child sitting and leaning with his body against the table with arms along the surface for easier movement with such support. Guide early visually directed reaching along a surface. In supine, reach sideways from child's body, along the ground. A side-lying board is helpful to bring hands into view for those children who persist in keeping their arms in abduction, extended bilateral or asymmetrical patterns and well back out of their view (see supine development in Fig. 9.68a–d, and in sitting and standing equipment).

(2) Once his hands are in front of him, the child can be made aware of them by your touch and songs, shining a torch on them, putting stickers of stars or pictures on his hands, playing with his fingers, putting thimbles, rings, coloured ribbon, bracelets or bells on the wrist and fingers. Continue guided reach along a surface at a table or in supine along floor, for severely visually impaired children.

Opening of hands

Opening of flexed hands are fully achieved at this level which is a necessary aspect for the development of release. Later active hand opening to grasp size and shape of an object will be needed. There may be a *total inability to let go of* an object placed or grasped with excessive flexion by the child after 5-month developmental level. See correction of whole

child's postures in all developmental levels, as these also correct arms and hands.

The following are suggestions:

(1) Gradually desensitise a child's whole palm by rubbing it with rough textures, especially sand, during play activities. Help him open his hands and rub his palms together, move his hands to stroke and touch his face and body and guide clapping hands, patting the table and making handprints in sand, soaped surface and with painted hands on paper. Weight bearing on hands on different surfaces, with or without stroking of the surface with one hand, integrates sensory and perceptual experiences. Later improve active hands held open by assisting interlocking of fingers in a clasp pressing together heel of hands. Children learn to do this alone if practised by them.

(2) Rhythmical shaking of a child's arm to relax it but without shaking all of him.

(3) Stroke the ulnar and dorsal aspect of the hand which activates flaring open of little finger and hands.

(4) You or the child may press the heel of his hand down on a firm surface combined with his weight bearing on that arm. Use a lower stool to place his hands open with your giving pressure (joint compression) through a straight shoulder and extended elbow (Fig. 9.205). Use a child's weight bearing on elbows and/or on hands to decrease hand clenching, within prone, sitting and standing development.

(5) Hold the child's upper arms rotating the limbs into external rotation. Children with less severity may only need to have the forearm supinated, so the palm faces up. The child actively turns his elbow into supination as far as he can to hold a toy, ball or see a picture drawn on his hand.

(6) Have the child's arms well away from his body. This avoids clenching in some children. Open the child's hand over a variety of textures such as velvet, rubber, wooden or plastic. *Do avoid textures or* toys which stimulate clenching, such as 'squeezy' toys.

(7) Open hands when child is prone leaning on elbows or hands, on hands and knees, sitting lean on hands and standing lean on hands. Open his hands by any of the above methods pressing the

heel of the hand down. Pull the thumb or fingers out from the base and not from their tips.

(8) Hands may open within the arm pattern of elevation–abduction–external rotation, or extension–adduction–internal rotation in techniques of creeping, rolling and reaching out in lying, and fully supported sitting during reach described in the next level.

Hand grasps

Begin developing hand grasps at this level and continue into levels 5–7 months according to capacity.

Use above-mentioned methods to open hands just before hand grasp development. Also, begin active grasp training before grasp reflex has fully disappeared.

(1) Place different objects before him so that he chooses what he prefers. Let him clutch materials and toys which are soft and easy to clutch. Start with objects of different sensations, for example beanbags, fur, velvet and suede objects, sandpaper, crinkling chocolate paper, shoe brushes, wooden, metal and natural objects. Use sand and water, dough, clay and modelling materials. Name these sensations for him as he feels them. Invite a child to have his hands in a bowl of dry beans or leaves, cones or other natural objects. Supervise a child in case small objects are taken to his mouth. Mouthing is useful for objects that cannot be swallowed!

(2) Depending on children's ages, offer teething toys, hoops, quoits (rubber rings), rattles, toy dumb bells, small balls, thick tubing with coloured liquid inside, cotton reels, sponge rubber toys. Avoid either squeezy or tiny toys.

(3) Have a variety of objects that fit into the whole palm of his hand, so they are not too big for his small hands. Grasping a cone with the large end on the side of his little finger often helps to overcome hand clenching (Fig. 9.203). Some children first learn to grasp soft objects more easily than hard ones or vice versa. At this level a child cannot grasp objects smaller or much larger than his palm.

(4) Light objects are often easier than heavy ones. Later strength increases with graded heavy objects.

(5) Place his hands around large hand grips, handles, bars, so as a result he can sit up, kneel up or stand up or enjoy a ride on a tricycle, swing, rocking horse or see-saw.

(6) Thicken handles of spoons, pencils, toys with rubber, hardened clay, wood, a rubber ball or attach handles from, say, screwdrivers. Use a cone to place fingers on the larger side so that they are opened up with thumb and index meeting. Reverse to fingers on the smaller side of the cone so that fingers and thumb are opened.

(7) Continue to look at what he is grasping as some children with cerebral palsy have persistent head turning away from what they are doing.

(8) Encourage the child to hold rusks or spoon in feeding. Hold his hand on the spoon handle. Encourage him to hold a piece of his clothing as you help him undress, to hold his sponge in the bath or hold his wet washcloth. If he has bent fingers, stretch them out onto a cloth between fingertips and thumb and progress to pulling off clothes, pulling up trouser tops.

(9) Besides placing objects of different shapes in his hand, make sure that he has had adequate mouthing experience to understand them. Help him to grasp and bring objects to his mouth to suck, lick, bite or chew, or to his nose to smell.

(10) Develop *grasp and press*, say, a bath sponge or large woollen pom-pom; *grasp and shake* a toy, rattle or maracas; *grasp and wave* a toy flag, ribbons, bells. *Grasp and drop* is present, but it is not grasp and release yet. *Grasp and pull or rake* one end of a soft cloth with a small toy on the other end which encourages the child to pull the toy towards him.

5–7-month normal developmental level

Common problems

Delay in successful reaching in all or one direction, voluntary grip, palmar grasp, and use of both hands, more accurate reach and grasp, taking weight on one or both hands. Dropping of the object is normal but by 7 months a child usually holds a second block in the same hand and does not drop the first. Delay in hand to mouth activities to *mouth* everything; in bilateral then unilateral grasp of his feet, to play with his toes.

Abnormal performance. There may be persistence of abnormal patterns from the 3–5-month level. Abnormal hand grasps, reaching actions and release are discussed below.

Reflex reactions. Saving reaction in arms down and forward is expected.

Treatment suggestions and management

Reaching actions

Reaching accurately depends on vision, proprioception and postural stability of trunk and shoulder girdle and counterpoising of the arm as well as perceptual abilities of direction and size of an object.

Range of motion and adequate strength of arm are relevant to a task.

Although these are discussed at this developmental level, the methods need to be continued at future levels depending on the tasks and an individual's difficulties.

There are various arm patterns, or individual joint motions, which can be found and which also correct abnormal synergies. Select those which are directly related to use of the arms *in function*. Basic arm patterns (mainly taken from PNF – Adler *et al.* 2008) which do this are:

(1) Shoulder flexion, elbow extension, pronation, hands open or grasp (Fig. 9.191).
(2) Diagonal, shoulder elevation–abduction–external rotation, elbow extension or flexion, supination, hands and thumbs open (Fig. 9.192) for reaching upwards, for example, to dress, brush hair with elbow flexing.
(3) The opposite diagonal to (2) is down into adduction–internal rotation, elbow pronation, hand closed (Fig. 9.193) or open for reaching downwards for object or self-care.
(4) Diagonal flexion–adduction–external rotation, elbow supination, flexed or extended (Figs 9.194 and 9.195) for example, touching face, mouth or hair in self-care including wash or wipe mouth, face and nose.
(5) The opposite diagonal to (4) is arm extension–abduction–internal rotation (Fig. 9.196), elbow pronation, hand closed, or open (Figs 9.196 and 9.197), for example, to reach into coat sleeve or pick up an object.
(6) Besides alternating diagonal patterns, useful arm actions are also alternating arm flexion

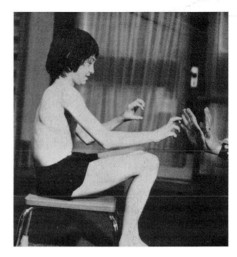

Figure 9.191 An individual boy attempting basic pattern of bilateral shoulder flexion with elbow extension and dorsiflexion of the hands. This pattern not only corrects many abnormal patterns as in Figs 9.187–9.189 but is functionally useful, for example shoulder flexion, elbow extension, hands flat or grasping support for sitting and standing well; in movements to reach for shoes or socks down at his feet, in pulling off a jumper over his head, reaching down to pull up pants or to push them down to his ankles. *Note:* Hands in poor anticipatory action.

with extension as in cleaning a mirror/window or wiping the floor or table top.

There are *many variations* on the basic patterns described above. However, they do not reinforce the patterns a child with cerebral palsy may already be using. They offer variety as well as to correct dynamic deformity.

Practical points

Positions. Carry out the reaching patterns in all positions given in gross motor levels:

0–5 months. Arm reach in side lying, supine, prone on elbows.
5–7 months. Arm reach in prone, supine, rolling and then reaching, or arm reaching to roll, lying reaching up against gravity. Reach with one arm in sitting while propped on the other hand.
7–9 months. Arm reach in crawl position, 'on hands' or in upright kneeling, with child supporting on the other arm.

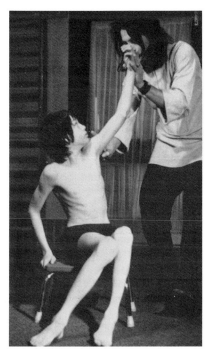

Figure 9.192 Arm elevation–abduction–external rotation corrects abnormal patterns in Figs 9.187–9.189 and is used to reach out for an object, to dress or brush hair (elbow flexion/extension).

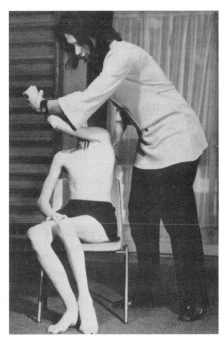

Figure 9.194 Arm pattern flexion–adduction–external rotation corrects arm patterns in Figs 9.187–9.189 and is used to reach for an object, touch own face, blow nose, dress or eat.

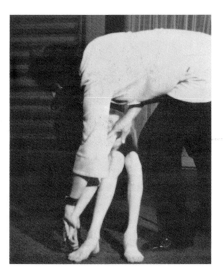

Figure 9.193 Arm pattern adduction–internal rotation corrects abnormal arm pattern in Fig. 9.189 and is used to reach down for an object, dress, wash and other functions.

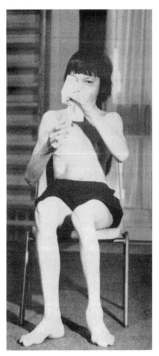

Figure 9.195 Arm pattern in use for wiping nose or face (from Fig. 9.194).

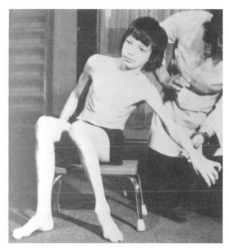

Figure 9.196 Arm extension abduction–internal rotation corrects arm patterns in Figs 9.187–9.189 and can be used for dressing, reaching out and pulling trolleys in play.

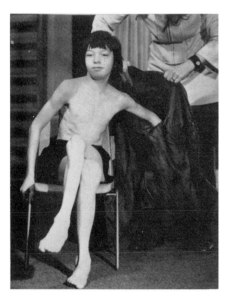

Figure 9.197   Arm pattern in Fig. 9.196 in use for putting on a jacket.

9–12 months. Arm reach while sitting independently, in upright kneeling or standing *holding* on with one hand.
Over 12 months. Arm reach in standing alone.

Reach, grasp and later reach and grasp and release of objects that interest child are practised in these positions. Trunk rotation with reaching must be in-cluded, especially if resistance is given to the child's arm movement, or heavy objects are lifted. Start in well-supported positions for success and progress to less support to challenge a child.

Direction of reach is first in midline, low down, then horizontal and forward at shoulder level, to the side, above him, and then behind him. This progression is easiest for most children. It uses gravity to help or challenge a child. However, active or supported postural control is needed.

Facilitation. Arm patterns can be facilitated with a variety of methods. For example:

(1) Touch, pressure stretch and resistance and good rotation of the child's shoulder girdle and/or trunk.
(2) The therapist may manually rotate the shoulder girdle, protract shoulders forward or retract shoulders backward to initiate automatic arm patterns in creeping and rolling techniques (see discussion on creeping patterns in prone development, 0–3 months and reflex rolling in supine development). This activates arm synergies and ranges of motion which may be useful for reaching for toys in severely involved children.
(3) It is preferable to develop reaching to grasp/touch food, for toys or take part in a play activity selected to activate specific arm patterns (Figs 9.191, 9.195–9.199).
(4) The child can be asked to concentrate on strengthening the arm for reaching, for example 'stretch your arm up and back', 'stretch your

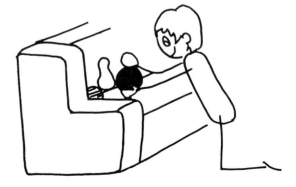

Figure 9.198 Both arms stretch towards toys and palms face inwards to hold toys. In this way, elbow extension, supination is encouraged and simultaneously corrects abnormal motor patterns. *Note* that the rest of the body is also in better alignment associated with a better arm pattern (synergy). Use of *both* arms corrects asymmetry particularly in hemiplegia.

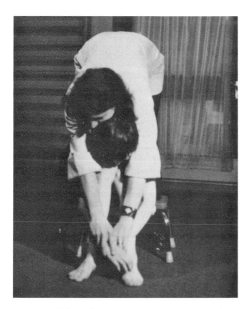

Figure 9.199 Bilateral arm patterns against appropriate manual resistance in diagonal patterns. Use to reach feet or floor for daily activities. Postural mechanism is also assisted.

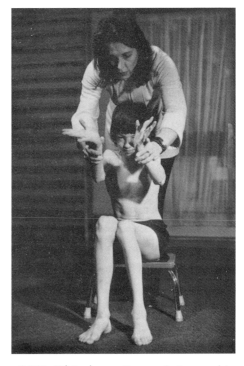

Figure 9.200 Bilateral arm patterns against appropriate manual resistance in diagonal patterns. Note facilitation of wrist extension.

elbow'. However, only draw his attention to the pattern once he is clearly working towards his interest (goal) for reaching or within chosen task.

(5) The daily activities of feeding, dressing, washing, bathing may use many desirable arm patterns including those described. Activities are carefully designed to be of interest to a child or older person.

Vision and arm reach. It is important to continue developing the child's visual abilities and to associate it with development of hand functions. A child's eyes need to focus, track and maintain attention on the object while looking from hand to object. Encourage a child to look at the hands and object and later a child looks at the object using proprioception to guide reach (Case-Smith 1993). Make sure his postural control is available and give support when necessary.

Unilateral and bilateral arm patterns need to be included in the programme. For example:

(1) Unilateral patterns such as moving one side only; leaning on one hand and move with the other; grasp a support with one hand and move the other (normal asymmetrical work) (Figs 9.192–9.197) and grasp or fix and steady an object with one hand to allow the other hand to manipulate it. Apply in daily tasks with all children, particularly in those with hemiplegia and dyskinesia.

(2) Bilateral patterns with both a child's arms in the same direction (bilateral and symmetrical) for support and for motion. This takes place to counteract abnormal asymmetry during function, involving the whole body (Figs 9.198–9.200). Use a child's less affected arm together with affected arm for symmetrical pushing of walkers, balls or grasping a stick. Activation of a hemiplegic arm takes place in such activities.

(3) Bilateral patterns with each arm in opposite directions (bilateral and reciprocal). This takes place in creeping, reciprocal arm swing, or motion using play equipment, pulleys or hand pedals.

(4) Bilateral patterns with each arm in a different direction, for example one sideways, the other forward (bilateral and asymmetrical), which is used in advanced perceptual motor training and

for highly complicated counterpoising activities and hand skills.

Abnormal hand grasps

(1) Abnormal grasp may be present in association with the total abnormal posture or only with the arm posture when the rest of the body functions well.
(2) Limited joint motion, weakness and problems with isolated finger, thumb movements are all found in abnormal grasps.
(3) Grasp may appear to be abnormal because it belongs to a lower normal level of development.
(4) Anticipatory grasp is distorted by inability to open clenched hands and by intellectual delay. Lack of experience in hand use also causes such delay. Proprioception, perceptual discrimination and cognitive abilities are essential for anticipatory shaping a hand according to an object's features and for fingers' force to be regulated according to different objects.

Treatment suggestions for some abnormal grasps

Grasp only possible in one position of the child's arm. Train grasp within all the corrective arm patterns (above, in different directions, and body positions). Movements to increase range, weakness and isolated finger and thumb exercises may contribute to hand grasp and release. However, activities directly related to tasks are more important and may well treat these problems at the same time.

Wrist flexion with palmar or pincer grasp or inability to grasp in this position (Fig. 9.201). Press the child's wrist down as he tries to grasp; place the object above the level of his wrist; ask him to lift his hands to the object (see Figs 9.200 and 9.203). Some children may need a wrist splint to train grasp with wrist in midline or extension (dorsiflexion). In some children with hypertonus, the wrist extension needs to be only at mid-position as there is excessively tight finger flexion with full wrist extension. This also prevents the child from opening his hands to release the object held.

The Lycra hand and wrist splint, or arm splint and a flexible splint encouraging midline and dorsiflexion, are used to decrease excessive palmar flexion. There are various hand and arm splints on the market requiring consultation with occupational therapists. Splints can be tailor-made with thermoplastic and other materials. They are pre-

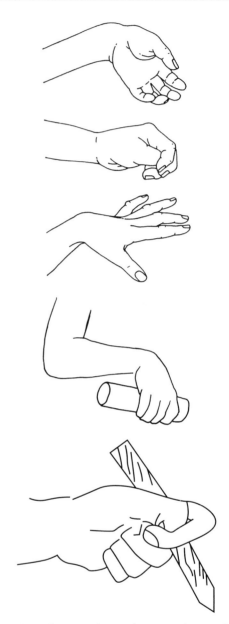

Figure 9.201   Common abnormal patterns of arm, wrist and hand.

scribed and made by paediatric occupational therapists. Clenched hands and flexed wrists may persist and make cleaning of hands difficult. BTX A and casting or splinting is mentioned in Chapter 11.

The use of glove puppets, hammering, lifting dowels out of holes, rings off a stick and similar activities may help to gain active wrist extension for grasp and release. In some cases, grasping with the wrist in

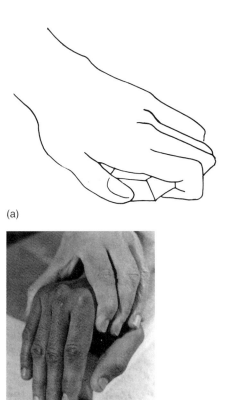

(a)

(b)

Figure 9.202 Abnormal grasp with excessive finger flexion and no flexion or even with hyperextension of metacarpo-phalangeal joint is being corrected by the therapist in (b) during lumbrical grasp and release.

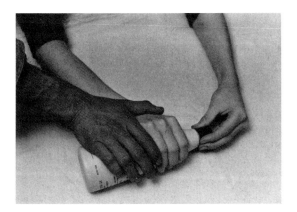

Figure 9.203 Overcoming excessive wrist flexion, overflex-ion of fingers by the task selected and the therapist pressing the wrist down. Press on a child's wrist as he grasps bars of walkers, spoons, cups and other tools.

extension may be achieved at the cost of opening the hand in this particular position.

Excessive finger flexion in grasp. With or without hyperextension of the metacarpo-phalangeal (m-p) joints (Figs 9.202 and 9.203). Place the child's hand over thick, larger objects such as bars and handles. Avoid the hand clenching onto squeezy toys. Hold the dorsum of the child's hand, lift his m-p joints and he or you can then press his fingers straight over the large ball, box or square bar. This may be done with the child's m-p joints pressing on the edge of a table as he tries to hold on to the edge, or the solid edge of a truck or box. Counteracting this abnormal grasp will prepare him for grasp with his fingers straight, using fingertips later. Grasping edges of cards or lids is one way of training this straight finger grasp.

Adducted *thumbs and ulnar grasp.* The adducted thumb may grasp or be useless. It can be seen with ulnar grasp (Fig. 9.201). In some children the ulnar grasp may result when the child tries to compensate for or avoid the adducted thumb. When the thumb is abducted, a radial grasp may occur. In other cases, the child grasps his fingers in mid-position with an adducted thumb. Adducted flexed thumbs (thumb tucking) may also accompany palmar flexion, or with excessive finger flexion (index curl grasp). The child should be encouraged to move his hand to-wards the thumb side, for example he pushes rolling toys away towards the radial side, brings a spoon-ful of food towards his mouth and other activities which encourage him to move his hand towards the thumb side. He may not manage this unless you hold his hand in midline during grasp. Hold the child's hand between his thumb and forefinger on one side and hold down the ulnar side as he grasps (Fig. 9.204).

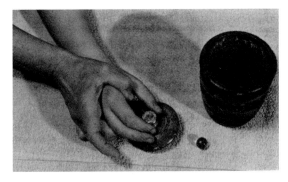

Figure 9.204 Guided abduction of thumb and pincer grasp.

The little finger and ring finger may be bandaged if the child does not resent such a procedure. Training grasping of objects with the radial side is then encouraged.

Check that the child is not given handgrips on walkers, handles and other supports which encourage an abnormal ulnar grasp. The handles at the sides of rollators or on crutches may do this. Avoid the angled spoons for those children where these utensils create an ulnar grasp.

There are splints to correct thumb positions designed and made by occupational therapists. For example, adducted thumbs may be held out with figure-of-eight thumb splints or made together with hand and wrist splint in a variety of materials.

Remember. To take an adducted thumb out of a fist or hand, never pull it by its tip or you may dislocate or sublux the m-p joint. Sometimes the other fingers flex more as you pull on the thumb. Rather turn the whole arm or forearm to face palm up to the ceiling and abduct the thumb out from its base. It is important to accompany this procedure with placing the child's hand over a toy, so teaching him a palmar or radial grasp. Some children can abduct their thumbs over the edge of a table with their hands pressed open on the top of the table. See 'Opening of hand' techniques; hand splints below.

Anticipatory grasp. The methods to reduce tight fingers and thumb contribute to opening of the hand to anticipate the size of object for grasping. More experiential learning is usually needed for practice with different sizes and weights of everyday objects (see developmental levels of 7–9 months). Check results of assessment tests for perception and cognition.

Inability to use both hands simultaneously. Although this is normal in many children under the 6-month developmental level, it may also be due to:

(1) Lack of head control in midline, so the child uses the hand that he can see; lack of midline head control in persistent head turning to one side. Head turn is sometimes easily overcome and may be spontaneous in babies.
(2) Asymmetrical tonic neck response to one side which is 'used' to reach to that side and when head turns away to grasp the object on the occipital side.

(3) Hemiplegia or greater involvement of one arm in any diagnostic type.
(4) Excessive spasms or involuntary motion on one side, in rare hemi-athetoids/dyskinesia.
(5) Sensory loss on one side especially astereognosis, two-point discrimination in the hand or visual field defect, usually found in some children with hemiplegia and tetraplegia.

During training of prone, supine, sitting and standing development check that both hands are given objects to grasp simultaneously or to grip for support. Use play activities which require two hands, for example play in water and washing, sand, clay, dough, larger toys, handles on bowls, rolling pins, sieves, sticks with dangling bells, broom, bicycle pump, toy concertina, small cymbals, maracas or toys which make a noise if pushed at both ends. Inability to grasp on one side will often result in the inability to hold with one hand and carry out an action with the other. Practise activities which include each hand in a different action, for example hold toy with one hand, carry out action with the other, winding a bandage or stabilising an object with one hand whilst the other is using various actions with that object. For example, stabilise a tin while the other opens the lid or lean on one hand to fix object during action with the other (Fig. 9.205). See developmental level for choice of play, use of hands in self-care.

Associated grasping or clenching on the child's affected side when grasping with the unaffected or the

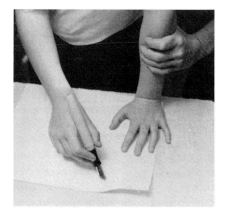

Figure 9.205 Support on more affected hand pressed open whilst child uses more skilful hand. Affected hand stabilises the paper or toy during use with the other hand.

less affected side. This is usually seen in the spastic type; associated *mirror* movements of the hand not in use are normally seen in very young children but disappear on normal development. If these mechanisms persist, they can prevent the child's transfer of objects from hand to hand and holding with one hand while using the other hand. Hold the more affected elbow straight with hand flat on the table while the other hand grasps. Try having the child lean on the more affected arm with hand open. Carry out joint compression to facilitate support on the more affected hand whilst the other hand is used by the child (Fig. 9.205).

Other parts of the body may also tense or assume abnormal postures during grasp. Check that these excessive motor activities are controlled as much as possible by the child with the assistance of the therapist. Assess whether better positioning or support with equipment for the rest of the body during hand function is needed. Motor tasks too advanced for an individual can increase excessive tension, grimacing, drooling or involuntary movements. Choice of developmental levels is important. See Fig. 9.206.

Involuntary motion disrupting hand use. Train conscious control of manipulation. With practice the involuntary motion is mastered by a child to a greater or lesser degree. The child, parent and therapist discover atypical ways in which control is achieved. Help the child by having him use his hands while leaning on his forearms, or reach for toys through a thin padded hoop which limits the excursion of the involuntary motion. Wide upright poles also limit his involuntary motion as he reaches between them for toys or objects. Use a dowel, stick, rubber ring for grasping and for important practice for maintained grasp. Maintained grasp with both or one hand also helps to stabilise the whole child. Select whole hand grasps in Fig. 9.206.

Note: All the patterns of grasp and release are also disrupted by visual loss, any sensory loss in the hands, cognitive delay, and by lack of visual, perceptual or perceptual-motor development as seen in intelligent 'clumsy' children (developmental incoordination disorder, dyspraxia).

Sensory loss of two-point discrimination in children predicts inability to adapt fingertip force to texture in manipulation (Lesny *et al.* 1993; Yekutiel *et al.* 1994). Gordon and Duff (1999) found that various impairments of grasp in children with hemiplegia relate more to sensory deficits than motor impairments.

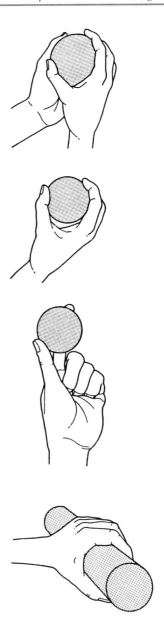

Figure 9.206 Grasp patterns.

7–9-month normal development level

Common problems

Delay in transfer from hand to hand, unilateral reach and grasp, grasp more than one block at a time, radial grasp, hand patting, banging, clutch, stroke, rake, scratch, bang two blocks together, release against a hard surface and use of hands in feeding and in holding on during sitting and standing.

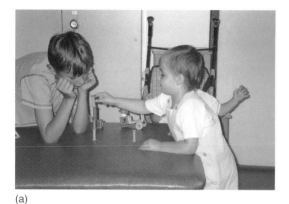

(a)

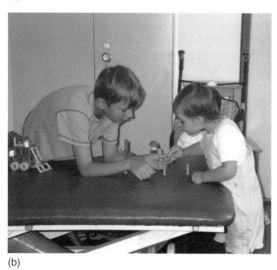

(b)

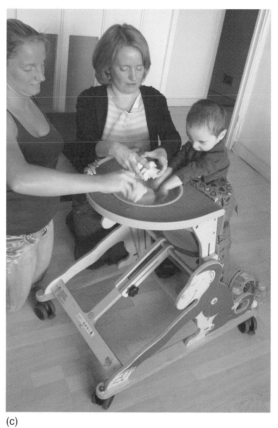

(c)

Figure 9.207   (a, b) Brother playing with sister (with cerebral palsy) activating pincer grasp and fine release. (c) Hand function during play in standing position. Promoting symmetry, hand opening, grasping toys of different sizes as well as socialisation. (Reproduced with the permission of Jenx, Sheffield.)

Scissors grasp (inferior pincer grasp) and use of fingertips may be delayed. Delay in anticipatory grasp in relation to size, shape, weight of object (9 months. See studies by von Hofsten & Ronnqvist 1988).

Reflex reactions. Saving and propping reactions are expected at these levels.

Treatment suggestions and management

(1) See methods above for reach, grasp and opening of hands.
(2) Train child's active grasp in feeding, dressing, washing, toileting (see Chapter 10). Begin training release by having the child release a block against a hard surface with the heel of his hand held down against the surface, or on his other

hand or on his body. Release may be impossible if hand opening has not yet been developed. See methods at 3–5-month level for training of hand opening.
(3) Ulnar grasp now develops into radial grasp.
(4) Transfer from hand to hand, using a firm rubber ring for palmar grasp and release. Then use a variety of objects. Practice banging blocks together and also holding on with one hand or leaning on one hand during unilateral banging, stroking, raking are particularly important for hemiplegia and for any child with asymmetrical function. Crude pincer grasp begins (Fig. 9.207).
(5) Play with suitable toys, dough, sand, water can involve transfer from hand to hand, grasping

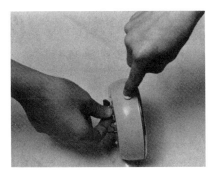

Figure 9.208 Developing index finger pointing and pressing and a fine pincer grasp during action of pull, push and later to turn object, as in screwing movement.

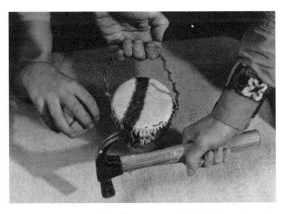

Figure 9.209 Some hand grasps to take hold of and to grip. Spherical with palm or fingertips only, hook grasp, cylindrical grasp. Others are lumbrical (Fig. 9.202), pincer (Figs 9.208 and 9.207) with sides and with tips of fingers. *Remember* to train grasps in vertical, pronated, supinated and other hand positions.

more than one object at a time as well as patting, banging, clutching, stroking, raking, scratching and release against a hard surface.

(6) Patting with open hands and other repetitive actions may become a persistent pattern in some children with severe learning problems or visual disability. Activities involving grasp and manipulation at the child's developmental level counteract these and other *mannerisms*.

9–12-month normal developmental level

Common problems

Delay in finger/thumb opposition and development of crude and fine pincer grasp, no protrusion of index finger. Delay in casting haphazardly and beginning to develop more control from 12 months. Delay of increasing control of accurate release into containers of different sizes and place peg in hole usually large. Delay in a child's searching for a fallen object, cast object or hidden object perceived immediately before disappearance (permanence of objects). Supination may not have developed. Delay in developing anticipatory grasp. Delay in improved shoulder, elbow and hand control. There may be delay in grasp and pull, grasp and push, and grasp and place using a variety of grasps and directions and containers.

Arm and hand saving and propping backwards is expected at this level.

Abnormal performance. There may be persistence of abnormal hand grasps, abnormal release and abnormal arm patterns.

Excessive avoiding reaction may prevent release becoming controlled as well as preventing main-

tained controlled grasp (casting toys is normal at this level of development but excessive hand splaying in extension is abnormal).

Treatment suggestions and management

Control of release

Release only possible if wrist is palmar flexed. The child may use his other hand, his chin or even his forehead, or a hard surface to press the back of his hand to obtain palmar flexion. Teach release with wrist in midline using a splint, manual support and active control by a child.

Release object against a hard surface after 11 months of age. These problems of release are discussed in the appropriate developmental levels below.

Release with thumb adducted and flexed in palm. Train a release with child's active hand opening together with thumb abduction following supination of the forearm by the therapist. Sometimes external rotation from the shoulder is indicated. Thumb splints may help. Isolated thumb abduction and extension is very difficult and is best acquired using larger objects placed in the hand.

Release with ulnar deviation can be improved if objects are released into container or dowel holes on the radial side of the hand.

Release with excessive splaying of the fingers, that is, hyperabduction with hyperextended m-p joints. A similar but less pronounced pattern is also seen in normal babies casting objects at about 11–15

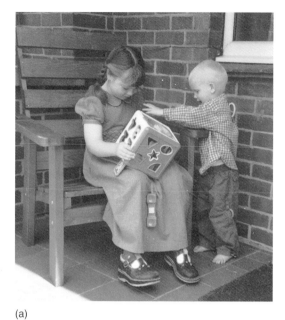
(a)

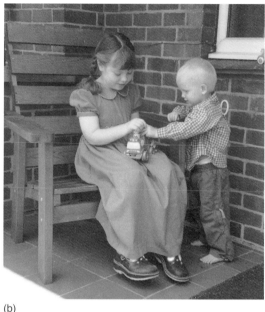
(b)

Figure 9.210   (a, b) Girl with right hemiplegia using both her hands as she assists her able-bodied brother.

months of age. In addition, this pattern is seen in excessive avoiding reactions in the hands of children with dyskinesia. There may also be plantar and/or a visual avoiding reaction with the avoiding reaction in the hands caused by tactile and visual stimuli, respectively. Grasp smaller objects and train release into a defined area or container. Hold the ulnar side of the child's hand and train release on the radial side and later with thumb and finger. Training a more precise release is closely allied with the training of pincer grasp (Fig. 9.207a,b).

Hand and visual avoiding reactions can be helped if one introduces the object slowly into the child's visual field and into his hands. Encourage him to maintain his grasp on a desired object to gradually assist him to become less sensitive to the stimuli. Avoid hand-over-hand method to maintain his grasp if he is sensitive. This is particularly unwise if a child is severely visually impaired and can lead to marked avoidance of touch on his hands. Allow to release in his own time with the reward of hearing an object drop. A light pressure on the dorsum of a child's hand helps release.

Conflict between grasp and release. This problem is seen in dyskinesia, when a person attempts to grasp an object but immediately withdraws his hand, splaying it open. This presents itself as a repeated involuntary motion in the hands. This con-

flict between the grasp reflex and the avoiding reactions in the athetoid type was described by Twitchell (1961). To break this disabling conflict, it is advisable to reinforce the child's active grasp or grip using your hand placed over his hand, or pressing an object gently against his palm with his wrist fixed on the table. Encourage maintained grasp for as much of the day as possible on bars, handles, in front, at his side, above or below him in his various situations during the day (Cotton 1980). When he is sitting in classrooms, toilets, at meals, in a buggy, place his hands to grasp bars. Frames or manual supported standing and walkers need to have bars for grasp.

Training of reach and grasp, especially grasp in supination and improving more accurate grasps.

Techniques in developmental levels above for reach and for grasp are now used to gain reach and grasp.

Problems in anticipatory reach and grasp formation and for force regulation can be due to poor understanding of the properties of an object. Perceptual and cognitive problems need assessment and intervention by psychologist and occupational therapist.

To develop fine grasp improve isolation of fingers and promote development of index finger action (see Figs 9.203–9.207a,b and 9.208).

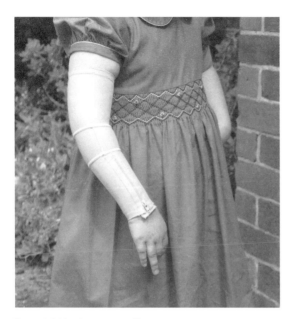

Figure 9.211 Lycra arm splint.

Use finger plays and action songs to isolate finger movements as, for example, 'walking' fingers on a table, pushing away an object using abduction of thumb, index or fifth finger are among many ideas which can be devised by you. Use *finger plays* particularly for index finger or middle finger in addition to other fingers.

Index finger approach to object, isolated finger pointing and pressing. If he cannot manage to isolate his index finger, hold his little, ring and middle finger flexed for him until he can do this alone (Fig. 9.204).

(1) Help the child to use toy telephones or ordinary telephones, using his index finger for dialling.
(2) Use index finger to press into dough, clay or sand. Later make lines and scribbles in sand.
(3) Put paint on fingertip and make dots and scribbles. A child enjoys popping soap bubbles with one finger.
(4) Press-studs on clothes should be attempted. Press small button or knob which obtains interesting sound or visual appearance as, say, a jack-in-the-box or other pop-up toys. Help him switch on radios, TV and electric lights. Press Velcro straps on clothes or his own orthoses.
(5) Use finger puppets.
(6) Practise on the keys of a piano, computer keyboard, cash register or with an abacus.

Finger pointing for communication and concentration in specific learning tasks in school is developed by speech and occupational therapists and teachers.

Pincer grasp. Begin with larger objects and then progress to smaller objects. Thumbs and all fingertips (Fig. 9.208) are used first before thumb and one finger, usually the index is used. (Crude and fine pincer grasp.) At first, steady the thumb against the table, and the child brings the index finger down to

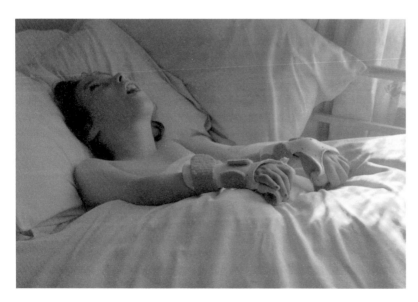

Figure 9.212 Hand splints.

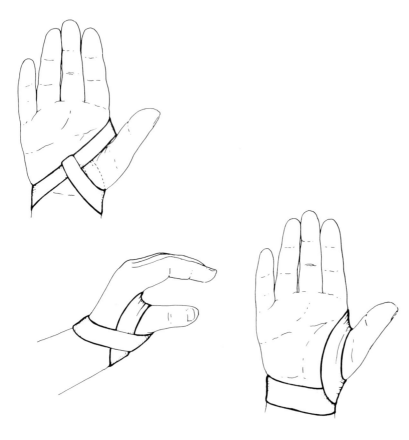

Figure 9.213 Thumb splint to correct adducted–flexed thumb. A cock-up wrist splint to midline may be incorporated if palm flexion is excessive. Figure-of-eight thumb splint at base of thumb and over the wrist in soft pigskin or simply a handkerchief may be adequate for babies and young children.

touch it imitating a pincer position. Then try lifting the hand off the support. Initially the grasp is with fingers and thumb and later index finger and thumb. Encourage raking small items towards him and into a container.

(1) Pick up pieces of cereals for young children, or small pieces of food or pasta and place in his mouth. The child may like to pick up buttons, wooden beads, marbles *under supervision* as he may pop them into his mouth to swallow them.
(2) Hold thick crayons and, if possible, pencils and thick chalk for making marks on paper or later writing with tripod grasp.
(3) Use toys with small knobs and of small size for fitting shapes.
(4) Hold small cup handles for drinking.
(5) Wind clock and turn its knobs, press alarm bell to stop, press doorbells. Various toys have knobs and buttons to press and turn. Use playdough, soft clay and with paint on the finger a child makes dots on paper.

(6) Begin screwing action with large screw-toys, large lids, etc. progress to medium and fine screwing later (usually around the 15th-month developmental level).
(7) Pincer grasp includes thumb tip to fingertip, thumb to index-and-middle finger together and a ('key') lateral thumb to index pinch. Pick a card out of its holder. Pull sticking labels off the surface and open small notebooks and wallets. Pull thick strings, ribbons pipe cleaners through large holes. For example, hold finger-to-thumb to create 'eye spectacles'.
(8) Develop a greater variety of grasps (Fig. 9.209 and your own ideas).

Continue training release. This involves dropping objects (beanbags) into container on the ground below his chair, in front of his chair, at the side and behind his chair. Help him look and see 'where it dropped'. Later encourage him to place small objects in smaller containers until he learns to fit a peg in a formboard and builds one block on top of the other. Precise release is required for building a tower of blocks as well as for gaining perceptual and conceptual adequacy. Building blocks may be made of sponge rubber shapes, wood, plastic or be household objects, boxes, tins or pots, to develop hand function in this developmental period.

Boyd *et al.* (2001b) have made a systematic review of many research studies on hand function, seating related to hand function, behavioural therapy, splintage and use of drugs.

Manipulation and perception/conception

Manipulation is by now integrated with perceptual development of:

(1) Space and depth in, say, well-coordinated reach and grasp activities.
(2) Form in placing a round peg in a round hole and similar matching.
(3) Size in placing objects into containers, according to size. Sorting objects of different sizes, shapes and textures.
(4) Colour and shape in use of matching toys (but not naming them), such as various posting boxes, mosaics and other sorting activities, jigsaws.
(5) Discrimination of soft, hard, scratchy, smooth sensations.
(6) Other cognitive and social activities such as wave bye-bye, point to visual stimulus, pat own face in mirror and smile at himself, and play pat-a-cake and similar games.

Manipulation becomes bimanual and later 'in-hand manipulation' in the third year of life with motor planning for novel tasks from $2\frac{1}{2}$ to 3 years in able-bodied children (Case-Smith 1993).

Perception, conception, perceptual-motor integration and fine motor manipulation continue to develop in such activities as threading large beads, smaller beads, other threading toys, scribbling, drawing, painting, pasting, using pegboards, formboards, draughts, jigsaws with knobs, using sewing cards, and a large variety of constructional toys, screwing toys, posting boxes and many more suggested in toy catalogues and by toy libraries and occupational therapists. Eye–hand coordination and rhythm, speed and precision of movement will need to be developed further after the basic arm and hand actions are trained.

Occupational therapists and teachers need to be consulted for appropriate activities for individual children, adolescents and adults with cerebral palsy.

Eliasson and Burtner (2008) have edited a book on hand function in children with cerebral palsy.

Splints and casting

Consult paediatric occupational therapists about hand splints, elbow back slab and Lycra splintage. Various materials as well as designs continue to be developed by them. Weekly casting associated with BTX A is mentioned in Chapter 11. Cosmetic splinting is weighed against associated loss of movement and of reducing the skin area for reception of sensory information (see Figs 9.211–9.213).

10

Motor function and the child's daily life

Chapter 9 has presented ways in which the child may develop various postures, maintain these postures or balance during movement, get in and out of postures, obtain various forms of locomotion and acquire the use of the hands. All these motor functions are not only developed in special sessions but suggestions include learning them in the context of a person's daily life (Levitt 1975; Tieman *et al.* 2004). This chapter reviews and adds details of motor function within self-care, perception, communication, speech and language, play and the emotional and social relationships involved.

It is also important to consider many recreational activities which can also be conducive to improved motor and sensory function, for example swimming, horse riding, skiing and so on (see Leach 1993) (see section 'Therapeutic motor activities' in Chapter 7). There is a growing amount of research studies on horse riding and swimming, showing their therapeutic value in cerebral palsy. These are given below. See Appendix 2 for addresses.

Motor function in feeding, dressing, toileting, washing, bathing, play and communication

Those below are of particular significance, although all motor functions are needed (see Levitt 1994).

Activate the motor abilities at a child's developmental stage, with and without equipment (see Chapter 9). See section 'Parent-child interaction' in Chapter 2 and section 'Emotions and learning' in Chapter 6.

Vertical head control, sitting on the floor and/or sitting on a chair of the correct size and design

Obtained by: holding the child's shoulders forward with your arm when a baby or severe child sits on your lap or next to you on his chair. In an older person, hold his shoulders forward with your arm for vertical head control in a forward position. You may need to support his chin. Later, face the child hold his arms stretched forward across the table between you, or hold him in weight bearing on his forearms. It is best if he can use his own support by either his grasping bars or table edge with both hands and straight arms. A child may be able to lean against a rounded edge of a table or onto his forearms on the surface. Bars or rails may be vertical or horizontal according to a child's ability. They are attached to the table, wall, bath, near the toilet/potty and stable toy shelves for daily activities (Figs 10.1–10.3). These positions are adapted for feeding, drinking, face washing, hair brushing, and pulling off top clothes. Positioning facilitates a child's use of vision, of hearing and for communication. Children are well positioned to socialise, including participation within music and other groups. When a child has the ability, he releases one hand whilst the other holds on or remains leaning on a surface for balance.

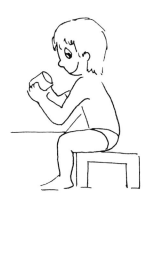
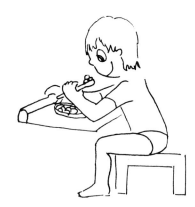

Figure 10.1

A child is also more able to play with toys as he stabilises himself on one arm and hand or just leans against a stable table. With improving balance, a child may sit astride his own chair and grasping its rungs for communication, play, dressing and feeding. Support may be needed for some children from behind by your sitting there and holding the child forward. They may reach a stage when they only need your stabilising hand at a child's pelvis. You may stabilise a child with your knees, or with your feet and knees, if you are sitting at a higher level to a child on a box or on the floor. In these positions a child can develop head and trunk control with or without using your or his own arm–hand support.

Sitting with support to the child's pelvis may be carried out with groin straps, diagonal strap across the hips or by firm pressure with an adult's hand in the lower area of the child's back, and later just holding his hips. The child can then carry out an activity whilst activating control of head, trunk and hands. Sitting on a cushion against a wall, in a corner of a wall or sofa and on a variety of chairs and boxes increases a child's experiences and used for those children who can function in all or some of them.

Remember to avoid slumping of the child or sliding down the seat during activities. Readjust the child's hips to be well back in a seat. Abnormal postures interfere with hand function, trunk and head control needed for daily activities (Fig. 10.3).

Standing or kneeling upright is used for painting, drawing, washing, toileting for boys, dressing and for many play activities. Sometimes eating and drinking is easier in supported standing. Standing at the levels of a child's peers increases communication and socialisation and increases visual and spatial experiences.

Obtained by: use of horizontal, sometimes vertical, rails on tables, walls, blackboards, easels, leaning against stable furniture and holding rungs of a chair. Standing frames are used initially, although more severe children may need them for many years.

Prone position or on hands and knees are other positions in which a child manages playing and

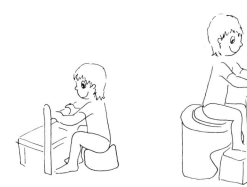

Figure 10.2

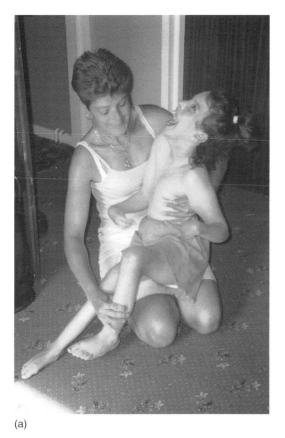

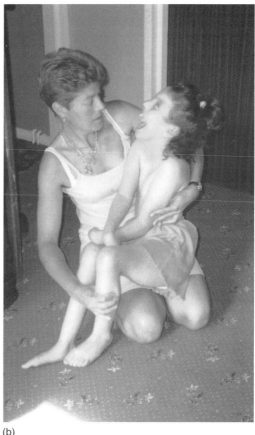

(a)   (b)

Figure 10.3   (a, b) Positioning for communication with postural alignment (see same child in Fig. 9.68).

communication with others on the floor, as well as when participating in dressing and drying after being washed. Head and arm control and partial rolling are activated for activities. On *hands and knees* may be needed for play with cars and trains, gardening, housekeeping activities, in sandpits and drawing or painting on the floor.

Obtained by: use of cushions, various sized wedges stabilised rolls, having a child over an adult's lap or arms. The adult is either on the floor, or has the child on a bed/changing table for washing, drying and dressing. Persistent use of kneeling positions is *not* advisable for those children who sit back on their heels during the activity or who have tightly bent hips and knees.

Use of the hands is obviously required for all activities and cannot be condensed unless a particular activity is discussed in detail. Hand function is associated with postural control (see Chapter 9).

Motor function and perception

All the training for motor function is also training perception. Thus, during the motor developmental techniques the therapist needs to recognise and involve the following main features:

Tactile and proprioceptive experiences with different textures, temperatures and feeling different shapes, sizes, weights, to develop stereognosis. Meanings of words become associated with these experiences of what is, say, smooth, hard, scratchy, knobbly, rough, hot and cold. These basic sensorimotor experiences underlie specific learning activities such as pairing, matching, sorting, brick building and other methods for perceptual and conceptual understanding in developmental delay (Stroh *et al.* 2008).

Recognition of the child's own body by tactile recognition during motor training as when touching his mouth, face, grasping his foot or clasping his hands, as well as touching others and sitting in close contact with parents and family members.

During motor training and other activities, a child can learn about his body parts by having his nails painted, putting on rings, bells, bracelets, make-up moustaches, earrings, ribbons, bandages, thimbles or play lighting up parts of his body with a torch. When handling a child in movement training, rub, stroke, use vibrating toys, ice therapy as well as words to draw attention to parts of his body.

Drawing attention to the child's body parts leads to an awareness of his own spatial relationships or body scheme, for example where are his toes? – 'in front', 'below' and so on. This is also involved with his body planes (Cratty 1970) and which part of his body is moving and in which direction. This is experienced through sensation and proprioception, but a child needs to be made more aware of what and where he is moving in perceptual-motor learning in occupational therapy and physiotherapy. Linking many sensations in motor experiences, especially in pleasurable play, is considered of importance by occupational therapists, psychologists and teachers. Some professionals call this 'intersensory development'.

Intersensory development is encouraged by associating the sensorimotor actions trained with hearing and vision. This is important in developing a child's hand function. During the exploratory play with toys and objects there is linking between what the child touches and feels, grasps, sees, listens, smells, and when still mouthing, tastes. Manipulation of objects with banging, throwing, squeezing, rolling, pressing and breaking are linking many senses. These actions develop perceptual and conceptual understanding such as:

Appreciation of the qualities of objects and of their relations to one another. Using both gross and fine motor activity, a child is gaining learning experiences to understand round, square, long, cylindrical shapes and discover which fits into which, which can be placed on top of which object and also which object is nearer, further away, behind,

in front of or next to the other. These perceptions and concepts are finely tuned in various selected activities in education and occupational therapy which interact with physiotherapy. The different therapists and teachers work together to offer activities to children.

Appreciation of the child's relationship to objects and space. These perceptual experiences also become involved with motor function. As the child learns to move through space, he is also learning to appreciate how far he is from objects, how to get into and out of things, how to get on top of, under, around, behind and learn many other relationships to objects and space.

Thus, the child finds out about his body parts, their relations to each other and also the relations of his body to objects and to space during gross motor development and fine motor development.

Development of praxia, motor planning or using movements appropriate to a motor task such as dressing, writing, using a pair of scissors or other implements. Although this depends on perceptual experiences and on the training of the neuromuscular system during motor development, a dyspraxia may be present on its own or together with perceptual problems (agnosias) in brain-damaged children. Specific teaching, or if dyspraxia is severe, cues for function without confronting the specific dyspraxia are provided by specialist, occupational therapists and specialist teachers.

Specialised perceptual and praxic training (including visuomotor training). This may be needed for many specific problems found amongst children with cerebral palsy with a primary motor impairment. Once again these problems may sometimes be even more disabling than the motor impairment. Referral for special assessment is essential to understand why a child is not progressing with physiotherapy methods. The general perceptual experiences are already included in the motor developmental training. This is not enough. It is also important to recognise that many children do not have these specific problems as perception and praxia *are also being trained within the activities of feeding, dressing, washing, bathing, toileting and especially playing.* The specialised therapy and education needed is discussed in other publications and advice must be sought from psychologists, teachers in special education, occupational therapists and physiotherapists working with developmental coordination disorder

(Ayres 1979; Fisher *et al*. 1991; Steel 1993; Lee 2004, among others*)*.

Motor function and communication, speech and language

The earliest communication between parent and child is within feeding behaviour. Therefore, the sections on communication and feeding need to be understood together as they are so intimately related. As this book focuses on motor function in cerebral palsy, the sections are only separated for clarity but not to neglect the integration of these functional aspects.

(1) It is well known that paediatric therapists need to develop appropriate ways of communicating with children. At first, a child with cerebral palsy needs to pay attention to achieving motor control without the distraction of verbal instruction. This is particularly relevant when a child would not be able to understand the language used. Language can contribute to the development of motor function, if the language used is appropriate to that child's developmental level. As outlined above, motor training becomes associated with body parts, movements and the purpose of motor functions, and other aspects of perception and conception. The development of communication, speech and language is also involved with all these aspects.

(2) From infancy, communication is associated with body movements within close contact with parents, such as nudging closer, turning away, patting parent's face and grasping a nose. Motor function during feeding, eating and drinking is outlined below. Rhythmic sounds with rhythms of movements in child with parent promote communication. In the section 'Development of communication – brief summary' given below, a number of movements are given of body, hands as well as of mouth, lips and tongue. Movements and postures developed in physiotherapy need to include those that assist communication.

(3) Motor functions and positions to promote communication, speech and language, eating, drinking, play and for other daily activities are all re-

viewed above. Although precise chewing skills are not a prerequisite for the acquisition of speech, eating and drinking develop the oral musculature. In addition, breathing exercises by a physiotherapist together with a speech and language therapist may be helpful for articulation. Relaxed breathing exercises to increase the length of expiration are used. Some physiotherapists trained in proprioceptive neuromuscular facilitation techniques have offered stimulation of the facial muscles with techniques of touch, pressure, stretch and resistance for older children and adults who are willing to accept them (Voss *et al.* 1985). Short periods of ice using the enjoyment of ice lollies reduce spasticity of tongues or mouths, while quick ice stimulation of the mouth muscles may help 'flabby mouths' and make the child aware of his muscles (Stockmeyer 1972). This sometimes discourages dribbling and helps mouth closure.

(4) Saliva control can normally be learned automatically, and drooling is seen in normal development until ages around 15 months. However, it is important to remember that saliva control in any child is more challenging when a child is tired, unwell, teething or engaged in physical activity, especially when learning to walk and when concentrating. Avoid telling a child to swallow. Children can be reminded to swallow or wipe their mouths when wearing towelling sweatbands on the wrists. The bands can easily be replaced during the day.

The development of speech and language requires special assessment, suggestions and treatment from speech and language therapists (Levitt & Miller 1973; Latham 1984; Winstock 2005; Stroh *et al.* 2008). See section 'Parent–child interaction' in Chapter 2.

Development of communication – brief summary

Speech and language development is very individual. The following is only a framework for most children:

0–3 months. Differentiated cries, eye-to-eye contact and expresses self with facial expressions and body movements. Makes sounds during kicking and feeding. Stills to noise. Smiles at parent.

3–6 months. Sounds vary, vowels predominate. Child gives clear signals of likes/dislikes. Anticipates food by opening mouth. Babbling begins, increasing intonations. Watches adult's lips. Turns to sounds and parent's voice. Laughs, squeals and annoyed screams. Excited limb motions as social responses.

6–9 months. Lip and tongue sounds. Syllables (ba-ba, da-da) with self-imitation. Actions anticipating being lifted. Uses voice to attract attention. Bounces on laps, showing pleasure and may indicate 'more'.

9–12 months. Double syllables, first word. Uses gestures especially pointing. Waves goodbye. Turns to sounds that interest him instantaneously. Continues vocalising to make personal contact. Imitates rhythmical sounds with movement. Playful turn-taking with familiar adults.

12–18 months. Understands more than expresses. Follows repeated adult's simple directions if given with gestures ('Give me', 'No', 'Arms up'). Responds to his name, single word and perhaps some meaningful words. Real object labels. Imitates sounds and intonations, develops baby jargon language.

18–24 months. Imitates adult speech (echolalia). Begins to imitate other children. Responds and discriminates sounds, responds to simple commands. Development of meaningful words and two or three word phrases. Has a growing vocabulary. Continues to love listening to stories, enjoys jingles and movements to nursery songs.

2–3 years. Simple short sentences to express self, especially likes/dislikes, many questions and verbal explosion. Gives own name. nursery rhymes, talks to himself during play and is using imaginative play which will increase with complexity after 3 years. Normal stutter, for example 'm,m,mummy'. Repetition of sounds and words. Unique dialogues.

Practical suggestions

(1) Follow the general guide of developmental levels and individual assessment by speech and language therapist and psychologist. This guides communication during motor training.

(2) Provide frequent opportunities for a child to initiate communication in any way that is possible for an individual child. Avoid anticipating a child's needs. Create situations that tempt a child to request for example, being swung again by you, have a song repeated or a musical toy wound up. A child may request 'more' of a favourite song, more of only a few bouncing or rocking actions, after only a few finger plays which are all deliberately given.

(3) Respond positively to all attempts at communication by a child, even when they do not appear to be deliberate. Give that child the benefit of the doubt. For example, if a sound could be interpreted as a word, say that word again to establish a likely meaning. Avoid fuss if a child's attempts succeeds.

(4) Avoid asking questions that require a yes/no reply. On asking 'Do you want milk or juice?' wait for a child to make his choice in whatever way he can. Help a child make the choice by saying, for example 'You are looking at the juice - so you want juice'. Accept eye gaze, gestures, reaching, pointing with whole hand or finger. A child may also vocalise. Give time and more occasions for a child's attempts to express his level of communication.

(5) Try to communicate with the child with noises (at first not too loud and sudden), songs, smiles, gestures; talk near the child and with face-to-face contact.

(6) Speak slowly and distinctly but not with exaggerated articulation, as in 'baby talk'. Wait for any response by a child and acknowledge them.

(7) Say names of familiar objects used during feeding, washing, dressing and playing, say what they are used for, and demonstrate and name parts of the body, and talk about child's own experiences. Parents are expected to let therapists know about their child's interests and experiences. Use language that he is able to understand, and stop when a child loses interest.

(8) Children need to be able to see your face in a good light during speech. Try to be at their eye level whenever possible and help with control of head and body. Check where you need to place yourself for children with visual impairments to hear or to see you.

(9) Enjoy and respond to a child's participation. However, do not pressurise a child to speak but create informal situations including play, for conversation, especially in groups.

(10) It is best not to fuss about the child's attempts to speak. Do not finish sentences for him if he can do so in his own time. Avoid giving an answer for him if he can say something.

(11) Explore *alternative and augmentative forms of communication* with experts. These may be photographs, symbols or signals. Respond to a child's 'low tech' communication methods, such as communication book or board as well as their use of electronic systems of communication. Learn about them from speech and language therapists or occupational therapists.

Development of feeding – brief summary

0–3 months. Rooting reaction, sucking-and-swallowing reflex. The mouth and gag are sensitive, having normal cardinal points reflexes. The tongue moves out and there is often an open mouth and dribbling. When sucking, the tongue moves forward and back together with the up and down movement of the jaw. A baby rests a hand on the breast or bottle, and sucks hands.

3–6 months. Sucking dissociates from swallowing as child transfers liquids for swallowing. All reflexes disappeared. Bite response followed by release. Takes liquids or later, liquidised food from spoon. Recognises bottle. Cup may be accepted for drinking. Experiences many tastes before textures. Mouthing hands, objects, clothes and later feet. Begins to temporarily grasp and suck a biscuit.

6–9 months. Takes mashed foods and semi-solids. Bites food if placed to sides of mouth, and sucks if centrally placed. Picks up and holds a biscuit, may drop it or crumble it in his hand. Around 8–9 months some guide mother's/carer's hand on spoon or cup to their mouth and can hold the bottle. Likes to feel food. Up and down jaw motion in chewing, tongue movements changing and less associated with jaw action. Swallows with mouth closed. Gags on new textures but gag response is much less sensitive. Babbles with mouthful of food. During drinking, loses liquids and tongue protrusion is slight. Mouthing continues to explore toys and objects.

9–12 months. Wants to control eating and drinking. Enjoys prodding, squeezing and smearing food. Finger feeds, and more varieties held in hand. Firmer foods are chopped, textures accepted and chewing with lateral tongue motion. Holds and drinks from bottle and with help holds, lifts and drinks from cup. Helps parent with filled spoon to mouth but cannot do this alone. Plunges spoon into food and bangs spoon on the table. Lips used to remove food from spoon held by adult.

12–18 months. Feeds self clumsily with a spoon and variety of foods increases. Uses spoon but turns it upside down before reaching mouth or within mouth. A child cannot scoop food so uses other hand to push food onto spoon with much spilling. Holds and drinks from cup, may bite on cup edge, often spills. Controls bite on biscuit. Chewing established. Lateral and rotary jaw motion. Pretends to feed another person and dolls.

18 months–2 years. Loads and uses spoon correctly, occasional spilling. Holds glass and cup for drinking without biting edge but may suck edge or tip cup and spill. Drops saliva or food while chewing. Understands what is edible and inedible. Begins straw drinking but bites edge. Imitates other children.

2–3 years. With small amounts, feeds self completely with spoon, later with fork. Pours liquids, obtains own drink from tap. Prefers little amount to drink, using one hand. May be fussy about food, have variable appetite and imitates other children about likes/dislikes and being independent.

3–4 years. Serves self at table, spreads butter, cuts food. Pours from different jugs. From 4 years onwards a child is learning to use knife and fork. A child learns to hold a fork with pressure by the index finger isolated from the others grasping the handle. There is increasing experience of new mealtimes in new situations. Enjoys help with cooking and more complex imaginative play such as with toy tea sets, dolls, shops, toy kitchens.

Practical suggestions (Fig. 10.4)

Although speech therapists and occupational therapists are the experts on the training of eating and

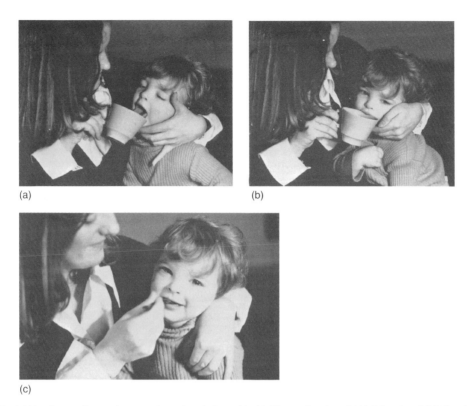

Figure 10.4   (a) Head extension and tongue thrust interfering with drinking and eating. (b) Holding the child's head upright and forward, supporting her chin and stroking under her jaw trains drinking. (c) Wait for the child to remove food from the spoon held below her mouth. Keep her head and shoulders well forward as she takes the food.

drinking, physiotherapists are very much involved as well. Feeding and drinking methods are part of the training of head control, sitting, hand grasp and release and hand-to-mouth action without balance loss. It is sensorimotor function integrated with understanding, communication, body image and perceptual function.

Such integration fundamentally depends on developing feeding, drinking and eating as a pleasurable experience for child and parent/carer. This has not been pleasurable from birth as there are usually feeding problems, particularly in premature babies and multiply impaired children. In the collaborative learning approach (see Chapter 2), mothers often choose feeding as the activity they want to improve and find less stressful.

Children with severe spastic quadriplegia or dyskinesia have most feeding problems. For different reasons, their hands cannot touch their mouths, hold an object for mouthing and cannot control head to use vision. They may be multiply impaired. Chil-

dren with spastic diplegia or hemiplegia physically manage early levels of feeding but are often asymmetrical in their actions. Poor sitting balance in all children with cerebral palsy interferes with eating and drinking.

Unhurried feeding period gives time for a relationship to develop and for a child to respond to being fed and later to develop eating and drinking. Give time for the child to accept new tastes and textures and participate by opening the mouth, taking food and to swallow. The speed of your feeding should be slower and similar to the speed at which his own early attempts will start. Being fed and later eating and drinking should take place in as social and pleasant an atmosphere of an unhurried meal as you can make it. Communication, including babbling or words often occurs during such mealtimes. Sitting at meals with the family and other children at school also motivates eating and drinking, and when imitation develops, a child's independence is enhanced.

Remember that making demands on self-feeding may compromise oral-motor skills and should not be at the expense of intake or safety. Recognise that in cerebral palsy a child has to manage more oral-motor, developmental and emotional difficulties.

When a child cannot imitate due to impairments of intellect or vision, or because the others are eating too fast for him to feed himself at the same meal-time, it is essential to have one-to-one therapy sessions. When a child and parent have much difficulty with feeding, or eating sessions with understandable anxieties, then one–to-one sessions are usually carried out by therapists with special experience. In any one-to-one sessions for child and parent/carer, the therapist settles them in a quiet, undisturbed situation so there is no response to distraction by, say, telephone calls or television. This allows for concentration on active achievements. Snack times are also particularly valuable for developing self-feeding. Naturally a child should join the family or others for the mealtimes, but be given something easy to do in the way of self-feeding or drinking.

Positioning for feeding needs to involve an upright position supported or, if possible, unsupported by special chairs or by the parent. Support is indicated when a child needs to concentrate on precise mouth control and coordination when learning to eat and drink. This support may not be needed on other occasions. Some children manage self-feeding more easily in a standing frame. Feeding positions are given in the first section above on motor function for all daily living activities. The child's head should be held by you or when possible by himself in a forward, chin in and upright position whilst taking food, during eating and drinking, especially on swallowing. Swallowing with the head back is more difficult and increases the risk of aspiration (food/fluid entering the airway). With the head upright, a child not only protects the airway but also allows active learning to eat and drink. Gently press a child's chest to help the head come forward and up, and if his head drops down, give minimal support under his chin. Elbows on the table are recommended! Leaning on a stable table activates shoulder girdle stabilisation which assists head stability. There is control of hand-to-mouth action as elbow steadies the arm on the table. Babies and young children with visual disability are also made aware of where they find the food and its smell and have the opportunity to search along the table surface for food when they are ready to do so. A child with vi-

sual or intellectual impairment can then understand that food does not come 'out of the air' but from a dish on a table. Gently banging the cup on a table alerts a child, indicating where to reach for picking up the cup of drink, when he can manage it.

If one upper limb is more disabled, then use that hand to hold a bowl, grasp a rail or place on the table. The better hand and arm is used for eating and drinking. This is much less frustrating than insisting on using the more disabled limb. When both arms are used, a child is helped to sit symmetrically looking at food in the centre, if he can use the eyes in that visual field. This avoids twisting of neck and body.

Mouth actions in taking the food, keeping the mouth closed during eating, chewing actions and swallowing can be facilitated by your hands, supporting under his chin. A speech and language therapist can teach how to stroke under the chin and along the neck to stimulate a swallow. Fingers may have to be held above and below his lips to stimulate mouth closure. Simply achieving mouth closure may lead to spontaneous swallowing. This technique needs careful supervision if a child is nasally congested and has a poor swallow as aspiration of food or fluid may occur. Wait for a child to bring the head forward and to take the food off the spoon offered below and in front of the mouth, and do not scrape the food and spoon off the top of his teeth.

Weaning from liquids to tolerate various textures, tastes through semi-solids to solids is most important and may take longer in some children with disabilities. Children who are visually impaired, or severely intellectually impaired, may be conservative about any change. Smooth, thick liquids are often easier to manage as they move more slowly and provide greater sensory experience within a child's mouth. Change from liquids to semi-solids gradually by adding to his cup of favourite drink, yogurts, custards, apple sauce or mashed banana. Later offer stewed or diluted crushed fruit *without* skin, pips or seeds and puddings. In the weaning process, the adult can spoon from cup of thickened liquid to spoon mashed food from a bowl. Mashed semi-solids enjoyed by a child may have to be mixed with textures of semi-solids and solids. A child who is fussy about textures, which is also normally present, may accept a preferred food with a new texture. There may be hypersensitivity and need additional methods to gradually normalise sensation. See discussion on hypersensitivity given below. A meal of ice cream and peas with mince and custard has been known to wean a child to solids. Weaning to solids is done to socialise and to improve nutrition. Introduce a solid he is able to hold and likes at snack time or during part of every meal from as soon as he is developmentally ready to manage. Offer him a baby biscuit to hold which dissolves easily in the mouth. Later, children may be able to cope with a soft pear slice, a small sausage or biscuit. This needs supervision as some children are liable to aspirate when chewing and swallowing is poor. Always introduce lumps in food so that food is of even consistency, rather than odd lumps in a smooth sauce, in the initial stages.

Gagging or choking. This may be due to gastro-oesophageal reflex. It is said that many children with cerebral palsy have gastro-oesophageal reflux which is associated with aspiration into the lungs. In babies, drugs and positioning are used and many overcome this by 18 months. Medical opinion is essential, especially for older children. When gag and choking occur in other children without reflux, calmly and quickly tip the child forward and down. Avoid banging him on the back. As gagging can be behavioural, do give small amounts of food and go slowly so that a child has time to make the decision to take the food and to swallow. The child may sometimes gag on foods he dislikes, to which he is allergic or if he has a behaviour problem. He may be reacting against a new person feeding him, an unfamiliar place, especially when in hospital, or he may be seeking the fuss and attention he gets from mother and others if he gags and vomits. Casualness in people's reactions and ignoring his 'performance' may stop this behaviour (see below). It also occurs in children with hypersensitive faces and mouths, which can be neurological or due to visual disability with fears, loss of body image and unfamiliar situations.

Hypersensitivity of face and mouth can be treated by gradual normalising the sensation with methods used and suggested by speech and language therapists. Guide a child's hands to touch parts of the child's body in a game and gradually touch his face and then mouth. Gently stroke his face with your hands or with soft toothbrushes and play with lipsticks and face paints, and sticking on moustaches or masks. Sensitivity is also normalised during the development of eating. It is helpful to use gentle wiping and washing the mouth area as well as guiding a child to wipe off food around the mouth. Remember

that desensitising the child's face is best done with his own hands rather than those of the therapist.

Gastrostomy and naso-gastric tube. Special feeding equipment is needed for children unable to take adequate food and fluid by mouth. A naso-gastric tube gives food to the stomach for a short time. It is also used to administer medications. However, it should not be used over time. Where long-term non-oral intake is required, a gastrostomy is usually preferred by medical consultants. It decreases negative associations by the child with his mouth and allows for the development of oral-motor skills. The gastrostomy tube is inserted through the abdominal wall directly into the stomach. The catheter is secured. When not in use, a button for a feeding tube is less obtrusive and is usually preferred. Parent and nurse are responsible for feeding a child via a gastrostomy and will advise therapists about handling and at appropriate times for the child. Nutrition is markedly improved so that a child has more energy for therapy. However, care is taken to avoid excessive gain in the child's weight.

Training self-feeding should begin with finger feeding so that the child feels his own fingers on his mouth, takes a small amount of food, learning how to manage early hand-to-mouth abilities and experiencing the texture, temperature and smell of the food. A child also learns to pick up food and place it in the mouth, and also doing so from different parts of his table. Food coming at him from unseen places does not encourage a child with severe visual impairment to feed himself. Use baby biscuits which dissolve easily and other foods he can safely munch and swallow himself. At first, he will push it all into his mouth and in time release with a finer hand control. Train finger feeding one item at a time and so finish each item before putting the next piece of food into his mouth.

Feeding with a spoon follows, with the therapist guiding hand to mouth whilst supporting a child forward to control any extension backwards or falling back. Special chairs may be needed for those children who need to concentrate more on difficult mouth control and swallow. Guide hand to mouth action from slightly behind and to the side of the child. Sit close to a child for emotional support and for positioning him in a good sitting posture with appropriate head control, as mentioned above. Guide his hand all the way from the bowl to his mouth at first. Feel at which point he seems to be actively moving hand to mouth, and let go at that part. For example, it may be that the active control is taken by the child when he smells the food near his mouth. Later it is a few more inches away from his mouth, then more until he carries through the full hand-to-mouth action. Grasping the spoon may have to be trained separately or it may be all he can do at first. Help a poor grasp with a special handle or thickened handle perhaps with rubber tubing, strapped on, but which can be removed, as grasp improves. Occupational therapists supply many different spoons to help individual children and older persons. See discussion on aids below.

Grasp, hand to mouth, taking food and eating are usually first achieved by a child. Later, scooping up the food on the spoon is managed. Use a bowl with sides to make this possible. Once again guide the child to scoop up food and select large, deep or small spoons to suit his ability. Use non-slip bowls, or have a non-slip mat on the tabletop. Scooping or spoon turning takes time to manage, so using a fork may be easier.

Guidance is done by *hand over hand*, that is your hand over his hand on the spoon or fork, or your hand alongside his hand on the handle, or by directing his elbow or his whole arm. Stiff, flexed and adducted arms may have to be held with the upper arm well away from the body to release tightness. On taking the food to his mouth, the child must be taught to keep his head upright and chin in, with trunk forwards, for swallowing and to prevent falling or extending backwards. Extending or thrusting into extension allows more abnormal jerking open of the mouth, gagging or choking, and may cause loss of hand grasp. If problems of extensor thrust, head and arm control are excessive, then at first, control of these basic movement and posture patterns will have to be taught without food and drink for easier learning.

Place a little on the spoon or fork at a time, quietly approve of anything active that a child does. Give some verbal information of how well an action was done, but do not distract his attention when he is concentrating. Your praise is not essential as he will gain the reward of getting his food by himself.

Behaviour. Behaviour varies according to a child's developmental stage, diagnosis, culture and temperament. For example, teaching eating needs to take account of a child's level of understanding, the relationships between him and objects, and between two objects such as spoon and food, spoon and bowl, as well as his physical ability (Kitzinger 1980). The outline of developmental levels above give some behaviours normally seen in children at different ages, and may appear later in the developmental delay of cerebral palsy. Feeding behaviour is changed by the special neurological problems and medical conditions such as gastro-oesophageal reflux. The suggestions given above for therapist and parent may help a child manage the development and medical aspects of children's eating and drinking, minimising stress in both child and parent/carer.

Remember the main points influencing a child's behaviour:

(1) Give opportunities for a child's choice from what is offered.
(2) Give time for a child's decision to take food or drink offered.
(3) Give small portions.
(4) Concentration is needed by a child learning to eat and drink. To help him, check positioning and give more physical support than in other situations. Make sure that the pressure of tables or positioning straps against a child's abdomen is not causing discomfort and even vomiting. Decrease distractions by other people, loud noise and minimise talking while a child is attending to eating and drinking. Occasionally mention about the food is made when a child is not concentrating on eating. Consider the length of the concentration span of each child. Usually this is about 20 minutes when you accept whatever a child has eaten without any remark. Leave a feeding session together with a child, so feelings of failure in mother or child are avoided. Mothers particularly need reassurance that development is positive no matter how slow.
(5) Naturally, a child is never forced to eat when there is refusal. There is neither need for persuading or cajoling nor using tricks to get food into a child's mouth when a child is not attending. An anxious and worried child can refuse to eat despite your good methods. He may push food away, turn away or cry, even throw food away. Remain as relaxed as you can and calmly put the spoon or cup down. Wait and try again slowly and calmly. Should refusal continue, calmly remove food completely and not as if he is being punished, so he does not eat at all. Hungry children may be more willing to learn to eat. During training of eating and

drinking, cooperation should be *expected* by you in a firm, matter of fact way.

(6) Find ways in which a child can help with food preparation, choose size of food helping and when more able, help to set a table.

Speech and language therapists and occupational therapists, as well as parents, carers and teachers have practical ideas on appropriate suggestions for preventing behaviour problems. When inappropriate behaviour occurs, psychologists and speech therapists should be consulted (Winstock 2005; Stroh *et al.* 2008).

Special problems. Speech and language therapists need to be consulted for floppy open mouths, tongue thrusts, gagging and hypersensitive mouths. When feeding, use of a polythene (unbreakable) or bone spoon which is gently but firmly placed at the middle of the tongue. If this is correctly done, a child may withdraw the tongue into his mouth and so he does not push food out with his tongue thrust. Head in midline and firmly held in the upright and forward is also essential. Bite responses are also best managed with non-metal spoons. Chewing development tends to decrease the early bite responses. Encourage an active bite with lateral tongue movement by slipping the spoon in at the side of the child's mouth between the teeth. Some therapists have occasionally used pleasant tasting ice lollies to reduce spasticity of tongue and mouth muscles.

Floppy mouths associated with dribbling are helped by training of feeding, chewing and general stimulation of the mouth muscles with touch or pressure. Speech therapists' opinions need to be obtained for all these problems.

Aids. Occupational therapists should be approached about the selection of utensils. Assessment must be made as to whether special utensils are necessary and if so, when a child no longer needs them. The following may be used:

Non-slip bowls, non-slip tabletops, high-sided bowls or suction bases for bowl or cup. Special feeding cups with weighted bases and with cut-out section at the lip so that the liquid can be seen. Drinking cups with spouts may be used before a child can cope with the lip of a cup. Straws are discouraged if their use perpetuates immature patterns and could lead to aspiration. Much later, straws are useful when hands are severely disabled to manage utensils but not to train drinking actions. Two-handled cups are advisable for a child's use of both hands and for chil-

dren with visual disability who need to learn about both sides of a cup, and also helps to avoid spilling. A more able hand is used for eating, while the more affected arm and hand are used to hold a dish or a bar. An inclined lip on a cup may help to delay the flow of liquid and let the child see it coming towards his lips. Thickened liquids in cups are easier to manage.

Spoons of bone, unbreakable plastic, with special handles, thick handles and inclined bent handles have to be selected for the individual child. Long-handled spoons, deep or shallow bowls of the spoon should be available to suit particular children. Unusual looking aids to feeding should be avoided until after a long period of training with other utensils has been attempted. A child's own abilities take time to develop. The bent or curved spoon is used by older children, if that becomes necessary. Some children find picking up food easier than using a spoon. Others manage a fork edge on a 'splade' spoon, or fork and knife on one implement or a fork and pusher. Much later, use of a fork and knife develops (see 'Development of feeding – brief summary').

Bibs which catch spills and are made of plastic are useful. Cover the floor with newspapers or a plastic cover to catch spills. Spills will decrease when the child is at the 18–24 months developmental level.

The development of eating and drinking involves patience, time and determination, but is worthwhile as independence in this area is something adults with cerebral palsy most appreciate having gained. Messing and spills are inevitable and carers or therapists, who cannot bear this extended *normal* phase of children learning to eat alone, should not be asked to take on the training of the children. If cleanliness is important, one should in any event train the child to wipe his mouth, wipe the table and help to clear up.

Parent–child relationships will be fostered by good methods used during feeding, as a child's difficulties can often create worries. A mother may feel more anxiety as she expects herself to cope. Support and explanations about the neuromotor problems and reassuring approval of any parent's coping abilities are essential. Any emotional difficulties of parents about feeding need sensitive management. At some stages, a mother may not feel able to take on the feeding training completely. A father can help and support his wife as soon as she is ready to learn to feed their child. All these suggestions are relevant to carer–child relationships during feeding.

Development of dressing – brief summary

6–12 months. Child was dressed in lying and is now supported in sitting, later supporting himself on hands. Child may put out arm or leg for dressing and cooperate in other ways between 10 and 12 months.

13–18 months. Postural control improving, so one or both hands are becoming free to take off socks or hat. Take off gloves, shoes, unzip around 18 months.

18 months–2 years. Cooperates more with undressing. Take off pants. Pull off T-shirt if placed on his head. Puts on shoes, hat. *Unable* to replace clothes. May sometimes help more with dressing.

2–3 years. Gradually able to take off all clothes. Confusion of back and front, right and left, top and bottom, two legs in one hole of trousers and so on.

3–5 years. Gradually able to dress self, becomes careless about details, such as tucking in shirt, which foot to put in which shoe. All buttons, laces, ties not possible until 6 years.

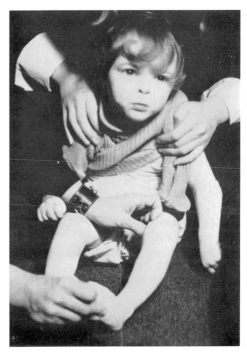

Figure 10.5 The child is held flexed for dressing and play. Tailor sitting is being obtained. Press beneath the big toe and bend hip and knee outward in order to overcome excessive leg extension–adduction for, say, a nappy change, sock removal and getting her into tailor sitting.

Practical suggestions (Fig. 10.5)

(1) Development varies greatly and too much must not be expected of the child. Dressing is not an easy task, involving the training of perception, motor planning, balance, eye–hand coordination, reach, grasp and release, steady with one hand whilst using the other movements, and as a source for speech and language development.

(2) Begin any dressing activity for the child, but let him finish it himself. If he can carry it all out himself, give him time and do not hurriedly do it for him if he is struggling to solve problems on his own.

(3) Vary stable positions for dressing to discover the easiest one for the child. He will be positioned and given just enough support, minimising dyskinesia and spasticity. Try to maintain symmetry of head and body, let him see your face and what is happening. For example, side lying may enable a child to dress, take off socks and shoes. Lying and bridging allows him to stabilise on feet while removing the lower clothes.

See the discussion on motor function and dressing as included in all daily activities above.

(4) Dress and undress for bathing, swimming and other purposes but not as an isolated exercise.

(5) Type of clothing: loose fitting garments, large sleeves and arm holes (raglan), elastic necks and waistbands, large buttons, zips with knobs, Velcro fastenings are required. Non-slippery materials are preferable. Tabs on front or top of shirts and dresses and back of boots are useful to guide the child. Avoid laces and small fastenings.

(6) Put the more affected arm in first. Use both hands, one to stabilise sitting or both to pull top clothes off over the head and pants/trousers down. A child can elevate one arm to receive clothes and then actively pull clothes down with the other arm. Arms reach to hips or knees, grasp trousers thumb on the inside, push trousers down or up.

There are many suggestions for an individual which can be made by occupational therapists, therefore consult them to advise on dressing techniques and clothing ideas.

Development of play – brief outline

This is the development of learning through play. This is closely correlated with development of communication, hand function, posture control, locomotion and the development of intersensory relationships and perceptual-motor control. See Chapter 9 and the therapy procedures which describe developmental levels in more detail, often within play. The section on hand function particularly has many suggestions for play. Play differs at different ages, but it is impossible to have it strictly classified as the child's personality, opportunities and intelligence affect this. Social and cultural backgrounds also affect play, and therapists learn much about this from the families of children.

Play is usually a synonym for exploration and experimentation and is a serious affair for the child. Play can also be relaxing, working out emotions, imitating reality in order to understand it in imaginative play, and obtaining satisfaction and development of the child's personality. It is often messy, dirty, untidy and destructive, as well as creative and constructive.

0–6 months. Visual fixation and pursuit, hand–eye coordination and bring hands to midline and grasp, drop, reach and grasp, touch and mouthing. Play with parts of body, mother's face, nearby materials. Finds pleasure in using all senses and movement to concentrate on exploratory play on his own. An attentive adult is nearby for safety but not guidance, unless baby shows need. This allows a baby's own discoveries.

6–12 months. Rolling, crawling, supported cruising and other gross motor activities to explore, strengthen body generally and enjoy moving. Hand function development continues using toys or objects. Investigates and experiments with increasing energy.

12 months–2 years. Solitary play but imitates another child or adult. Uses large equipment, swings, balls, toys on wheels to push and pull. Sand and water play. Enjoys small objects such as shells, pebbles, buttons, but needs supervision as child often takes them to mouth until 15 months of age.

2–3 years. Rough and tumble play. As above, only with more perceptual and conceptual ideas. Begins imaginative play ('Let's pretend'). Solitary and parallel play.

3–4 years. Plays with other children. Imaginative play, dressing up feeding dolls. Less energetic activities such as looking at books and play with more complex constructional toys.

5–6 years. Games with rules, arts and crafts. 'Tricks' with body and hands.

Practical suggestions

(1) There is less spontaneous play due to the difficulties in cerebral palsy. Give helpful positioning, guidance and support to use what abilities he has to enjoy learning from play.

(2) Select objects and toys in a size he can handle and those he can understand, but especially those that interest him. Use his communication for him to choose between two toys for play.

(3) Show the child how to use a toy, but wherever possible, see if he can find things out for himself.

(4) Do not interfere with any child who is concentrating on a play activity unless absolutely essential. Before helping, recognise that a child needs his own time and speed to reveal his abilities and initiatives when there are difficulties of understanding, memory, visual and other impairments.

Techniques for carrying the child correctly (Figs 10.6–10.11)

(1) To stimulate head control.
(2) To correct any abnormal postures.
(3) To suggest easier ways for a parent/carer to carry a child with cerebral palsy.

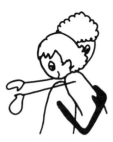

Figure 10.6   Both the arms are over the adult's shoulder for symmetry, straighten back and raise head. Keep the legs apart and hips flat if necessary in spasticity. Bring tight arms away from their habitual positions next to the child.

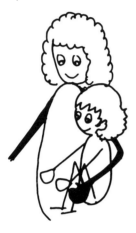

Figure 10.7   For head control and correcting an excessively extended child, help bring hands down and together helps control an athetoid or floppy child.

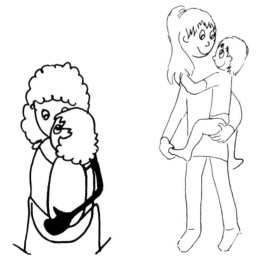

Figure 10.8 and 10.9   Use of both arms, eye-to-eye contact, separate tightly adducted legs or very extended legs. Move the child to points around the adult's hips to find the most corrective posture of legs for him.

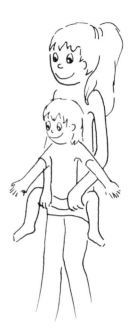

Figure 10.10   Head and trunk control, if the child is moved slightly away from the adult's chest. Correct extended–adducted–internally rotated legs.

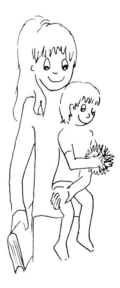

Figure 10.11   Stimulates greater head and trunk control for floppy and other children. Hold child at chest and under his armpits and/or under his buttocks as well.

Management of deformity

A deformity is an abnormal position of a part of the body. In cerebral palsy and other developmentally delayed children, abnormal positions rarely appear in only one part of the body due to biomechanics. The positions and movements are initially limited by the action and lengths of muscles and soft tissues in cerebral palsy, though joints may have full ranges.

Most babies with cerebral palsy do not have deformities, though these may be anticipated by their preferences for postures and movement patterns. Deformities become evident with growth and development, especially when weight bearing becomes present. Explanations have to be given to those parents who may be confused as they were correctly told that the brain lesion will not increase. The deformities are anticipated and treated, as they can be progressive.

Each deformity may be mobile or dynamic, that is *unfixed*, which means that passive or active correction can take place. Deformities can be mild and do not restrict some children or be a serious problem in others. Dynamic deformities are less during sleep and absent under anaesthesia. Some or all deformities may have become *fixed* or contractures when there is adaptive shortening of muscles, tendons and other soft tissues (Lin 2004). This leads to joint and bony changes. The range of motion is limited in a contracture, so full passive or active correction cannot take place. Fixed deformities remain during sleep and under anaesthesia (Graham 2004).

Dynamic deformities can coexist with contractures, particularly in older children. This may be contributing to the same joint position or be dynamic in some joints with contracture in other joints in limbs. A primary deformity in one joint can lead to deformities in other joints due to the biomechanics of movement and posture. For example, equinus of the ankle can cause compensatory hip and knee flexion, though hip and knee are not necessarily deformed on ranges of motion. Deformities and contractures vary with the degree of severity of stiffness, weakness and immobility of a child.

It is necessary to point out that in the literature the words 'deformity' and 'contracture' can be used interchangeably without always clarifying whether either is fixed or unfixed. The definitions given above are kept throughout this book to avoid confusion.

Preventing, minimising and, if possible, correcting of deformities with conservative therapy and daily care are particularly important. This avoids secondary soft tissue and structural muscle and joint changes. Early therapy and ongoing daily management prevent or minimise secondary impairments, disability, discomfort and pain. A number of medical and surgical treatments are also available together with physiotherapy.

Although this chapter focuses on the musculoskeletal features, they cannot be separated from the developmental and neurological aspects. Remember that 'neuronal mechanisms are a part of bio-mechanical strategies but are themselves constrained by bio-mechanics' as stated by Dietz. The therapist needs to consider the postural mechanisms, *abnormal postures and movements* in developmental motor functions as these are linked with the causes of deformities. Chapter 9 offers practical suggestions, treatments, activities, orthoses and equipment within the motor developmental functions in lying, sitting, standing and walking.

Causes of deformities and aims of therapy and management

(1) Immobility.
(2) Hypotonicity.
(3) Hypertonicity.
(4) Weakness – general or specific.
(5) Co-contraction and synergies (movement patterns).
(6) Abnormal reflex activity.
(7) Asymmetry.
(8) Involuntary movements in one repetitive pattern.
(9) Growth factors.
(10) Biomechanics.

Some of these causes are interwoven and their relationships are discussed.

Immobility

General immobility is associated with persistent posture and very few, if any, movements in a child. The causes may be due to:

■ *Physical impairment* of hypotonicity, hypertonicity, weakness with limited ranges of motion, a few abnormal, inefficient movement patterns, impaired postural control with prolonged abnormal postures. The combination of dystonia and spastic hypertonia causes more severe immobility.
■ *Other causes* such as sensory loss (mainly blindness), severe perceptual-motor defects, especially those related to space and body image, emotional problems, especially if the child is fearful or withdrawn, severe intellectual impairment, social deprivation and malnutrition.

Most of these reasons tend to create lethargic, unmotivated children, who prefer to be immobile.

When many of the above causes of immobility combine in the same child, deformities are most likely to occur. Therefore, immobile children who have severe multiple disabilities are particularly prone to their deformities becoming contractures.

Partial or even very minor immobility of children compared to their able-bodied peers happen in mild-to-moderate disability. Some of the more severely involved children can acquire a few abnormal postures and stereotyped movements for partial mobility.

Aims. Therapy, special equipment including orthoses and adapted environments aim to enable children to become more mobile. The degree of mobility depends on the severity of the condition. The aim is to use interesting playful activities to motivate actions and as much appropriate mobility as possible throughout the day.

Hypotonicity

The floppy baby or very young child with hypotonia may be due to many neurological causes other than cerebral palsy. Hypotonic babies or very young children with cerebral palsy may become hypertonic, dyskinetic or ataxic as they develop. They are initially immobile and may sometimes be left lying for long periods in one or two positions, which can create deformities. For example, the *frog position* of the legs in prone, supine or with the child propped up on pillows in the half-slumped sitting position may all lead to deformities especially in the spine and hips. Anterior subluxation or dislocation of hips may be found in such cases.

A common characteristic of most floppy babies is the absence of all or some of the normal postural mechanisms. The neck, trunk, shoulder and pelvic girdle muscles are not being activated by these mechanisms, and are weak and hypotonic. Hypotonia is not always associated with total weakness. Fair, though weak, voluntary movement may be present, but it is not enough to make the child mobile. Without the presence of postural mechanisms a child cannot get out of his few positions during the day and night. Postural control is therefore absent or poor, preventing reliable function.

The baby with ataxic cerebral palsy has hyper-mobile joints and may later develop some postural mechanisms being able to sit, stand and walk un-steadily and with a delayed development. There are common abnormal deformities such as sitting with legs in *frog position* and round backs; standing with round backs, lordosis, hyperextended knees (*back knees, recurvatum*), valgus knees (*knock knees*), varus knees (*bow knees*) and pronated feet (*flat feet*). Children who develop spasticity retain trunk hypo-tonia with stiff limbs. Children who become dyski-netic retain hypotonic trunks with fluctuating tone, in trunk and/or limbs. They have similar deformi-ties as in ataxia due to a variety of causes (see sec-tions 'Spastic cerebral palsy', 'Dyskinetic/dystonic cerebral palsy' and 'Ataxic cerebral palsy' in Chapter 1).

Aims. Train postural control, strengthen and correct abnormal postures with equipment where necessary.

Hypertonicity

Historically, spasticity was considered the most im-portant cause of deformity. Currently there is still a focus on 'spasticity' by some physiotherapists and also in many studies on the use of botulinum toxin A (BTX A), usually with physiotherapy. There are different types of hypertonicity and spasticity needs clarification, as spasticity can need therapy for stiff-ness, weakness or incoordination of muscle acti-vations (see below). Focus on spasticity includes the use of baclofen (Albright & Neville 2000; Lin 2004) and neurosurgical selective dorsal rhizotomy (Peacock & Staudt 1991; McLaughlin *et al.* 1998).

Types of hypertonicity. The dystonic-dyskinesia type of cerebral palsy is less liable to have deformi-ties owing to fluctuating tone. There is a persistent type of dystonia together with spasticity, as well as a specific rigidity type in post-traumatic cerebral palsy, which do cause deformities. In these children a *lead-pipe* rigidity is felt on stretching throughout their joint ranges. Many workers focus on deformi-ties in the spastic type as it is the commonest type of cerebral palsy and most liable to progressive de-formities. In the spastic type, there is an abnormal reaction to rapid stretch (a velocity-dependent hy-peractive stretch reflex), described by neurophysiol-ogists, and also called a *clasp-knife* spastic reaction.

This physiological test of spasticity is not associ-ated with abnormal posture which causes deformi-ties (Lin 2004).

The creation of the deformities is, however, dependent on the neurological and orthopaedic (musculo-skeletal) views. Deformities are associ-ated with immobility in habitual abnormal posi-tions, stiffness (Brown 1985), muscle shortening and muscles overlengthening. There are other important aspects that need consideration, such as the recog-nition of aspects of abnormally coordinated move-ments (abnormal synergies), weakness and ineffi-cient muscle work, and especially in compensation for absent or atypical postural mechanisms. These causes together with growth and biomechanics are discussed below.

There is a tendency for spastic muscles to shorten, which will cause *one aspect* of the deformity (Tardieu *et al.* 1982; Dietz & Berger 1983; Huf-schmidt & Mauritz 1985; Cosgrove 2000). Short-ening hypertonic ('hypoextensible') muscles pull the joints into abnormal motor patterns involving the whole child or at least of the whole limb. Shortland *et al.* (2002) and Fry *et al.* (2004) have used ul-trasound to study muscles in spastic cerebral palsy, and one finding was that weakness of muscles may contribute to muscle shortening and atrophy. They have included research on muscle length in these children. Akeson *et al.* (1987) consider that mus-cle contracture is related to length changes whereas stiffening of joints is more related to movement de-privation. At first 'hypoextensible' muscles with or without hypertonic stiffness can be overcome in a young child but later it can become fixed. Although one joint with its muscles may be more deformed than the others within a motor pattern, it is im-portant to *check each joint* as well as observe the *pattern of abnormal posture and movement*.

Muscle imbalance. There is a common assump-tion that spastic muscle is strong with a weak an-tagonist (Bobath & Bobath 1984; Reimers 1990). This is called a muscle imbalance, which is assumed to lead to deformity. Although some orthopaedic workers still talk of the muscle imbalance, they un-fortunately say that the spastic muscles are *strong* and the antagonists are *weak*. This is rarely so. It is the strong *pull* of the short spastic muscle that is strong, and not the spastic muscle work itself. Once spasticity is decreased, spastic muscles often reveal weakness. The antagonists of the spastic mus-cle groups are working at a mechanical disadvantage to the tight pull of the stiff, short spastic muscle groups. Therefore, the antagonists cannot shorten to stretch the spastic agonists. As antagonists cannot counter the pull of the spastic muscles, they appear too weak to do so. In time they really become weak from disuse and inability to be active through their full ranges. It is necessary to prevent deformity by mobilising and lengthening the spastic muscles and strengthening them and their antagonists. As full a range as possible is needed for all muscles.

Ross and Engsberg (2002, 2007) have investigated the relationship between spasticity and strength and also found that there was no 'muscle imbalance' at a joint. They also found that the degree of spasticity (velocity-dependent resistance to passive stretch) had no relation to the amount of strength in that muscle. They consider that 'muscle weakness, and not spasticity may be a prevailing impairment' in cerebral palsy and that their research on the individuals with spastic diplegia showed more involvement distally than proximally in the legs. There was little to no significance of spasticity with function, but strength was correlated with a number of specific variables in functional measures.

The impairment of weakness is further discussed in the next section.

Aims. The therapist and especially those involved in daily care aim to carry out correct management of the abnormal postures and abnormal movements which appear *in function as a priority*, as well as maintain the elongation of short muscles and soft tissues in selected orthoses and equipment. Encourage a variety of active postures and movements in daily motor functions. See aims for strengthening below.

Weakness – general and specific

(1) General weakness is present in hypotonicity and when there is absence of the postural mechanisms. Poor postural control causes weakness in all types of cerebral palsies as they are not available to activate the muscles.

(2) Specific weakness is the weakness of the spastic muscles and of their antagonists. Spastic muscles may usually only act in their inner range, and antagonists in their outer range, but not in the rest of the range. This varies with the severity of the condition.

(3) Asymmetrical weakness occurs in hemiplegia on one side of the body and in asymmetrical diplegia or tetraplegia. In the bilateral cases, greater weakness may be of one arm or leg on different sides or on the same side of the body. One side of the trunk can be weak.

(4) Short weak spastic muscles are initially inelastic ('hypoextensible'). In animal experiments, a muscle immobilised in a short position is associated with a loss of 35% of sarcomeres; conversely, if a muscle is in a lengthened position, the number of sarcomeres can be increased by up to 25% (Tabary *et al.* 1981). Tabary *et al.* (1972) and Tardieu *et al.* (1982) showed that there is reduced activity of the weaker, shorter, inelastic spastic muscles.

(5) Gough *et al.* (2005), in their critical discussion of theories underlying BTX A, draw attention to the importance of weakness rather than muscle fibre length in their research. In children, Lieber and Friden (2002) also did not find decreased muscle fibre length in fixed flexion deformity of the wrist. Shortland *et al.* (2002) in studies of fixed deformity of medial gastrocnemius in children with spastic diplegia found decreased fibre diameter and shortening of the aponeurosis secondary to muscle atrophy rather than short muscle fascicles. The studies of Fry *et al.* (2004) indicate that fixed deformity might relate to muscle atrophy rather than muscle fibre length changes. The decrease in muscle belly length has a relative increase in tendon length. These studies support the importance of weakness in children with spastic diplegia. In previous studies, the inefficient muscle action was associated with the electromyograph showing abnormal contraction in spastic muscles (Tardieu *et al.* 1982; Young & Wiegner 1987).

(6) Assessment of strength of a muscle group on the couch may not relate to its action in function. For example, shoulder girdle muscles may work well in crawl position but not in a muscle test on the couch. Back extensor muscles may be well activated in prone but not in sitting or standing. Extension of the elbow is greater when a child reaches out for a desired object than in muscle tests. This can also be observed when a muscle is active in lying but not in a gait analysis which is more complex (McMulkin *et al.* 2000). Strengthening procedures are used within functions as well as in active exercises and active

movements against resistance for specific muscle groups. In less severe older and ambulant children there has been evidence that strengthening exercises do improve function (Damiano *et al.* 1995a,b; Andersson *et al.* 2003; Dodd *et al.* 2003).

(7) Engsberg *et al.* (2006) in a pilot study on 12 children in a 12-week strength programme with 3 sessions per week found the following: The majority of subjects increased ankle dorsiflexion and plantarflexion separately and together compared to the controls. The Gross Motor Function Measure score for the dimension of walk, run, jump increased. They also measured quality of life, and that improved significantly in child reports and parent reports about the child.

Aims. Considering the discussion points above, the clinician aims to strengthen spastic muscles and their antagonists in as full a range as possible and improve bilateral strength in asymmetrical distribution of weakness. Postural mechanisms need to be developed in active motor activities for the whole child to avoid both specific and general weakness. Developing fitness in leisure activities includes strengthening.

Abnormal co-contraction and abnormal synergies

The abnormal postural mechanisms or their absence lead to abnormal postures against gravity. The normal postural mechanisms are discussed in Chapter 5. In Chapter 9, there are practical therapeutic suggestions for assessment and activation of postural mechanisms within all developmental functions. Compensations result from absent or poor postural mechanisms and may activate excessive co-contraction to maintain balance. The legs appear to be stiff and straight similar to the positive supporting action seen in normal infants. There can be compensations which use a variety of abnormal postures for balance such as those mentioned above in hypotonic ataxia and the examples in Chapter 9 in all antigravity postures.

The abnormal postures are also combined with abnormal movement synergies, which include coactivation (co-contraction) and abnormal recruit-

ment patterns (Tedroff *et al.* 2006). These abnormalities are not due to hypertonicity but due to motor control problems (Shumway-Cook & Woollacott 2001). The postural co-contractions and coactivation in movements are also seen in early normal development or early stages of learning a new motor skill. They do not necessarily create deformities but the persistence of co-contraction in cerebral palsy can lead to limitation of range of the muscles.

There are also abnormal synergies with the difficulties in isolated muscle action seen in lack of selective motor control. For example, a child with spasticity cannot easily dorsiflex an ankle without also flexing hip and knee. Muscles for grasp may not be activated without flexion of wrist and elbow. If a particular movement pattern is used repeatedly for daily functions, then this may cause deformity. In some individuals, persistence of such movement patterns in individuals has also been related to abnormal reflex patterns discussed in the next section.

Aims. Provide a variety in motor patterns within active developmental functions and active exercises, as well as improvement with specific treatments. Develop postural mechanisms within developmental functions.

Abnormal reflex activity (see Table 8.3)

These activities may be used by individuals with dyskinesia or spasticity. There may be persisting infantile reflex patterns or pathological reflex reactions. It is not the reflex *as such* that lead to deformity but the recurring unwitting stimulation of these patterns by those handling a person with cerebral palsy. Children or older people may only be able to move by repeatedly using reflex patterns as the only resource available to them. They learn to activate specific abnormal reflex patterns in their efforts to function. This perpetuates the reflex patterns which lead to deformities. However, not all children depend on a strategy of moving by activating reflexes, and are not being dominated by any reflexes. Examples of reflex patterns are:

Asymmetrical tonic neck reaction (ATNR) may be used by turning the head to the side of a more useful arm for it to reach for a toy with reflex arm extension. A subsequent head turn away from this extended arm obtains a reflex flexion on the occipital side of the head. This arm flexion brings the toy to midline. Another example is of a child with asymmetry, walking with head to one side to stiffen reflex leg extension for stance and head turn away from the extended leg to allow it to bend for stepping. The persistent ATNR to one side creates asymmetrical limb postures by head turning which may lead to deformities in the limbs, a scoliosis and/or a torticollis. Extensor postures are associated with ATNRs, so head flexion in midline enables limitation of the ATNR. In some cases, 'windswept' legs which are associated with persistent ATNR to one side can later lead to hip subluxation due to the flexion-adduction on the occipital side. This abnormal positioning is combined with the effect of gravity.

Symmetrical tonic neck reflexes is rare but may occur in some very severe cases. Immobility and lack of treatment may lead to deformities within these patterns, or in remnants of them.

Reflex stepping may aggravate hypertonic plantar flexors, adductors and extensors if this reflex is used to 'walk' the child frequently. However, the flexion phase of stepping can modify the pattern although the equinus of the ankles, reinforced by reflex stepping, may persist.

Excessive supporting reaction or antigravity reflex may be overstimulated by, say, *baby bouncers or inappropriate walkers* and increases the deformities of the legs, especially equinus and extensor-adductor postures.

Active use of total flexion reactions, withdrawal reflexes in kicking, during rolling, crawling, kneeling. The withdrawal reaction which repeatedly combines hip–knee and ankle flexion rather than a variety of synergies including the hip flexion, knee *extension* and ankle flexion needed for future walking. The repeated use of flexion in all these movements or postures tends to flexion deformity.

Use of total extension reactions as in using the extensor thrust in active kicking, when bounced on the feet in standing, in order to achieve rolling and creeping with abdomen on the floor, may lead to deformities into these patterns of extension.

Aims. When reflex reactions persist in some children, use methods to modify them. As suggested in earlier chapters, the specific methods for development of motor functions will spontaneously decrease or overcome early reflexes. Train a variety of functional motor patterns so that infantile patterns of reflexes need not be used.

Asymmetry

See abnormal postural asymmetry in prone, supine, sitting, standing and walking development (Chapter 9). Deformity may be due to:

(1) Asymmetrical distribution of hypertonus with muscle transformation and asymmetrical weakness.
(2) Excessive weight bearing on one side of the body, arm or leg associated with asymmetry of postural stabilisation. Using only one hand or limb when the other is more impaired develops postural adjustment (counterpoising) more to one side.
(3) Asymmetrical development of tilt, saving and rising postural mechanisms.
(4) Asymmetrical use or persistence of an abnormal reflex, particularly the asymmetric tonic reflex reaction.
(5) Asymmetrical growth of legs mainly in hemiplegia and marked asymmetry in diplegia.
(6) Hemianopia (of visual field), absent visual acuity on one eye or deafness in one ear, which can augment asymmetries above.

Aims. Correct excessive asymmetry. Develop normal symmetrical and asymmetrical motor functions. Use raise on shoes to adjust unequal growth of lower limbs. Check raise by placing different thicknesses of small books under the shorter foot to establish when pelvic adjustment takes place with bilateral weight bearing.

Involuntary movement in one repetitive pattern

Any repeated flexor spasms or involuntary dyskinetic kicking with hip and/or knee flexion, or a flexor involuntary repeated pawing of a leg, may give rise to tightness in the knee or hip. Miller (2007) reports loss of standing for transfers due to knee flexor deformity in young adults or adolescents with athetosis (dyskinesia) combined with spasticity. Similarly and less commonly, children have repetitive extensor spasms or rotary involuntary movements, which may create tightness. Older people with dyskinesia may use muscle tension to control involuntary movements which result in tense abnormal postures with muscle pain.

Aims. Reduce tightness. Treat pain.

Growth factors

There are four main factors which cause or aggravate the development of deformity:

(1) The mechanisms of growth and deformity have been of interest to a number of workers (Graham 2004; Cosgrove 2000; among others). Reduced activity is mainly due to weakness, poor balance and abnormal selective motor control rather than the spasticity (Graham 2004). Activity is needed to provide the frequent stretching which contributes to muscle growth. In mild deformities, muscles and soft tissues do grow but not as fast as the bones. Therefore, muscles grow abnormally slowly in relation to bone, depending on the amount and variety of movement experiences. Botulinum toxin injections are used to maintain muscle length during growth and delay surgery (Cosgrove *et al.* 1994).
(2) The specific bony structure of the hip does not change as it normally would with growth due to abnormal tone, abnormal posture and non-weight bearing. The neck of the femur remains in anteversion and the shaft/neck angle of valgus does not decrease. This is part of the reason for hip deformity and dislocations (see further discussion on hip dislocation).
(3) Spurts of growth in children and adolescents are linked with increase of deformities. The unequal growth of bone and muscle in hypertonia as well as increase in height and especially increase in weight seem to bring on deformities. Usually there would also be less mobility, as older children need to spend longer hours at their studies.
(4) The difference in leg length due to growth results in asymmetry and compensatory deformities. The difference in leg length in hemiplegia creates various abnormal gaits, discussed below.

Aims. Monitor posture and movement throughout the lifespan of a person with cerebral palsy. Treat when indicated, particularly during growth spurts. Therapy needs to increase activity and take care to include stretching of limbs and trunk.

Biomechanics (see sections 'Abnormal postures in standing' and 'Abnormal gaits' in Chapter 9)

The biomechanics related to deformities are as follows:

(1) The spastic muscle groups, particularly those that flex one joint and extend another, such as hamstrings, rectus femoris and gastrocnemius act on bony and joint levers. Abnormal limb alignments result which may not be corrected, especially with weight bearing. In time, they become established producing bony torsion and joint subluxation. The muscle actions are then even more ineffective. Bony torsion or joint subluxation reduces the muscles ability to generate an effective moment (Graham 2004). Stiff soft tissues including muscles, bony and joint abnormalities impair the biomechanics of gait (Gage 1991).
(2) There is an effect of one joint deformity on the whole limb and the whole body in the biomechanics of short spastic muscles and weakness. For example, equinus can increase hip and knee flexion in standing. Equinus of one foot can produce an apparent leg length with associated asymmetry of the pelvis and secondary postural scoliosis. More examples are given in Chapter 9 in the subsection 'Abnormal postures in standing'.
(3) Section 'Development of standing and walking' in Chapter 9 discusses the view of the author that initially it is the poor postural mechanisms and not necessarily the limb deformities that are the primary cause of instability with biomechanical compensation. Some orthopaedic workers who assess children who already have deformities find biomechanical causes of balance problems due to the limb deformities. However, the important clue is the presence or absence of the postural mechanisms of postural stabilisation and counterpoising (postural adjustments). In some children, the posture may have normal alignment in quiet postures up against gravity without movement. When voluntary movement is used, these children cannot balance due to lack of counterpoising and compensate with abnormal postures. These biomechanical compensations for

poorer balance can also take place during both quiet postures and postural adjustments. Therefore, abnormal body alignments are seen during quiet postures against gravity as well as during hand function and leg use in crawling and walking.

These abnormal postures, if uncorrected, can further disturb balance due to increasing abnormal alignment with growth. Green *et al.* (1995) have observed abnormal biomechanics in lying, sitting and standing. Butler and Major (1992) and Farmer *et al.* (1999) have observed biomechanics in upright postures. Gage (1991, 2009) discusses biomechanical problems in gait analyses.

Biomechanics of limb movements are affected by moving in relation to gravity.

Aims. Improve postural mechanisms particularly stability and counterpoising of limb motion. Improve postural alignments and weight bearing both actively, with orthoses and equipment. Apply the biomechanics for movements and strengthening involving use of gravity for assistance, eliminating gravity for neutral actions and increasing muscle actions against gravity for strength (see Chapter 9).

Deformities and gait

For a review of deformities in different topographical types and orthopaedic surgical procedures, see Samilson (1975), Sussman (1992), Cosgrove (2000), Graham (2004), Horstmann and Bleck (2007), Miller (2007) and Gage (2009), among others. Surgeons have different views of surgery and the follow-up rehabilitation, so the physiotherapist will cooperate with an individual orthopaedic surgeon.

Assessment of gait for surgery is based on instrumented 3D gait analyses or, if not available, with observational gait analyses. These analyses are carried out together with other examinations.

Gait analyses for conservative therapy without surgery are discussed in Chapter 8. See Figs 9.164–9.170 for gaits and therapy suggestions.

Upper limbs. The aims of BTX A injections or orthopaedic surgery are for function of hands, cosmesis and hygiene (Cosgrove 2000; Graham 2004; Horstmann & Bleck 2007).

Orthopaedic surgery. Procedures are for wrist flexors, or stabilisation of the wrist joint, lengthening of pronator teres or other muscles. Occupational therapy is used in either the follow-up of surgery or in prevention of deformity and development of function. There is an overlap of occupational therapy with physiotherapy. Arm deformities and function are discussed in this chapter as well as in Chapters 9 and 10.

Spastic hemiplegia

The upper limb deformities are shoulder girdle protraction, shoulder flexion, adduction and internal rotation. A few may develop subluxation or dislocation of the gleno-humeral joint. There is tightness of the pectoralis major and subscapularis. There is elbow flexion with pronation. The tight flexors and pronators together with very weak supinators are present and may occasionally lead to subluxation of the radial head. The wrist and fingers are flexed with thumb flexed, adducted in the palm. The metacarpo-phalangeal joint may be a secondary deformity in the thumb. Wrist ulnar deviation rather than radial is more common. In individual gaits, a hemiplegic arm may also be retracted and hang down straight with elbow pronated and does not swing or be held in the arm position above without swing. A very young child or one with mild-to-moderate involvement will only show the flexed arm pattern on running or jumping. Early therapy usually prevents the arm from becoming more severe.

The lower limb usually begins with a dynamic plantarflexion deformity, which becomes an equinus contracture together with a smaller, shorter limb as the child grows. Equinus gait or 'toe-stepping' may at first have a straight hip and knee with a minimal limp. Later if severity increases or in more severe cases, equinus is accompanied by hip–knee flexion with adduction–internal rotation of the affected leg. Compensation for the equinus may be a vaulting action to assist with clearance. Compensation for equinus on the affected side can also be hyperextension of the knee or use of valgus of the foot to obtain a plantigrade foot. Miller (2007) reports that some children with hemiplegia are 'toe-stepping' on both the hemiplegic side and the unaffected side to avoid a limp.

A gait in hemiplegia may have the affected side retracted with weight in front on the other leg. A momentary stance on the hemiplegic side only allows a short step with the other leg.

Gait is affected not only by weakness but also by inadequate length of plantar flexors in swing phase and stance phases. Below-knee plaster (casting) or orthosis has been used in the early stage. A hinged ankle-foot orthosis (AFO) with or without an injection of BTX A is used for the early dynamic phases. Casting together with BTX A may be another option. These procedures delay surgery until a child is well over 6 years. Depending on severity, surgery may be a lengthening of Achilles tendon (z-plasty) or gastrocnemius slide. In more severe cases there is co-contraction of short hamstrings with quadriceps and equinus, valgus, varus and foot problems. For the hip, knee and foot deformities there are various surgical procedures according to the severity of the hemiplegia (Graham 2004), which are followed by solid AFO or ground reaction AFO. However, many children with hemiplegia achieve walking without walking aids and following conservative physiotherapy. They may or may not develop fixed deformities later.

Spastic diplegia

Generally, the walking of children with diplegia is much slower than in able-bodied children, and their choice of velocity is most efficient but in later years their inefficient walk leads to fatigue (see subsection 'Prognosis for walking' in Chapter 9). Deformities may be mild, not interfering with walking, but if more severe may lead to deterioration of walking.

Upper limbs. There may be persistence of arms held up in the air in toddler 'high or medium-guard', or in a 'tight-wire walking' position as well as excessive arm saving reactions. In early independent walking, reciprocal arm swing is absent. Abnormal postures of both arms in the hemiplegic-flexed pattern are mentioned above.

Lower limbs. In the *toe-stepping gait* in young or mild diplegia, there is initially a toe walk in equinus with a normal or stiff knee extension and mild internal rotation of hips. *Toe first* and not the normal heel strike on initial contact following the leg swing is common. With arms in high guard a child can walk fast on toes and falls rather than stop. This is

managed with ankle-foot orthoses and physiotherapy to gain balance and control. Walking with a plantigrade foot becomes possible in this case.

Knees may overflex on swing and on weight bearing. Hip and knee flexion may occur to allow a plantarflexed foot (or equinus) to swing and clear the ground, and once on the ground, hip and knee flexion occur to push the heel to the ground. However, as mentioned above, there may instead be equinus on initial foot contact with hip and knee straight. Lack of heel strike after swing may be compensated by flexion of hips with hyperextension of the knees to press the heels to the ground in pronation. This is usual with extensor patterns or excessive antigravity support as the forefoot strikes the ground. Hyperextended knees if untreated in middle childhood may cause much knee pain in adolescence and a wheel chair may later be needed (Miller 2007). Miller suggests a calf-length articulated AFO that limits plantarflexion to assist hamstring strengthening over time to counter the knee hyperextension. Hyperextension can be treated with operations for equinus if that is the cause.

A child may become stiffer with spasticity and the equinus and varus increase. In these cases, BTX A injection is used to tolerate the ankle-foot orthoses and physiotherapy continues together with passive stretching and strengthening exercises for feet and legs as well as balance training.

A diplegic gait that is more common is presented in the following pattern. There is hip flexion–adduction–internal rotation with knee flexion and equino-varus, or feet flat with valgus. In diplegia the hips may adduct and legs cross when the child is supported, and adduct, internally rotate and flex when the child is walking independently. A wider base of the feet is achieved with flexed closely adducted (valgus) knees as the child cannot balance on the small base created by adduction of the legs. Feet may also be in valgus to overcome equinus.

There may be a '*jump gait*' of hip and knee flexion with equinus on initial foot contact followed by hip and knee extension during stance. This has a jump-like appearance. Graham (2004) may manage this gait with articulated orthoses. The equinus may be apparent and secondary to hip and knee flexion, so BTX A is *not* used for plantar flexors.

In the '*crouch gait*' the ankle is excessively dorsiflexed with increased hip and knee flexion. These children may have been toe walkers with straight or mildly flexed hip and knees before becoming an adolescent with a crouch gait. BTX A and various surgical procedures are used by different surgeons. Ground reaction AFOs may be used in milder crouch gaits before surgery or following surgery. With increased severity the flexion contractures are seen together with bony torsion deformities and joint problems in hips, knees and feet due to the biomechanics of walking (Graham 2004). Damiano *et al.* (1995a) have markedly improved crouch gait with strengthening exercises against resistance for quadriceps and hip extensors. Presumably the deformities are then largely dynamic.

Various operations are recommended to overcome hip–knee flexion in crouch gait, such as hamstring and psoas lengthening and correction of bony deformities if present. Ground-reaction ankle-foot orthoses may follow some operations on muscles and soft tissues in less severe cases.

Surgery is suggested when there is increased knee flexion in both foot contact and mid-stance phases of gait, together with a markedly increased popliteal angle on physical examination. Surgery is usually used for fixed knee flexion deformity. Examples are partial hamstring tenotomy, hamstring slide, hamstring transplants, with various lengthening procedures and transfers of other muscles. Surgery to lengthen short hamstrings has been used when hamstrings create a kyphotic sitting posture in older people. Post-operative physiotherapy may include knee splints range of motion exercises, strengthening of both extensors and flexors of hips and knees. Treat the hamstrings for two-joint muscles. Rehabilitation teaches a child to move with his 'new legs' and work on extension. Weight bearing depends on the advice of the surgeon.

Many children with diplegia have asymmetry between the legs of individual weak muscle groups but pelvic asymmetry and scoliosis may not always be present. However, when scoliosis is present, it is due to unequal weight distribution and/or difference in leg length. There may be limited mobility in hips, pelvis and lumbar spine. Backward tilt of the pelvis with flat lumbar spine may be present in some children, or excessive forward pelvic tilt with lumbar lordosis. There may also be round backs (kyphosis) with lordosis and the hip flexion. Spasticity and deformity are more in the psoas, hamstrings, rectus femoris and gastrocnemius. Postural malalignments may be secondary to limb problems or persist from abnormal sitting postures and poor postural mechanisms against gravity.

The pelvis often rotates abnormally in all 'spastic gaits'. The rotation may be backwards, so the leg appears *retracted* and behind the other. Usually the front, more able leg takes more weight. However, there may be the situation when a back leg may take more weight and allow the forward leg to step, take its momentary weight and then transfer on to the back leg, which only has time to take a small step and *cannot* get in front of the forward leg.

If the child takes a step, his stiffness may be so great that he has to lean back to push his leg forward. He has an antero-posterior jerky walk. Lateral 'waddle' is associated with spastic adductors and weak abductors. It is also involved with inability to stabilise the pelvis or to adjust the trunk when counterpoising in standing on one leg. The trunk and head may lean forward to help overcome stiff spastic extension or use much head and trunk mobility to counter the lower body stiffness to maintain balance (postural control). Orthopaedic surgical procedures are indicated for excessive hip extension with abnormal pelvic tilts (Sussman 1992; Horstmann & Bleck 2007).

If a child has an early gait which is efficient, this is frequently maintained until adulthood. If the child is struggling to walk and just managing with much flexion, then retaining walking is less likely. Weight gain and prolonged sitting will also decrease the future likelihood of walking with or without crutches, sticks and other aids.

Spastic tetraplegia (quadriplegia)

This type is usually more severe with weakness, loss of selective motor control, retention of infantile reflexes, muscle imbalance, abnormal posture and general spasticity. The whole body is much more involved than the other types of cerebral palsies. Deformities of limbs, position of pelvis and trunk, and abnormal weight transference are similar to spastic hemiplegia and spastic diplegia usually with greater asymmetry and severity. The leg deformities can be accompanied by unilateral or bilateral hip dislocation, pelvic obliquity and scoliosis. As hip problems are frequently encountered, there is further discussion below in the subsection 'Hip flexion–adduction–internal rotation'.

Bone density problems. In severe diplegia and tetraplegia, there are more bone density problems due to poor nutrition and some medications for epilepsy, and there is less likelihood of weight bearing and independent standing and walking. However, there are some who will continue to use a walker until 12–13 years (Miller 2007). Older children are encouraged to use standing frames and well-supported walkers to maintain weight bearing for transfers, general fitness and possibly for bone density problems. In early childhood, standing frames are needed followed by well-supporting walkers. If there is mild-to-moderate flexion in hips and knees and correction of deformities of feet, this allows standing, transfers and, in individual cases, stepping in fully supported walkers, or with less support but in forearm-supporting walkers. The legs are sometimes more severe than the arms, so hands can be used with special controls for electronic communication equipment and electric wheelchairs. Children with tetraplegia may have good cognition, so focus on education and hand function warrants more time than the training of walking. However, there are adolescents who continue household walking with an appropriate walker for that environment. Surgery for knee flexion contractures is suggested by some surgeons for community walkers rather than for predominantly wheelchair users. Knee flexion surgery is discussed above.

Surgery for feet in all types of cerebral palsies depends on the other joint deformities. BTX A injection for plantar flexors with and without casting has been mentioned in this chapter, which delays surgery until children are over 6 years old. Surgeons may carry out lengthening of Achilles tendon (z-plasty) for gastrocnemius and soleus shortening or gastrocnemius slide. Surgery for varus or valgus may also involve tendon transfers. Surgery for equinus may be associated with surgery for other joint deformities. Post-operative physiotherapy may follow plasters, and strengthening is the main aim. Use of orthoses varies as how long a period they are worn in times of the day as there may be very weak muscles post-operatively, needing active strengthening. Several older children with more skeletal maturity may have various types of triple arthrodesis and some have peroneus brevis lengthening for valgus and transplants for equino-varus or varus. Various foot problems such as forefoot deformities are also treated by surgeons (Miller 2007). Post-operative physiotherapy for feet emphasises strengthening and training of standing and gait with correction of foot posture.

Therapy and daily care

Many of the aims based on the causes of deformity given above in points 1–10 suggest methods which overlap and interact with each other. Methods give consideration for the aims of immobility, abnormal tone, co-contractions, movement synergies, weakness, abnormal reflexes, asymmetry, repetitive involuntary motion, growth and biomechanics.

Conservative treatment methods are usually favoured in young children as their growth may decrease the need or delay the needs for surgery. In addition, conservative physiotherapy avoids potential risk of surgical overlengthening, infection, scarring and perhaps anaesthetic problems (Jefferson 2004).

Methods suggested are the following:

(1) Positioning to stretch muscles in equipment and orthoses (braces) was used by Phelps (1952) and has become traditional with designs by many workers. However, the positioning equipment and orthoses have improved over the years. Today, a 24-hour postural management programme is planned which includes:
   (a) Frequent changes of a person's posture. Use different postures through 24 hours with and, when possible, without equipment for prone, supine, side lying, sitting and standing. This avoids stretching only one group of spastic or dystonic muscles.
   (b) Correct positioning of each part of a person's limbs and body for alignment and symmetry, and regularly check these alignments. Educate others to participate in these regular checks.
   (c) Selection of equipment to maintain postural correction during use of hands within daily activities and for a child's speech and language, visual experience and social interactions.
   (d) Bone density is assisted (Stuberg 1992). At least 30–60 minutes daily or 3–4 times a week in standing frames are recommended for muscles, joints as well as for bone density (Stuberg 1992). Select orthoses, splints and equipment according to age and severity. See details in subsection 'Aims of standing equipment (frames)' in Chapter 9.

(e) Selection of equipment for positioning during sleep, provided there is no contraindication such as seizures, vomiting from gastroesophogeal reflux, threats of aspiration and breathing problems, excessive opisthotonus and nocturnal hypoxaemia (Martin *et al.* 1995). The bed needs to be correctly tilted for these problems without causing the child to slip down in bed. Tardieu *et al.* (1988) found that stretch needs to be maintained for 6 hours daily to have an effective increase in muscle length. They use the soleus as an example. This can be obtained when the child is relaxed at night in positioning equipment or splints depending on the child's condition and family views. The 6 hours need not be continuous in all cases.

Night-time positioning equipment or 'sleep systems' is available on the market. They include Symmetrisleep (Goldsmith 2000), Chailey lying boards (Pountney *et al.* 2004), Dreama by Jenx (Hankinson & Morton 2002) and models by Moonlite (Collins 2007). In a survey of the value and design of Night Time Postural Management equipment (Polak *et al.* 2008), Snoooooooze (Peacocks Medical Group) and Sleepform (Leckey) are also added.

Aims of night time positioning are for better sleep, reducing deformities especially of hips, to avoid surgery for pressure relief, comfort and less need for repositioning a child at night and to reduce pain. As night positioning is part of 24-hour postural management it has the same consequences for a child's function in all areas in daily life.

(f) Conservative physiotherapy with 24-hour management is difficult for some families, and careful education and support of families and carers is most important. Explain the importance of postural management programme to parents and carers, educate and support them.

(2) Train a variety of functional motor patterns within daily functions. Techniques for all the aims mentioned above are presented within daily functions in Chapter 9 in the sections 'Treatment and management at all developmental levels'. Chapter 10 reviews motor function

in daily life activities, which includes positioning to avoid deformities as well as enable a child to function.

For example, in selected functional activities of interest to a child, such as reaching out and up for a toy or reaching and turning to touch a friendly person, there is a simultaneous correction of flexion. Games, action, songs and playthings are more motivating to activate and strengthen muscles. During activities, place desired objects or playthings which use stretching, bending and turning actions of limbs and bodies.

(3) Manage the biomechanics of deformity with treatment procedures, orthoses and equipment. Use functional activities to activate postural mechanisms for better biomechanics.

Postural management is individual and can be guided by the Gross Motor Function Classification System (GMFCS) giving criteria for the level of function (Palisano *et al.* 1997). Levels IV and V start postural management earlier than Level III with early activity more easily emphasised from Levels I–III. Although there is a recommendation that children in GMFCS Levels IV and V should start postural management soon after birth and in sitting at 6 months (Gericke 2006), this is controversial. The diagnosis of cerebral palsy is 'far from clear' in the early months (Neville 2000) and may not be firm before 12 months (Nelson & Ellenberg 1982; Touwen 1987) and even later. A child may have a variance of normality and identification may take time (Bax & Brown 2004). In addition, the GMFCS is only stable from age 2 years (Gorter *et al.* 2009).

Specific goals for postural management and postural control are given at each developmental level in Chapter 9. However, people in GMFCS Levels IV and V may need to use equipment for deformities which is beyond their developmental levels in sitting and standing.

Additional methods and comments which augment those in Chapter 9 are the following:

(1) *Ice treatments* (cryotherapy) to whole limb or on the spastic muscle groups to decrease spasticity or to stimulate a muscle action depending on application (De Souza 1997; Shumway-Cook & Woollacott 2001).

(2) *Prolonged stretch to spastic muscles* in correct positions in plasters or moulded orthoses and postural equipment. There are bivalved plaster

casts as night splints which can be removed for activities during the day. The positioning for stretch is usually routine in school and home for medium to severe cases (GMFCS Levels III–V).

(3) *Gentle manual stretch* given together with 3–4 minutes of maintained ice treatments. It is more effective if stretchings are given as assisted active or active movement. Very young children as well as older individuals are easier to stretch in warm water at bath time or in hydrotherapy. A regime for manual stretching with hold in the stretch for 40–60 seconds and 3–5 repetitions for each movement is given 1–2 times per week (Fragala *et al.* 2003) or daily by other physiotherapists. This is added to routine positioning in different types of equipment. As tissue damage due to immobility needs to be considered daily range of motion (ROM), and change of position is important especially in severely affected children (GMFCS Levels IV and V).

Such children also like stretches and ROM as they prevent muscle cramps and their limbs and body positions are changed (Pin *et al.* 2006). After daily manual stretches, people with cerebral palsy report feeling looser and more able to carry out an activity (Soames 2003). Stretching is also helpful before positioning a person in equipment and before the application of orthoses. Always give *slow gentle stretch* as forced stretches can tear muscles and soft tissues and quick stretches stimulate physiological spasticity.

Manual stretching or slow rhythmic passive ranges are not prolonged enough for changing muscle length, but maintain length obtained after 6-hour stretch at night or spread between night and day according to family needs.

(4) *Passive ranges of movement* in as full a range as possible and with knowledge of normal ranges in infants and young children. Infants are normally more flexed than older children. Passive ranges of motion are mainly for flexibility of joints but soft tissues and muscles are also stretched. Procedures to lengthen spastic muscles are not possible if joints are stiff from immobility or only moved in a limited range. The passive ranges of motion need to be carried out slowly for soft tissues and joint flexibility. As already mentioned, passive ranges of movement are less likely to overcome problems of muscle length than prolonged stretch.

Note: Stretchings and ROM need to be worked out with parents and others involved directly with a child or older person. Parents, carers and a young child enjoy the slow rhythm and song with the touch associated with interactive communication during passive stretchings. It is easily done during dressing, nappy changes and at bath time and during swimming. Parents and carers need to report any pain, discomfort and change in ranges to a therapist.

There is some evidence though limited by rigour in studies of the changes of spasticity or change in ranges of movement following short-time stretching and ROM (Pin *et al.* 2006). Pin *et al.* (2006) prefer sustained stretch, as do Tremblay *et al.* (1990), particularly in standing equipment. Pin *et al.* (2006) recommend more rigour in research on stretching. Pountney and Green (2006) state that 'cohort studies provide limited evidence to support 24 hour postural approaches', and as postural management programmes have limited evidence they recommend more research.

(5) *Activation of antagonists and agonists* assists the correction of deformities. This takes place in strengthening exercises for short- or over-lengthened muscles.

Exercises are given below in this chapter for:
- Active and full range of movement of antagonists to hypertonic muscles, especially in middle and inner ranges.
- Active and full range of movement of hypertonic muscles, especially in middle and elongated ranges.

(6) *Holding a corrected position.* This takes place passively with orthoses, special seating, standing frames and lying equipment. Passive positions may give a sensory picture of body image but not an active learning experience of body image. Motor learning needs to be more active for better effect (Chapter 5). A child and an older person are trained to actively hold the correction. Manual assistance may first be given and withdrawn as the child shows ability to do this alone. Follow with manual resistance to trunk and pelvis with method of 'hold and relax' (Knott & Voss 1968; Levitt 1970b). In addition, such active control needs to be translated into a daily activity. A child often prefers to practice holding a position for the duration of a rhyme or song. Active limb movements need

to be stimulated through play in order to correct head and body postural adjustments as well as limb positions in purposeful activities.

(7) *Rotation and diagonal movements* have been observed to decrease spasticity and dynamic shortening observed in the straight flexion and extension ranges (Knott & Voss 1968; Adler *et al.* 2008).

(8) Treat asymmetry in hemiplegia, diplegia or quadriplegia which may lead to various deformities, and if walking with or without equipment/aids then present asymmetry creates abnormal gaits discussed below.

Symmetrical and alternate weight bearing on legs is emphasised in therapy together with both upper limbs and hand grasps forward. Strengthening of the hemiplegic leg or in bilateral conditions, both legs especially of gastrocnemius for push-off and dorsiflexion for heel strike on initial contact is important. In a particular gait, strengthening of weak hip, knee and arm muscles on one or both sides, as assessed in gait problems.

(9) *Additional methods are* vibration techniques used either to activate muscles or reduce spasticity (Rood 1962; Hagbarth & Eklund 1969; Eckersley 1993). Electrical stimulation to antagonists are claimed to decrease the pull of agonist spastic muscles. Repeated contractions of spastic muscles followed by an active contraction of the antagonists was used for increasing ranges (Rood 1962; Stockmeyer 1972). This method sometimes helps mild-to-moderate cases.

Use of plasters (inhibitory or tone-reducing casts)

Indications for below-knee plaster (tone inhibitory casts) for dynamic (unfixed) deformities are the following:

(1) When child pulls up to stand on his toes only, or continues standing on toes.
(2) When child stands with heels down but walks on toes.
(3) When child is ready for standing and walking but cannot balance on deformed feet which are in either equinus, varus or equino-varus. When

sitting balance is poor and feet are habitually in plantarflexion or with feet twisted inwards, so they cannot be used for stability.

(4) To prevent any of the above becoming fixed deformities.
(5) To delay orthopaedic surgery in young children as surgery results may be unpredictable in a delayed developing nervous system.
(6) To train a better walking pattern using the proprioceptive responses and body image of weight bearing with the heel down and the possibility of heel strike on stepping forward, made possible by the corrective plaster. The plaster also correctly moulds the feet with toe flexion reduced.
(7) To stretch short tight muscles and connective tissues. There is then also correction of overlengthened antagonists so that a child can tolerate orthoses. Lengthening of short muscles aims to improve movements, postures and gait.

See casting together with BTX A discussed below.

Collaboration with parents is essential for good results, thus explain the purpose of the plaster or thermoplastic splint to both parent and child who can understand. The importance of their help and encouragement for their child is essential to make sure the child wears them. Discuss with parents and teachers when times are convenient for application of splints. Show parents and carers home exercises and the training of standing and walking.

Materials for casting. Various materials are available such as plaster of Paris (POP), glass fibre casting bandages with polyurethane resin and other synthetic materials. POP is easier for moulding the foot, while other materials dry more quickly allowing weight bearing. Gloves must be used for all materials. There are various methods of applying plaster casts used by orthotists working together with physiotherapists and some physiotherapists independently apply plasters (Levitt 1977 and Jones 1993 in earlier editions describe techniques of plaster applications). Experience is needed to get adequate but not excessive stretch, corrected position and avoidance of skin pressures.

Use a series of casts for those children who do not maintain correction. Have a short period of exercises and weight bearing before the next plaster is applied. The period between plasters has been from 1 to 2 weeks to as long as 2 years in different cases. Cottalorda *et al.* (2000) applied plasters weekly for 3 weeks, which achieved results for equinus. Therapists prefer short periods as weakening of muscles can occur with long immobilisation. Initially a cast for a few days may be used before applying a series of casts to continue further improvement of position.

The athetoid (dyskinetic) type of cerebral palsy have involuntary movements which either preclude wearing a plaster or for not more than a week at a time. BTX A is preferred for dystonia rather than plaster casts. However, the weight of the plaster cast seems to help the development of stability. Casts are usually followed with an orthosis. Phillips and Audet (1990) have used knee plaster casts in adolescence. BTX A injections are used together with plaster casts. There are various studies mentioned in the section on botulinum toxin injections.

Miller (2007) points out that new materials such as thermoplastics can be correctly moulded to limbs and sole and have the same effect as plaster casts for prolonged stretch and corrections. Miller (2007) has heard from parents of the inconvenience to them and their child of the need to have a series of plasters, so many weeks of childhood may be spent in casts, with difficulties in dressing, washing and general lifestyle. Orthoses made from thermoplastic materials are preferred by him.

Aims for below-knee orthoses are like those for casting in addition to other aims for deformities above.

Exercises in plaster or orthoses. Emphasise extension movements of the knee and hip, and back (see Figs 11.1–11.10), for example straight leg lift backwards, knee stretching in sitting, side lying extension. Weight-bearing exercises after 3 days. Standing weight shift from leg to leg sideways and forward and back. Shift the pelvis forward over the weight-bearing foot, counteracting hip retraction. Sitting stretch up and stand up 'tall'. Stand walk as much as possible, with weight distributed on to both sides equally. Tilt reactions in standing on sponge to increase weight bearing through the leg in plaster or orthosis.

A long leg back plaster slab from hip to ankle is used and is removable for washing and exercises, with movements in water.

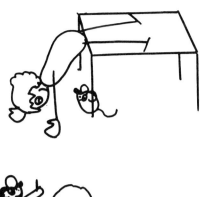

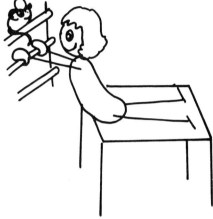

Figure 11.1 Bend over edge of mother's lap, large ball or couch, raise up and bend down again. Hold rungs and 'walk up' for level of hip extension. Keep legs apart and turned out if necessary. Child raises head and trunk up in association with hip extension. Initial support may be given by the mother's hand on his chest. Avoid abnormal extensor thrust, excessive lordosis.

Upper limbs. Yasukawa (1990) looked at the effect of casting for elbow and wrist flexion and pronation deformities in hemiplegia. Boyd *et al.* (2001b) mention casting in their review of upper limb dysfunction. Lannin *et al.* (2007) critically reviewed casting in children and adults but found insufficient high-quality evidence to either support or abandon this practice in more severe cases. There are serial and drop-out casting for adults with 5 or 10° less than full range of elbow extension with forearm in neutral. However, compliance of children and adolescents is poor and caution is advised for severe cases of spasticity, due to myositis ossificans, skin breakdown and sensory deprivation in the hands.

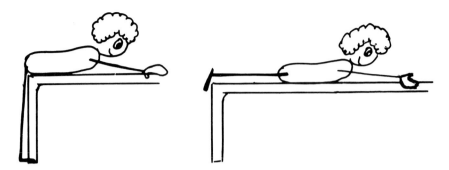

Figure 11.2 Child's legs over mother's lap, edge of bed, large ball or roll. Bring legs down to floor (hip flexion) into bed (hip extension). Hold knees and thighs apart in external rotation to encourage hip extension-abduction-external rotation if required. Raise *one* leg at a time to control lordosis (Fig. 11.6). Child may grasp side of table or both his arms are held elevated-abducted and externally rotated by adult if abnormal flexion in arm and trunk is present. Use these movements when getting up on to bed/plinth *or* getting out of bed.

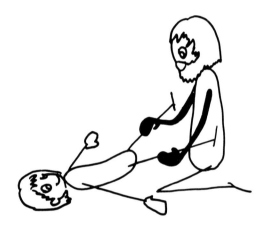

Figure 11.3 Legs of child held in abduction-external rotation. Active raise of child's hips into extension. *Avoid* use of lordosis to do this. Legs may be on lap of therapist, on low stool or with his feet flat on the ground for 'bridging' the pelvis into extension. Manual resistance may be given to anterior superior iliac spines to augment extension. Obtain flexion by asking child to bend knees to chest, and then repeat hip extension activity. Use this action during play, dressing and washing.

Research studies

There are many recent research studies on casting, which usually accompany studies on BTX A (see below). Bertoti (1986) has researched casting without BTX A comparing casting to no casting in a randomised controlled trial. According to the review of many research studies by Blackmore et al. (2007), this study was rated highly as II and found that casting improved stride length, whereas dif-

ferences in other gait components were not significant. McNee et al. (2007) studied short-term serial casting in children with spastic cerebral palsy. Their results showed increased passive and dynamic dorsiflexion and changes in some elements of gait. They state that the dorsiflexion with straight knee and functional changes were small and short-lived. However, Cottalorda et al. (2000) have found serial casting to be more positive for children who were toe walking. Plantigrade feet were obtained in these children.

There is also the view that the aim of casting to reduce shortening is not always supported by evidence (Pin *et al.* 2006). Shortland *et al.* (2002) found in their research that the spastic muscle weakness was the main problem. The shortening is due to the aponeurosis secondary to muscle atrophy.

If casting needs to be applied so that tolerance of orthoses is assisted, then a short period of casting for a week is recommended. To avoid weakness, active exercises are important for periods after casting and when orthoses are removed for a period after school or during weekends.

Botulinum toxin A

BTX A injections are often used as treatment for spasticity and dystonia. Multilevel injections are used (Scholtes *et al.* 2006), though focal injections are more common. Lower and upper extremities are treated. More recently, trunk muscles have sometimes been injected.

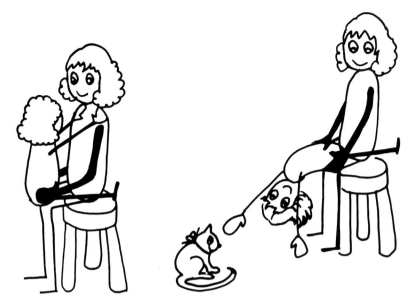

Figure 11.4 The child actively stretches down and comes up to sitting with or without grasping your hand. For babies, you may use the large ball or roll. The child may also bend sideways to the floor for scoliosis correction.

BTX blocks the release of acetylcholine in the nerve endings at the neuromuscular junction. There is a reduction of spasticity of the individual muscle injected which commences between 24 and 72 hours. Muscle relaxation is most evident after 2 weeks following injection and disappears between 3 and 6 months and may sometimes last longer. Re-peat injections are indicated but may be limited as long-term damage is not yet known (Gough *et al.* 2005).

General clinical recommendations for BTX A:

(1) Usually spastic hemiplegia and diplegia are preferred but tetraplegia is also selected for limbs.
(2) The candidate responds best when full joint ranges are present on static examination,

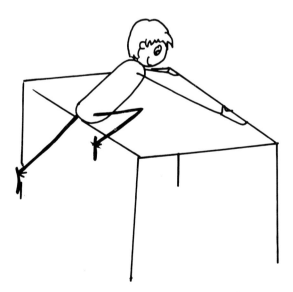

Figure 11.5 One knee held bent to chest during hip extension of the other leg to counteract lordosis. Carry this out in side lying or in prone. Also flex-abduct-externally rotate extended leg for action of those agonists.

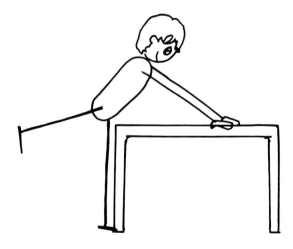

Figure 11.6 Child leans forward onto ball, table, roll, during active hip extension of each leg. Lordosis is more easily controlled this way. Next, flex the leg so that foot reaches high bar or even table.

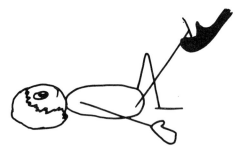

Figure 11.7   One knee flexed to chest or flexed with foot flat. Press other leg into extension into adult's hand, sponge rubber surface, soft couch. Child's hips raise into extension with his weight on one foot. Full flexion of each hip should be carried out actively if required. Arms straight, and hands pressed flat or grasping edge of bed.

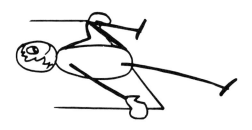

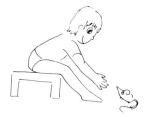

Figure 11.8   *Activate agonists and antagonists* and full range of active hip and knee motion. Use of arm extension is incorporated in these exercises.

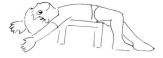

Figure 11.9   *Activate agonists and antagonists* and full range of active hip and knee motion. Use of arm extension is incorporated in these exercises. Use hip flexion to manage socks and shoes.

though dynamic shortening of spastic muscle takes place during activity (Eames *et al.* 1999). Fixed contractures need BTX A together with other treatments, but bony deformities of torsion cannot be altered.

(3)   Frequency of injection is at intervals of 6–12 months and at a minimum of 3-month interval.

(4)   Parents and child need to know that their postoperative participation is most important. They need to be told the aims of injection and that it is given with a local anaesthetic with a mild sedative, or maybe under a general anaesthetic. Multilevel injections of BTX A usually need an anaesthetic. With a local anaesthetic, 2-hour rest is given post-injection so that a child can overcome his sleepiness before he returns home.

(5)   Explain that a child will have an initial feeling of weakness of an injected limb. If in a lower limb, a child may begin falling due to weakness and the change in his body image using a different base, say, plantigrade feet or more abducted thighs. The physiotherapy programme in which all participate improves all this and maintains the correction of deformity as long as possible.

The aims of BTX A

Selection of cases continues to be studied and the physiotherapist's view is expected by the team. The report on BTX A by the Association for Paediatric Chartered Physiotherapists (APCP 2008) is prepared in the United Kingdom for evidence-based practice.

Selection is based on identification of the specific muscles causing a child's main functional difficulty.

Examples of aims include use of calf injections for dynamic equinus and hamstring injection for dynamic knee flexion greater than 20° during gait. There are aims to improve crouch gait, scissoring and equino-varus and valgus. Aims of injections in adductors are to avoid hip problems and in adductors together with hamstrings to improve seating and for ease of care in severe conditions.

In the upper limbs, aims of injections are used for tight thumb adduction, abnormal wrist position or elbow flexion. Aims include improvement of function and cosmetic appearance and to counter marked asymmetry of limbs.

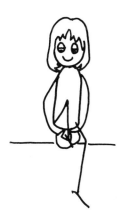
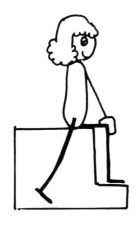
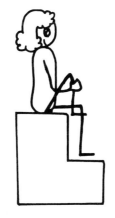

Figure 11.10 *Activate agonists and antagonists* and full range of active hip and knee motion. Use of arm extension is incorporated in these exercises. Use these movements during dressing/washing.

The specific times for BTX A are:

- When a child pulls to stand and cruises, particularly with 'on-toes' pattern.
- When a walking (ambulant) child is at a plateau in walking skills, is losing balance, is continuing to have falls and a gait pattern is not improving.
- When a child wishes to progress to pedalling a bike (tricycle), climb stairs with less support, kick a ball and try other motor skills involving a better base for postural stability and counterpoising.
- When a short muscle or muscles need stretching to allow improved posture and movement.
- When spastic adductors and plantar flexors limit transfers and base for sitting or walking.
- When spasticity blocks nappy changes, hygiene of perineum or difficulty in washing tight hands.
- When there is pain or painful spasms.
- When high-energy expenditure is causing poor endurance or decreasing distance walked in a specified time or decrease in motor repetitions.
- When there are anxieties of child, adolescent and families concerning appearance of gait.
- When there is difficulty applying orthoses and skin intolerance to them. Serial casting may precede or follow the injection with BTX A.
- When surgical intervention needs to be delayed in young children as growth changes results of surgery. BTX A can maintain muscle length during growth.

Injections are used in diagnosis before surgery and as analgesic for pain and spasm immediately after surgery. Reduction of spastic shortening of a muscle group shows the likely post-surgical biomechanics in the individual. The degree of surgery is also optimised following injections with continual physiotherapy.

Research studies and reviews of BTX A

There have been more than 100 studies to establish its effectiveness since around 1993 (Cosgrove *et al.* 1994). There is a large multicentre study by Baker *et al.* (2002) and Koman *et al.* (2001).

Bjornson *et al.* (2007) carried out a randomised controlled trial, which included parent satisfaction measures and electromechanical measures of joint range among the 14 separate measures of outcomes. Physiotherapy continued throughout the study of 33 children with spastic diplegia at GMFCS Levels from I to III. The findings were that despite mechanical and physiological improvements the families did not perceive meaningful changes in their goals and in societal participation. Therefore, clear goals for BTX A treatments need to be confirmed with families and child.

Jefferson (2004) has a helpful detailed review of 24 studies.

Lannin *et al.* (2006) have carried out a systematic review of research on therapy after BTX A and found only three studies of a good enough design (Levels of evidence II and III). However, these studies did not produce significant findings and more research is needed.

Simpson *et al.* (2008) in an assessment of 80 studies find only four research studies in Class I (American Academy of Neurology criteria), plus one on adductor spasticity and one on the analgesic effect of BTX A in Class I. Their list of studies in their review is of interest to the clinician for evidence-based therapy.

Upper limb studies of BTX A

These include research by Wallen *et al.* (2007) who investigated the outcome of BTX A and occupational therapy (OT) in the upper limbs. They found that BTX A with OT accelerated attainment as shown by the Goal Attainment Scale and the Canadian Occupational Performance Measure. However, the Melbourne Assessment of Unilateral Upper Limb Function, QUEST, PEDI, the Child Health Questionnaire and ranges of movement did not show any significant effect of either BTX A or OT alone or together.

There are studies by Fehlings *et al.* (2001) in hemiplegia showing functional improvement using the QUEST and parent report. Friedman *et al.* (2000) showed functional gains with OT, and they also assessed the appearance and ease of management of upper limbs by carers. The study was rated IV (Lannin *et al.* 2006). Speth *et al.* (2005) found that the wrist dorsiflexion gains after BTX A were clinically useful, but no statistically significant results were obtained for supination and function. They report that the Melbourne and PEDI measures were not sensitive to effects of BTX A. Both the treated and untreated groups were on intensive OT, and as functional differences between both groups were not great, it seems to me that the OT was achieving more than BTX A.

Corry *et al.* (1997) found that BTX A injection in the upper limb of children with hemiplegia significantly increased active elbow and thumb extension, reducing tone at the wrist and elbow. There was a modest functional change and in some cases a temporary deterioration.

BTX A and casting

Blackmore *et al.* (2007) have carried out a systematic review of casting on equinus in cerebral palsy. They reviewed 22 research studies which examined the effects of casting, either alone or in combination with BTX A. They concluded that 'there is no strong and consistent evidence that combining casting and BTX A is superior to using either intervention alone'. They also found that there is no evidence that casting before BTX A has any different effect from casting after BTX A.

Glanzman *et al.* (2004) in a retrospective analysis of serial casting, BTX A and combined treatment for spastic equinus found no significant difference between casting with or without BTX A. Both improved the range of movement of the ankle to a greater degree than did BTX A alone. Corry *et al.* (1998) compared BTX A with stretching casts and found that they gave equal results but that BTX A was quicker, more convenient and lasted longer.

Marshall *et al.* (2007) in a systematic review of treatment strategies for motor impairment found strong evidence for serial casting. They found moderate evidence for casting being as effective as casting with BTX A. All the studies reviewed were of people with acquired brain injury.

The studies of Gough *et al.* (2005), Fry *et al.* (2004) and Shortland *et al.* (2002) suggest that short spastic muscles are weak and need strengthening rather than in need of reduction of spasticity with BTX A.

Daily management following injections

In the management of BTX A, Graham *et al.* (2000), Ubhi *et al.* (2000) and Eames *et al.* (1999) all recommend using BTX A together with physiotherapy and orthoses. Physiotherapists suggest the following methods for the goals set for therapy with BTX A. This is based on the Association of Paediatric Chartered Physiotherapists (APCP) survey in the United Kingdom (APCP 2008). Dumas *et al.* (2001) report a consensus of 62 paediatric physiotherapy experts in the United States and Canada, which included a ranked importance of various direct interventions following botulinum injection(s) for lower limb spasticity in cerebral palsy. These are similar to many of those used in the United Kingdom. It seems that BTX A does not change the goals and methods of paediatric physiotherapy but offers a transition phase of intensifying training of motor control and function. Some therapists increase sessions whereas others continue twice-a-week sessions just pre-injection (O'Neil *et al.* 2003). The report by APCP (2008) states that one cannot be prescriptive, leaving decisions to individual physiotherapists based on their assessments.

Physiotherapy consists of the following:

(1) Daily range of motion with stretches and maintained stretch in day orthoses and night splints.

Night splints immediately after injection worn for 6 hours or more (Tardieu *et al.* 1988). Orthoses may be increased initially and decreased from, say, AFO to hinged AFO to dynamic AFO to supportive shoe with insole. Increased activity of leg muscles is enhanced with such progressive decrease of support.

(2) A sleeping system for postural correction depends on each child (see discussion on night-time positioning above).

(3) Strengthening injected muscles which appear weak or very weak after injection, their antagonists and postural control muscles.

(4) Among many other individual physiotherapy programmes are activating motor control with targeted motor training, constraint-induced movement therapy, neurodevelopmental therapy, walking and gait training, functional training of activities of daily living, use of stairs, inclines, tricycling, climbing and therapeutic horse riding. There are also motor learning and relearning approaches and especially home programmes. Combinations of techniques are usual (Dumas *et al.* 2001; O'Neil *et al.* 2003; APCP 2008). There is 'insufficient evidence either to support or refute' therapy interventions nor for specific interventions after BTX A in children (Lannin *et al.* 2006).

(5) Re-educating gait pattern and gradually decreasing support that walking aids provide (see Fig. 9.174e).

(6) Checking that postural alignments in sitting, standing and lying are correct.

(7) Training of daily living activities and functional locomotion is highly recommended as desired by parents, for example get in and out of chairs, of car, put on shoes and socks, walk in community. Impairment improvement may not result in functional improvements (O'Neil *et al.* 2003).

(8) Home programmes and regular monitoring of parents, carers and school staff for daily stretching, strengthening exercises and use of postural management equipment. Their comments are especially important for choice of methods and progress. General weakness or other unexpected symptoms should be immediately conveyed to the medical consultant.

(9) Activities such as swimming, horse riding and gym clubs become beneficial once specific treatment regimes are established. Horse riding is frequently recommended after BTX A for adductors.

Selection of strategies, frequency and timing of therapy depends on the individual's response to BTX A. Decisions of therapists depend on their assessments of impairment and function following injections.

Outcome measures

Outcome measures from some of the many studies include measures of impairment, activity and participation in daily life. Measures are usually used at pre-injection and 2 weeks, 6 weeks and 3–4 months post-injection. This varies in clinical settings. Measures used at 3–6 weeks post-injection and 3–6 months or more were made for long-term functional changes (Slawek & Klimont 2003). It seems that long-term measures are not necessarily used once injections have worn off. They found support for other studies which continue to confirm that long-term improvements remain once injections are no longer used and spasticity has returned.

Review of outcome measures (see section 'Current measures used in cerebral palsy' in Chapter 8)

Impairment measures include goniometry for joint range, video gait analyses and other observational gait analyses, tests of strength, of selective motor control and of stiff, spastic muscles and soft tissues. Pain scales and other pain measures are used in more severe non-ambulant children.

The activity measures may be Gross Motor Function Measure, Goal Attainment Scale, video gait analysis, Gillette Functional Assessment Questionnaire and PEDI for ambulant or non-ambulant children. Pain measures are usually used for non-ambulant children, which may well interfere with activity. There are a number of upper limb functional measures such as QUEST and MACS.

Participation measures are Quality of Life (QoL) and Canadian Occupational Performance Measure. Energy expenditure measures have also been used (physiological cost index; Butler *et al.* 1984). However, the accuracy of heart rate in children is normally variable and not helpful for energy.

The APCP in Britain have a pack on outcome measures (APCP 2005) and a pack on outcome measures in evidence-based guidance for physiotherapists (APCP 2008).

The reports and diary by parents, carers, school assistant and child are important in evaluation of progress.

Review of deformities

Although the deformities in the whole child have been discussed above and in Chapter 9 in the context of developmental training, this review may be helpful in giving additional attention to each joint. Nevertheless, as already emphasised, no joint is seen in isolation for assessment, treatment and management.

Hip flexion–adduction–internal rotation

One component may be greater than the others. The shape of the hip joint may be abnormal; for example the acetabulum is shallow, neck of femur anteverted, subdislocation and dislocation may occur in time in bilateral cerebral palsy (Hiroshima & Ono 1979; Sussman 1992; Cosgrove 2000). The excessive pull of adductors, internal rotators and even minimally shortening flexors causes the hip to migrate laterally until it dislocates. This process may take 3–4 years or up to 6 years in non-ambulant children. Migration over 15% in children not walking 10 steps at 30 months should be referred to an orthopaedic surgeon for surveillance (Scrutton & Baird 1997). X-rays are essential by 30 months for children with bilateral cerebral palsy. Scrutton *et al.* (2001) in their studies found that none of 69 children who walked alone by 30 months had a hip problem, 8 of 52 children walking between 30 months and 5 years had a hip problem and 109 of 202 children unable to walk at 5 years also had hip problems.

Hip subluxation is diagnosed if migration is between 33 and 80% and dislocation if over 80%. Hip dislocation 'may be silent' (Graham 2004) as there is not always obvious abnormality in function and the clinical picture.

Hip subluxation or dislocation is common. This is associated with deformity in hips, pelvis and spine,

may cause pain and interfere with standing and daily care. Delayed weight bearing in standing is significant in causing dislocations (Phelps 1959). Scrutton and Baird (1997) and Scrutton *et al.* (2001) monitored hip migration and found that children who did not walk by 5 years had a one in two chance of hip dislocation. Late sitting or walking together with hypertonus, asymmetry and no weight bearing in standing are risks for hip dislocation. Gudjonsdottir and Mercer (1997) clearly describe the development of hip and spine deformities for clinical work.

Therapy and daily care

Prevention of hip dislocation

At birth the hip is normal in children who will be diagnosed as cerebral palsy. Positioning of a neonate and premature infant is needed as part of general development care for neonates and premature infants (Grenier 1988). Excessive hip abduction, external rotation and flexion or hyperextension needs special attention in very young, unwell babies. Positioning reduces the risk of subluxation/dislocation and uses mid-range positions of shoulders and hips, well supported but not restrictive of movement. The positioning is carried out by nurses and parents under supervision of physiotherapists in hospital and home.

Positioning in supported standing is essential from around 12 months of age (Gericke 2006), when a child prefers an abnormal hip posture (with flexion-adduction-internal rotation) during the night and day. This is particularly when the preferred posture is combined with delayed development of weight bearing in standing. Hypotonia or hypertonia and dystonia/dyskinetic conditions with marked asymmetry and scoliosis are associated with unilateral hip dislocation. Hypotonia and lack of weight bearing may have an anterior dislocation from hip–abduction–external rotation.

All children at risk of hip subluxation or dislocation need positioning in a variety of well-aligned positions and upright supported standing for weight bearing through hips, straight femurs and plantigrade feet. Hip abduction is important in the growing years in order to develop location of the femoral head in the acetabulum. An hour of weight bearing 4–5 times a week, usually in correcting standing equipment, is advised by Stuberg (1992) to improve joint and bone growth as well as bone density. However, studies by Caulton *et al.* (2004) on increasing bone density through standing have not been conclusive. Standing needs to be accompanied by nutrition and consideration of drugs used for epilepsy.

Positioning in lying equipment at night or during the day needs to take account of sleeping problems and medical problems of sleep hypoxaemia, seizures or gastroesophageal reflux, problems such as vomiting, swallowing and respiration. Side lying with correct abduction and body alignment is also used if supine or prone is not useful for any baby or child.

If there is any pain and decrease in a child's hip ranges of movement, there should be referral to an orthopaedic surgeon immediately. It is interesting that a study of pain in 29 adults with spastic quadriplegia revealed that 71% of 38 dislocated hips were not painful, 11% had intermittent pains and 18% were painful (Knapp & Cortes 2002).

Conservative positioning and physiotherapy in early treatments for children at risk of hip dislocation may prevent or delay surgery. This may be combined with BTX A injections with and without surgery if hip migration continues, pain increases and clinical/functional examinations suggest further procedures. Positioning in all positions needs special care when one hip is subluxating or dislocating. Prevention of hip displacement and wind-blown posture will prevent or minimise the associated scolioses.

Positioning. Prone lying straightens hips with gravity, assisting pulling pelvis down, legs apart on conical-shaped pommel, in prone wedges, prone lying or supine positioning equipment, standing frames, in sitting with legs apart, or with external rotation, sitting in chairs with pommels and corrective symmetrical hip–knee adaptations; stand or sit straddling equipment of rolls and horse riding for special disabilities are helpful. When carrying these children, position their legs apart, slightly turned out and pressing a child's hip flat. Use thick nappies or padding in milder cases. Extension–abduction is a most therapeutic position (Goldsmith *et al.* 1992; Goldsmith 2000; Hankinson & Morton 2002; Pountney *et al.* 2004). Positioning provides a maintained muscle-tendon soft-tissue stretch preferably when a child is relaxed and asleep. This is usually accompanied by daily manual passive stretch and active holding of position by the individual and exercises, mentioned in this chapter.

Abduction padding/wedge are used in all positions; abduction splint used in standing and walking; and abduction in night splints or lying frames. Some mild conditions of cerebral palsy learn to correct internal rotation with the use of *twisters* (Fig. 9.166) and others BTX A with the SWASH (standing, walking and sitting hip) orthoses in standing and walking (Boyd *et al.* 2001a; Fig. 9.174e). There is not yet adequate evidence for the SWASH together with BTX A injections as experience is limited. The Rifton Dynamic Stander (Fig. 9.155g) and Rifton Pacer Gait Trainer with abduction adjustments (prompts) at hips and lower legs are also used (Fig. 9.171a).

Positioning of legs in lying with extension-abduction of 20–30 degrees avoids a risk of subluxation (Hankinson and Morton 2002). However, some standing frames need more abduction. Recently Gough (2009) and Pountney and Green (2006) have stated that more research is needed on the benefits of 24-hour postural management. Gough pointed out that, for all deformities, there is no rigorous research to support 24-hour postural management with equipment. He quotes studies of pain, sleep disturbances, extra demands on parents and carers, and poor quality of life of children when using 24-hour positioning equipment. He calls for definition of a subgroup of children who would benefit from this postural management.

Ice treatment (cryotherapy) to reduce hypertonicity together with active-assisted movements. This is usually used in older children, adolescents and adults (De Souza 1997), as explanations for therapy and subsequent cooperation are more available at those ages.

(1) Apply towels wrung out in chopped ice and water to adductor surface of leg for 3–4 minutes. In addition, place the child in tailor sitting or over a roll *while* the ice pack is tied on to his thighs. Repeat applications of ice packs. Carry out active abduction movements as well.

(2) Wring out rough towels in chopped ice so that ice flakes cling to the towelling. Roll the whole leg from groin to feet in the towel for 3 minutes. Carry out leg movements with corrective rotation in the hip during and after ice application as well as positioning. Repeat to gain results.

(3) Bags of special gels which can be frozen and frozen peas in a towel are also used.

Active exercise to antagonists.

(1) See developmental training for active hip extension, hip abduction, hip external rotation in functions such as lateral cruising, creeping, rolling from prone to supine, active extension in 'standing tall', in stand and reach overhead. Counterpoising techniques using leg extension, abduction, external rotation (Figs 9.37, 9.38) in four-point kneeling and in standing, squatting with external rotation or sitting rise to standing up straight, half-kneeling with front leg held in external rotation in rise to standing, and maintain abduction-external rotation-extension in lateral weight shifts.

(2) Other examples are given in Figs 11.1–11.10. Emphasise the movement of the antagonists to the deformity, for example the extensors and the abductors in hip flexion or adduction deformities or in both.

Remember that range of motion and stretch of a child's hip flexors may rock the pelvis, increasing lordosis. Therefore, in assessment, positioning and in exercises, stabilise the pelvis as shown in Figs 11.5 and 11.6. Observe correction of hip flexion without hyperextension of thoraco-lumbar spine. This hyperextension is the compensation for hip flexion deformity.

Active exercise to agonists and antagonists. See developmental training of creeping (flexion and extension of legs). Counterpoising techniques in crawling positions and standing positions include stability with movements. Standing active bending down to floor/low table followed by stretch of hips to upright standing. Avoid hyperextension of spine during exercises for hips.

Orthopaedic surgery for hip deformities and dislocation. This is for muscle imbalance and relocation of the femoral head in the acetabulum. There are many different views and the surgeon involved will advise. All team members need to know what the objectives of the surgery are. Surgery may be soft tissue surgery in younger children whose hips are not as severely migrating out of joint as others (Cosgrove 2000). Soft tissue surgery includes muscle, tendon and connective tissue lengthening, transfer or releasing of adductors, flexors and proximal hamstrings (Turker & Lee 2000). Tenotomies and myotomies are treatments frequently chosen as muscle transfers were controversial. Bony surgery includes reconstruction of proximal femur and acetabulum, femoral and/or pelvic osteotomy and arthroplasty (Miller 2007). Soft tissue releases with bone surgery may be used as well (Cosgrove 2000, Graham 2004, Horstmann & Bleck 2007). There are potential risks of surgery, and it is best undertaken at a specialist centre where a surgeon is experienced in paediatric orthopaedics.

The surgeon will advise on weight bearing and the post-operative rehabilitation. There are strengthening exercises for antagonists to the deformities and good postural management to prevent recurrence of malalignment (Turker & Lee 2000). Post-operatively the child will need to learn how to use his different body in function and how to prevent further surgery as far as possible.

Outcomes of surgery vary as they are difficult to compare due to heterogeneous subjects and different combinations of procedures and assessments used (Stott & Piedrahita 2004 – an American Academy for Cerebral Palsy and Developmental Medicine evidence report). Young *et al.* (1998) found windswept deformity in 54% of a follow-up of young adults despite surgery for the hip. However, Graham (2004) and Miller (2007) have experience of having to carry out 'salvage surgery' in people with hip displacement which did not have earlier soft tissue surgery and who used excessive compensation for function which became disadvantageous over the years.

Surgery presents a difficult consideration for child and families as it causes family disturbance. Such family and child stress needs careful consideration as part of the professional team's assessment for surgery.

For further reading on hip dislocation prevention and management, contact Association of Paediatric Chartered Physiotherapists (see Appendix 2).

Hip extension deformity

Therapy and daily care

Hip extension is corrected together with the associated knee extension or flexion and plantarflexion.

Positioning. Chairs to increase flexion and symmetry (see section 'Evaluating a chair for a child' in Chapter 9). Correct carrying of young children in flexion positions. Use some hip flexion with straight knees and plantigrade feet in standing and keep arms forward to counter body extension. Use tailor sitting, squatting and crook sitting for extended hips and legs.

Active movements of flexion and of flexion and extension, use mid position of joints during developmental training of creeping, crawling and standing. In Fig. 9.167, there are methods for training walking with a simultaneous correction of excessive hip extension with knee flexion in walking (see Figs 11.1–11.10).

Note: To overcome excessive extension of head, trunk, hips and knees, it is important to flex the child at his head and shoulders *and* at his hip joint. Hold his head and shoulders, hold under his knees and flex him 'into a ball'. His extensor spasm, thrust or constant extensor hypertonus decreases in this position. This may be easier in side lying. Try different positions for flexion. Medications to reduce spasticity and dystonia are available. *Orthopaedic surgery is used* (Sussman 1992; Horstmann & Bleck 2007). Drugs reduce hypertonus.

Knee flexion deformity

Therapy and daily care

Knee flexion is often associated with hip flexion with internal rotation or adduction and with either dorsiflexion or plantarflexion as described in 'Deformities and Gait' above.

Positioning. Prone lying with straight knees or sitting with straight knees on the floor or in a floor seat. If the back rounds and pelvis tilts back with straight knees, use an inclined leg support with a raised floor seat or with a special chair. Postural equipment in lying positions, in prone standing or in upright standing provides correct posture.

These positions together with the use of knee gaiters use maintained stretch, and manual stretches keep length achieved. Passive full ranges of flexion and extension of hips and knees help to maintain joint flexibility.

BTX A has been used for stiff hamstrings.

Splintage. Knee gaiters, knee splints, soft knee night splints or 'immobilisers'.

Plaster back slabs and thermoplastic back splints from hip to ankle may be useful for day- or nightwear.

Ice treatment to whole leg (see discussion on hip flexion above).

Active movements for knee extensors and hip extensors and for knee flexors. See developmental training for hip and knee extension and exercises in Figs 11.1–11.10. Active sitting with pelvic and trunk positioning in postural control may prevent a need for a hamstring lengthening to correct a round back. Post-operative physiotherapy to strengthen hips and knee extensors and flexors, and development of balance is important. Re-educate walking and other functions.

Knee hyperextension deformity

Therapy and daily care

This may be associated with hip flexion or secondary to plantarflexion and valgus. Therefore, combine therapy with procedures either for hip flexion or for plantarflexion or both based on assessment of the muscle, tendon and soft tissue tightness.

Positioning. A standing frame needs to align knee posture and sometimes allow some flexion. If hip extension is present with knee hyperextension, then vary postures such as sitting on different sized boxes, on chair, side-sit, upright kneeling avoiding excessive lordosis, and crook-sitting in the corner of a sofa with back supported and weight on buttocks. If a child is standing already, stand with knee pieces preventing hyperextension; use shoes with higher heel to throw child's weight into knee flexion posture, *if* his plantar flexors are not shortened.

Splintage. Knee pieces which lock with knee in midline, but allow knee flexion motion may be necessary in some older children during the day.

Plasters, orthoses or ice treatment for plantar flexors if the plantarflexion is the cause of hyperextended knees.

Passive stretch and movement. When hyperextension may be due to tight plantar flexors, maintain passive stretch of these muscles in orthoses or standing frames (see technique for equinus below).

Active movement of knee flexors and the dorsiflexors of ankles if tight plantar flexors are present. *Active work for stabilisation of pelvis*, which is often the cause of hyperextended knees. See crawling development, standing development for pelvic stabilisation. Use upright supported kneeling. Train holding hips in bridging position in supine. Teach *bear walk with knee control and flex knee in stepping* (Fig. 9.169).

Equinus and equino-varus deformity

Therapy and daily care

This may be toe walk on its own or associated with hip and knee flexion. There is too early a heel raise after mid stance and persistent plantarflexion on the swing phase of gait. Feet are not flat in sitting and make putting on of socks, tights and shoes difficult.

Positioning. Prone lying with feet hanging relaxed over edge of wedge or pillows and not in plantarflexion, position child in prone standers and upright frames with heels down; sitting in chairs with heels flat on the ground; standing feet held flat on ground; standing in boots with raised soles. See suggestions for passive stretch and active dorsiflexion below.

Splintage and orthoses. Use various ankle-foot orthoses either solid, encouraging dorsiflexion or dynamic orthoses. Mild-to-moderate conditions may correct with special boots and insoles strap to keep the child's heel down in his boot. The strap should be wider and padded as it crosses the front of his ankle. Orthoses are usually worn post-operatively. Orthoses are discussed in section 'Development of standing and walking' in Chapter 9.

Plasters (see examples of inhibitory cast and postcast splint, Figs 11.11 and 11.12). Thermoplastic splints may be preferred by orthotists and by Miller (2007). See above for discussion on casting and BTX A for dynamic deformities.

Ice treatment to whole leg or the ice pack to plantar flexors only. Quick ice stimulation to dorsiflexors once relaxation and lengthening of plantar flexors is gained.

Passive stretch and movement. Hold the knee flexed with one hand, and grasp the heel and foot with your other hand. Gently dorsiflex foot as far as possible. Hold in dorsiflexion as you passively extend the child's knee. *Do not evert* the child's foot as you push it up into dorsiflexion. Stretch must be slow and maintained. Ask child to hold foot up in dorsiflexion with you. Also stretch with inversion if valgus is compensating for equinus.

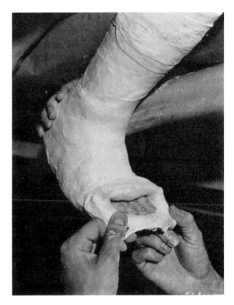

Figure 11.11

Suggestions for passive stretch of plantar flexors, hamstrings, including active dorsiflexions:

(1) Child stands and leans forward to wall to stretch plantar flexors and heel cords.
(2) With child's legs apart, knees straight and feet pointing forward, help him actively push both

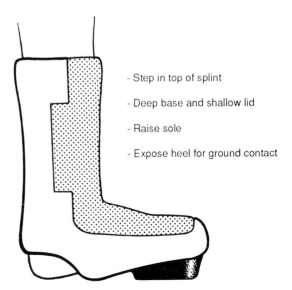

- Step in top of splint

- Deep base and shallow lid

- Raise sole

- Expose heel for ground contact

Figure 11.12   Post-plaster splint (removable) (day or night splint).

his feet into dorsiflexion. Control knee hyper-extension (recurvatum) if it occurs.

(3) Stand and lunge forward keeping heel down and back knee as straight as possible; half-kneeling lunge forward on front foot. Push balls under the front knee.

(4) Sitting heels on small inclined footboard obtaining dorsiflexion; stand with heels down, child facing up on small inclined board during classroom/play activity. Knees straight or with gaiters.

(5) Bear-walk with heels down; stand on hands and feet with toys on low table.

(6) Standing on tipping board or rocker, slowly tipped back with child's heels held down (Fig. 9.181).

(7) Walk on heels if possible. Raise the soles of his shoes, or remove heels off his shoes (heels down in Figs 11.2, 11.6, 11.7 and 11.10).

(8) Child is reminded to sit in a chair with heels down and to squat with heels down. Slow rise from sit/squat to stand with weight forward.

(9) Stimulate creeping patterns for dorsiflexion. Other leg flexion patterns may do this (see Fig. 9.37).

(10) Brushing, quick icing to dorsiflexors following passive stretch to plantar flexors, and during backward tilt in point 6.

(11) Striking heel of foot on surface stimulates dorsiflexion. Use in context of gait training.

(12) Walk up inclined plane or ramps with heel down on surface. Slow stair ascent and descent keeping heels down. Ascend two steps at a time to stretch hamstrings.

(13) Draw faces on child's feet, and ask him to dorsiflex or raise his feet to look at the face, or to touch a toy, use toe puppets and create similar games of your own.

(14) Child to practise heel strike in walking. Attach flat squeezable toys to the heels of child's shoes which create a sound on heel strike. There are trainers with lights in the heels on heel strike. These amuse a child and motivate the *heels down* action as a biofeedback during stance and step.

(15) If method is known, use Proprioceptive Neuromuscular Facilitation (PNF) pattern of hip flexion-adduction external rotation, knee extension, foot dorsiflexion, synergy of muscles. The child is in sitting over edge of bed or in supported standing. Use stretch, touch, pressure and resistance to muscles in this pattern (Fig. 9.162b).

(16) Check dorsiflexion in equipment such as wedges, and equipment for postural management.

Older children can use these exercises on their own after supervision has been given by therapists.

Valgus feet (pronated)

Valgus may be secondary to plantarflexion, or tight peroneal muscles and the forefeet may be everted with medial prominence of the talus.

Positioning. Have hips and knees turned out with weight on outside of feet using supporting shoes, also during the round sit on the floor, with hips externally rotated with feet in varus. Correct equinus in sit and stand if present as valgus is often overcompensation for this.

Splintage and bracing. Correct shoes or boots with inside raise, inside the shoe or outside on the sole or both; use moulded foot support to inner side of feet; below-knee orthosis; flare the heel or sole on the inner side so that it juts out slightly at the base. The position of the feet should be carefully monitored during the growing years.

Ice treatment. Occasionally may be used for reducing tone of spastic plantarflexion and for spastic peroneal muscles. Quick ice to dorsiflexors to active them just before exercises.

Plasters (casting) or moulded orthoses if equinus needs therapy.

Passive stretch as for equinus, emphasising some inversion.

Activity. As for equinus, but emphasise inversion (see Figs 11.13–11.16). Tap the bone at the heel and malleoli on one side to activate inversion, just before active attempt by a child.

Varus feet

See equinus for treatment above and Figs 11.14–11.16; tap bone at heel and malleoli all to activate eversion before strengthening exercises. Plasters, splintage and orthoses may be used with adjustment to the opposite side to that used for valgus. Train stand and walk with corrected feet.

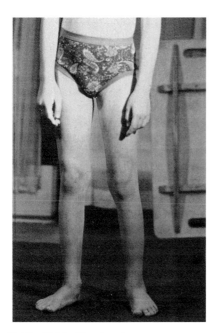

Figure 11.13   Child with valgus feet.

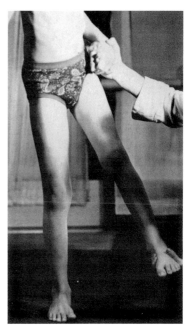

Figure 11.15   Stand, tip the child on to outside of his foot to provoke action of foot muscles to correct valgus. Child may move his pelvis laterally against your hand to obtain inversion of feet, backwards for dorsiflexion, forwards for plantarflexion.

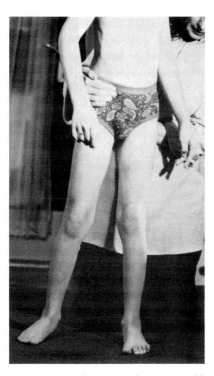

Figure 11.14   Rotate pelvis to stimulate action of foot muscles to correct valgus. Rotate against your manual resistance at the hip in front and behind.

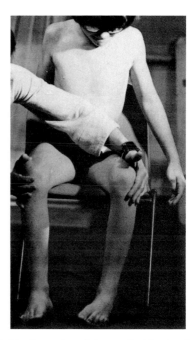

Figure 11.16   Correction of abnormal adduction, internal rotation or valgus feet. Press his knees outward against your hands or the therapist turns his knees outwards for him. This may be done in sitting, in standing or in squatting positions.

Varus causes instability with tendency to sprains and strains of the foot.

Clenched toes or everted toes

These disappear with correct weight bearing and balance training. Heel must be on the ground and equinus treated. 'Flick' toes up as child takes weight. Use sponge or felt to hold toes corrected while balance develops. Excessive toe flexion occurs if standing is too early for the child. Incorporate toes into plaster or orthoses. This avoids clenching.

Arm deformity

Orthopaedic surgery reviews are mainly on hemiplegia. Function of hands, cosmesis and hygiene (Cosgrove 2000; Horstmann & Bleck 2007) are main aims.

Shoulder flexion–adduction–internal rotation, elbow flexion, wrist flexion and ulnar deviation and hand and thumb deformities

Chapter 9 on the development of hand function and developmental training includes the following:

Positioning. Elevation of arms, extension of elbows, wrists and hands on tables of different heights during play and other activities, using his hands. Shoulder and arm retraction and asymmetry is corrected.

Activity of the arms and hands to correct dynamic deformities. In positioning and in developmental training of gross motor function, for example developmental training of creeping, crawling and counterpoising, sitting and counterpoising arm elevation, arms over large ball during training of standing, arm elevation in standing and counterpoising. There is also active correction of *shoulder retraction and active* movements and correction of posture (see Figs 9.101–9.106, 9.185–9.200).

Splintage. Lycra splints may help to correct deformity during developmental training (Fig. 9.211).

For *flexed elbows* with dynamic deformity, elbow gaiters are used and need to be well padded in forearm area. Do not force into splint.

For wrist and hands. In mid-position with thumb abduction or hand-cone with a mid-position splint. Wrist and hand splint for maintained grasp may assist a child with dyskinesia. Thick thumb spacer (made of foam), thumb splints finger spreader and opposition splints prevent deformity and assist hand function. See hand splints in Figs 9.212 and 9.213 as examples.

Many new splints and materials are regularly being designed and occupational therapists need to be consulted.

Passive stretch and motion. The whole arm and hand need a gentle stretch as one pattern. Avoid any forced stretches of elbows as this is dangerous. Slow, very gentle passive ranges of motion of each joint to maintain existing mobility is used. The pronators are in particular need of gentle stretching together with activation of the weak supinators with elbow bent and with arm extended.

Ice treatment of the whole arm, together with active motion, is used to decrease stiffness of spasticity.

Deformities of trunk and neck

Trunk and neck deformities are associated with pelvis, legs and arms, and are incorporated in positioning of the whole child in the day and during sleep. Windswept hips, pelvic asymmetry and scoliosis are seen together but which is the primary cause may be unclear (Figs 9.68a–d). Figures 11.1–11.10 show the active strengthening of neck, trunk and pelvis to counter deformities. See figures of equipment in all sections of Chapter 9, particularly section 'Evaluating a Chair for a Child', which correct head and trunk as well as the whole child. Twenty-four-hour postural management for the whole child includes minimising deformities of neck, trunk, and pelvis. Special seating is essential for functional positions in school, for access to computers, for eating and drinking and for communication. Check that seating pads give three-point correction of scolioses at sides of trunk and pelvis.

To minimise or correct scolioses, position a child in side lying, observing correction with either a straightening of scoliosis when lying on side of convexity or on side of concavity. Raise hips and legs to stretch concavity. Correct side flexion with rotation.

Passive stretch in side lying with arm elevated. Rotate hips and shoulders in opposite directions to stretch trunk muscles in young children using a slow rhythm (Fig. 9.61).

Orthopaedic surgeons recommend special seating as well as trunk orthoses or body jackets, though in some cases breathing is difficult for a child and there may be skin breakdown. Body orthoses are for kyphosis, for scoliosis and to give extra support for sitting in a child who cannot manage this (Terjesen *et al.* 2000; Miller 2007). Some experts have devised various operations as well, mainly in adolescence. Surgery is considered when scoliosis and other joint contractures interfere with comfortable seating. This is usually in adolescence and in people in GMFCS Levels IV and V. This is major surgery which is explained by the surgeon to the family and individual with cerebral palsy. A skilled, experienced surgeon with nurses and therapists in the team is best. It may take up to 12 months for recovery and rehabilitation.

General considerations related to surgery

The physiotherapist should understand the aims of surgery and help the surgeon prepare the child and his family for surgery, if that has been recommended. *Their cooperation is most important.* The child and family and an older person with cerebral palsy need to have information and understanding of the following points:

(1) The surgery is not a cure, but an episode in the total rehabilitation programme. The degree of drive and *sometimes* intelligence of the child affects the results of surgery.
(2) There will be a setback before the ultimate progress is more obvious.
(3) How to look after the child in plaster. How to apply any splintage or orthoses to maintain improvement by surgery.
(4) Generally how to help with post-operative details of home rehabilitation. There will be new demands on home therapy, which the family need to consider as that is important for follow-up therapy to help regain function. Families

need to stipulate who will be able to do this before surgery is undertaken.
(5) Families need support so they can try and maintain confidence and an encouraging atmosphere for their child.

It is best if the child's own physiotherapist can be the one to treat him before the operation and follow up in the home or centre. Otherwise, she and the parents should at least introduce the child to the hospital environment, meet some of the staff and the physiotherapist involved. Generally, let the child know what is going to happen and what will take place at the hospital. Possible psychological disturbance due to surgery and its associated hospitalisation must not be ignored, as it has been known to affect children for years and also hamper the physical advances gained by the surgery.

Surgeons have their own pre-/post-operative protocols and periods of immobilisation and orthoses. Guidelines are presented for physiotherapy but may need modification according to the surgeon.

Pre-operative physiotherapy

Hips, knees and feet

(1) Train all muscle groups *not only* the antagonists to the deformity.
(2) Train all postural mechanisms for postural control and balance. Results of surgery depend on activity of these mechanisms, or as many of them as possible.
(3) Obtain measurements of a child for any splints or orthoses ordered for the child's use postoperatively when indicated.

Post-operative physiotherapy and care

This depends on the surgeon and orthopaedic nurses.

Hip and knee operations

In plaster
(1) Check that child's head and trunk are kept in alignment. Discourage sacral sitting.

(2) Carry young child over your shoulder keeping his hips flat with your hand.
(3) Change position from bed to sitting on chair with board for legs, in plasters. Weight bearing in plasters is important and permission to do this must be obtained as soon as possible.
(4) Use prone board on wheels with wide board for legs. Keep hips flat with a band across them. Place ankles on roll of towels, pillow under chest.
(5) Plasters may be split after knee operation.
(6) In plaster, carry out extension movement of head, arms and back. Check positions during sleep with leg plasters, with the nurses or surgeon.

Out of plaster
(1) There is splintage for knees to control any flexor spasms. Medication may be used.
(2) Treat pain and swelling, dry skin as for all post-operative cases.
(3) Gentle movements in as much range as possible. Emphasise improved motor patterns, which are new to the individual. He will take time to adjust to a new body image.
(4) Continue balance training whenever possible and preferably in standing. Therefore, place the child on his feet as soon as possible with surgeon's permission.
(5) Gently obtain hip and knee flexion by sitting on increasingly lower and lower chairs, over the edge of pillows and in exercises.

(6) No unrelieved sitting is to be resumed following surgery for flexion.

Harryman (1992) gives techniques following orthopaedic surgery.

Foot operations

Foot operations may be followed by long leg plasters, including the foot or below-knee plasters.

In plaster
(1) Train standing as soon as possible with surgeon's permission. Walking in plaster must be emphasised. Correct pelvic-trunk alignments.
(2) Extension exercises for hips and knees in all positions are required, especially in sitting rise to standing.

Out of plaster
(1) Below-knee orthosis may be recommended by the surgeon.
(2) Active dorsiflexion encouraged (Figs 11.14–11.16).
(3) Continue training postural balance mechanism in pelvis and trunk in all positions, especially standing.
(4) Plantarflexion and push off should be trained, if possible.

12 Therapeutic group work

Children's need for group activities has long been recognised in the habilitation of children with disabilities. Such children are often isolated from their peers. Owing to motor disability, they may not be able to run up and join a group of children, put an arm round a friend or even push away an annoying child. Parents may find it difficult to bring their child into contact with other children whether able-bodied or disabled. Children need group treatment for contact with other children, sharing an activity with others, feeling part of a group and responding to competition and cooperation. Group work in special or inclusive education as well as in therapy offers opportunities for the child's social and emotional development.

Groups have been used in a variety of ways:

- *In speech therapy* for stimulation of communication and development of speech and language.
- *In occupational therapy* for perceptual training, for play involving perceptual motor function, for recreation, social interaction and learning to play a game involving rules and taking turns and so on.
- *In physiotherapy* for training children with a specific diagnosis to carry out a set of exercises, for games involving gross motor activity, for swimming and activities in water, and various sports for disabled people. Circuit

training groups have benefits (Blundell *et al.* 2003).

As the aims of these different therapy groups overlap, it is possible to carry out *interdisciplinary groups* of two kinds:

Playgroups, including toy libraries, adventure playgrounds, special or ordinary nursery schools, opportunity groups or nurseries, are orientated to each child's developmental levels and special problems. The therapists may advise or themselves work in the group setting, stimulating a few or occasionally all the children with play activities which involve gross motor, fine motor, perceptual and speech and language activities. The therapist may be in the playroom or nursery, relating to one child with specific problems and may or may not also bring in other children in the same activity. Classroom assistants are trained to position and handle children appropriately.

The children may all be in the same room and may or may not feel themselves to belong to the same group in all activities.

Songs, storytime, percussion band, games and music are well-known sessions when all the children carry out the same activity. Therapists are, therefore, working closely with teachers, psychologists, childcare staff, nursery nurses and nurses in the therapeutic playgroups and classrooms. Parents are often present in playgroups including therapeutic goals for their children. Children's siblings may also participate in playgroups or games with them.

The structured group works to treat or train a specific area of function. These groups integrate the gross motor, fine motor, perceptual, speech and language activities, but with more focus on any one of these areas. This focus may be on the major disability of the children in the group, for example motor problems in cerebral palsied children. The focus may be on a specific area of function in one group session, whereas the focus will be on another area for that same group in other group sessions.

These structured interdisciplinary groups in Britain have been influenced by the ideas of Petö, Hari and the work of physiotherapist Ester Cotton (1970, 1974, 1975). Dorothy Seglow (1984), a physiotherapist, introduced mother–child groups and a teacher Titchener (1983) evaluated such a group. Many others have developed 'Peto Groups' in Britain (Russell & Cotton 1994). See section 'Conductive education' in Chapter 3 (Hari & Tillemans 1984; Cottam & Sutton 1988; Hari & Akos 1988).

These groups may not follow the full system of the Petö approach, which involves very much more than a group session or group sessions. From studies with the staff of The Cheyne Centre for Children with Cerebral Palsy, these structured interdisciplinary group sessions for multiply disabled children were invaluable and often essential for such children (1969–1979).

Some of the main observations are:

(1) Individual sessions sometimes create too much pressure on an older child and aggravate the normal or abnormal rebelliousness in a child. In the group, such children often cooperate because all the other children present are doing what is expected of them.

(2) The one-to-one relationship in individual treatment may be too similar to the one-to-one relationship in the mother–child situation. This is normal in children under 3-year developmental level. Children with physical disabilities, however, are often over this age and need to relate to their peers, *even though* their physical function may still be under a 3-year developmental level.

Although a child may need some private tuition in his school life and some disadvantaged children and children with very severe learning disabilities may still need this one-to-one relationship, many more need to 'grow out' of it emotionally and socially. Perhaps some of those who refuse to cooperate may be protesting at the dependency felt on being handled by the therapists all the time in this one-to-one situation.

(3) In the group, children follow a programme and imitate the other children. Imitation helps the children with partial hearing loss or learning disability to understand what is required of them. In addition, the children in groups are observed to instruct and help each other carry out the programme of work.

(4) Speech is stimulated as the adult's concentration on all the children seems to take off the *pressure* on one child to speak.

(5) Concentration of the children who are working at their own pace is great. The attention span is far longer than in individual sessions; children work hard in groups lasting one and a half hours whilst in individual treatment for only 20–40 minutes.

(6) The programme consists of integrating essential aspects of physiotherapy, occupational therapy and speech therapy together with group work. It is planned by the team but carried out by one therapist and one or two aides or assistants. In this way a number of children are helped at the same time with economy on staff and on time spent getting children to and from each therapy department, as well as on time required to establish rapport with each different professional.

(7) Physiotherapists, occupational therapists, speech therapists, teachers and nursery nurses welcome interdisciplinary groups, as they can then see the total child and the relationship of their specialty to those of the others in his total function. On planning and using the structured group session the different disciplines are enabled to share their knowledge with one another so that practical integrated group activities can be created. Different disciplines have then to clarify their main aims with each child and make certain that they are understood by everyone in the planning of the programme and in its execution. It is not possible for each

professional to convey all her expertise to the other different disciplines, but rather to learn how to discover the overlap of her particular discipline with others. In this way the overlap becomes a practical achievement and enriches the teamwork.

General management of groups

Number of children. This varies according to the numbers of children in each centre, school or unit, from whom selections may be made. No matter how many children are in a group, they must be *involved* and preferably participating.

Staff. One staff member leads the group with another assisting her. The assistant should be from another discipline. If the children are all severely disabled, more help may be indicated. However, the adults present must be kept to a minimum, or their one-to-child relationship rather than a child-to-child relationship may occur. The leader may alternate with her assistant each week or alternate days in conducting the group.

All assistants need to work according to the leader's action and not divert the child's attention away from the group by private conversation with them or with each other.

Venue. The group is best done in the child's own classroom or where there are no unfamiliar distractions and a coming and going of adults or other children.

Arrange children during the group session so that they can see the leader of the group at all times and also so that the children see each other. Semicircles or L-shaped seating arrangements are best, but the positions will change in a class with particular motor activities and walking exercises.

Length of sessions should be planned for 1–2 hours depending on the children's ability to continue participating and the programme of work.

Frequency. Group sessions are best done daily or three times a week depending on the aims of the group programme. Some aims only require twice a week. The main object is that the children work together for not less than two or three times a week so that they know each other and develop a group dynamic.

Behaviour. If a child refuses to join in, make sure that the programme is not too difficult for him. If it is not, let him watch for a while, ignoring him. The other children may be given a particularly pleasant activity, or they may occasionally be told 'Let's do that again for so-and-so to try as well'. Other ideas may be offered by the parent or team members who know the child. However, if non-participation continues or if the child seems oblivious to other children and cannot imitate others, the group cannot 'carry' him indefinitely. He may not be ready or not suitable for group treatments, and this is not always obvious in the beginning.

Children with behaviour problems may become disruptive to the group. Hyperkinetic children may be particularly difficult. However, try a trial period of partial sessions with the group, increase to full sessions and the techniques above. Restless children may settle down and join in with the others. Finally, good selection of children and programme planning makes organised management easier.

Selection of children

The basis for selection varies and ideas are still developing. The early days of group treatment both for staff and children seem to be easier if the disparity between the children is not great. A group with children who have hemiplegia and are at the walking level and at approximately the same chronological age and have intelligence forms a group which works well. Such a group is best for inexperienced staff and for those professionals beginning group work. The hemiplegic group might enlarge itself to encompass other diagnostic types of cerebral palsies who have asymmetry. Mental levels of children may be varied. A variety of developmental levels among motor developmentally delayed children may be contained in one group. The following points influencing selection may be helpful.

Problems of children

Motor problems

Selection of children according to diagnosis is not usually helpful. Select the children according to their problems. Although it is difficult to generalise them, motor problems are usually some or all the following:

(1) Head control – postural stability, particularly in the upright position.
(2) Head and trunk in midline, symmetrical arm and leg postures.
(3) Head and trunk counterpoising so that arms and legs can move into various asymmetrical postures or movements.
(4) Grasp to hold on, and grasp and release.
(5) Corrective movements and postures for any recurring abnormal positions of any joints, for example in spastic or athetoid conditions, elbow flexion, shoulder retraction, hip extension or semiflexion, adduction, knee flexion, equinus feet.
(6) Form of locomotion.
(7) Ability to sit or stand.
(8) Ability to rise from the floor or from a chair.

It is possible, say, to have a *pre-sitting group* with a selection of motor activity building up to sitting, prone to hands and knees, and weight bearing on feet with trunk support (see developmental channels in Appendix 1, 0–6 months level). It is possible to have a group on *sitting and prewalking* with activities taken from the channels of development of 6–12 months (Appendix 1) or an ambulant group, 12 months and over (Appendix 1). The motor abilities selected for training will depend on the children with these problems. It is obviously essential to have individual assessments to plan for the problems. The other impairments and disabilities in the child should be considered, although motor problems are primary.

Age of child

Children should be around the same chronological age, as their developmental levels alone will offer a range of children. It is sometimes an unhappy situation if a large boy aged 11 with a developmental level of, say, sitting equal to about 6–9-months normal level is in a group with 3-year olds also at this developmental level.

Cognitive level

The cognitive level should not cross too wide a spectrum. Some prefer keeping intelligent children in one group, whilst others find it useful to mix as the cognitively impaired child will imitate the intelligent child in carrying out the motor activity or other activities that do not demand high intelligence. Intellectually disabled children may also be better at movement than, say, children with severe physical disabilities, and intelligence as, say, in dyskinesia. The programme, therefore, allows each child to demonstrate his assets and abilities.

Personality and behaviour

Personality of the children is rarely a consideration unless a child is excessively disruptive and management ideas for behaviour fail (see above). A child's emotional and social stages of development influence whether he or she is suitable for a particular group.

Other disabilities

Deaf, partially sighted or children with severe visual impairment may find it more difficult to join a group if the focus is on the motor disability. However, again some children with partial hearing loss and some children with partial sight have responded well to groups through imitation, lip reading or augmented visual clues, as well as the fact that a good group session focused on problems other than specific hearing and severe visual problems. Children with profound intellectual impairment may be too oblivious of the group dynamics being used and remain in their own world, and be unsuitable for such group work.

It must be remembered that factors for selection are still being explored by those working with groups in therapy and education.

Whatever the basis for selection the 'answer' to the best way to select children finally rests on whether group programmes of work can be created by the staff and on the ability of the leader of the group to weld her group of children together, so they work together and there is a group spirit.

The programme

(1) It is essential to have this prepared before the group commences.

(2) It can be modified once used and *must* be changed as the children change and progress.

(3) The group leader needs to have the programme in front of her so that she does not delay and lose any group impetus and collaboration gained. She must know 'what comes next' to maintain group concentration.

(4) The programme should not be too long, but it is better to spend more time on each item. The items are after all only chosen because they are to be trained and repetition is needed. Time is given, so each child can be active.

(5) Occasionally, have an easy item already achieved, as well as items *just beyond* the capacity of the children. If the children experience a successful achievement, this motivates them further.

(6) Use action songs to carry out motor activities for the children; as they use the same songs each time, their familiarity is often appreciated. For many children, the programme should contain familiar elements, songs, the same assistant and leader, the room, the time of day or days of the week and the general outline. However, the activities must gradually develop and change and not remain so predictable that the children do not progress or become bored.

Items of the programme

The programme and its further modifications need to be assessed and reassessed not only by the group leader, but also together with the other professional workers in the centre. Ongoing consultations are necessary to make sure that the items selected for the children motivate *all* the children and that any child is not 'carried' as a non-participant for too long.

Select items from the treatment suggestions in the chapters on developmental training and the problems of deformity. Give preference to those items which do not depend on holding or handling the child, or there may be too many adults required. The presence of many adults disrupts the growing child–child relationships in the group. Select items

which are at first easy and become more difficult as the children develop in the group programme. In addition, such selected items may be used in groups to allow some children to function better than the others. This motivates the others to work towards these more advanced levels, which they can observe in their peers. In this way the therapist can have children at different levels of motor development in one group. She must have components selected, so they *build up* a particular motor function.

For example

All the children sit around a large table. Children at 3–6-months developmental level of sitting will have to lean their trunks against the table and grasp a horizontal bar attached to the table or grasp a slatted table. The children from 6–9-months level do not lean against the table, but only grasp the support, and the children from 9–12-months level, who can sit alone, do so with their hands at their sides or on their laps. All children may sing or use language and visual activities while practising sitting.

Similarly, standing may be modified from standing leaning on arms or against the table with grasp support, stand and grasp, and stand alone.

Also prone lying raise head, prone lying raise head and rise on to elbows, and prone lying raise head and rise on to hands can be included simultaneously. With careful planning and assessment of the children, many more examples will be found.

All motor activities must be associated with perceptual experience of direction, spatial relationships, colour, body awareness, various matching activities in relating shapes, sizes, textures as well as speech and language, social awareness and of course the fun of children working and playing together (Fig. 12.1).

Music and movement, songs, action songs, fingerplays and any other children's songs and music are enjoyed in group work. However, as with the other activities, these are modified to relate to the children's levels of development and interest. Imaginative activities such as 'Pretend you are a tree in the wind' or 'Let's wave our arms like birds' which are used for children's groups are not advisable unless the children understand them and are at the 'let's pretend' level of play development. This is about the level of understanding of normally developing 2–3-year olds.

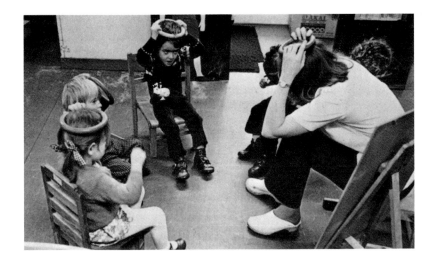

Figure 12.1

Children's group games and party games may also be adapted and used in group work. Whatever items are selected, they *must not* be random but selected according to aims of therapy with each child. There will be aims of therapy which cannot fully be realised in the group sessions, or not at all. *Individual sessions* will be necessary for the children. However, if a child has the items well chosen for him in the group, individual sessions may not be essential for him, for a period.

It is not possible to give programmes for groups, as these must be composed around the children themselves. However, the following are necessary for groups:

(1) Start and end with a dressing activity, for example taking shoes and socks off, or taking a cardigan off.
(2) Fetch and put away any equipment for the group.
(3) Use gross motor activities for one session, integrating this with perception and language activities.
(4) Use hand classes for a session, integrating this with perception and language activities.
(5) Have a meal or tea for the group in order to include feeding training and washing hands.
(6) Suggested group games for walkers and non-walkers. These may include crawling hand ball, passing ball or objects in sitting, throwing bean-bags into large containers, obstacle course, cro-

quet, ring toss, deck quoits, carpet bowls, shuffle board, rolling balls on the table or floor, ping-pong with the ball attached to a high horizontal wire for ball retrieval and other play activities. Board games need to have large counters or handles on the draught pieces or holes for the pieces and other adaptations. (Catalogues of adapted playthings are available from organisations for children with disabilities.)

Summary

Interdisciplinary group work is valuable in the treatment of cerebral palsied and motor delayed children. They require consultations between staff:

(1) To assess children's functions in all areas before and *during* group sessions.
(2) To plan, monitor and progress the items of the group programmes.

It is best for one person to carry out the programme with perhaps other professionals occasionally assisting but *not* interrupting during the group session itself. Adjustments of the programme can be discussed after the session is over.

Teachers and therapists depend on each other to create dynamic group sessions and therefore need to work closely together.

Appendix 1: Developmental levels

Function	0–3 months	3–6 months
Prone		
Supine		
Sitting		
Standing Walking		

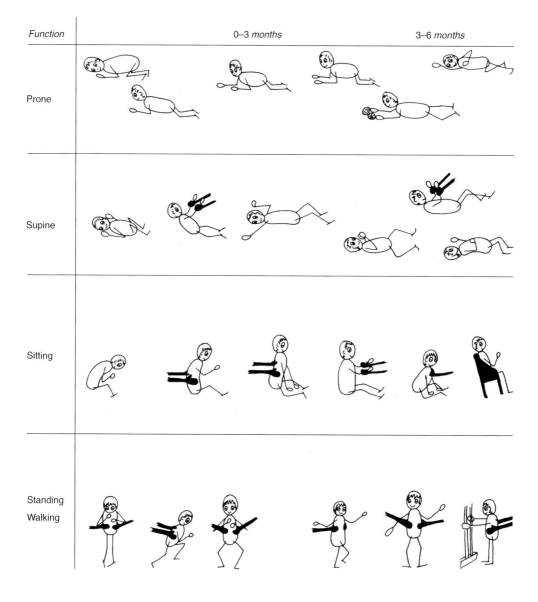

6–9 *months* 9–12 *months*

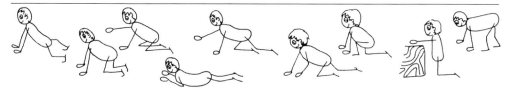

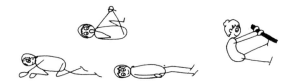

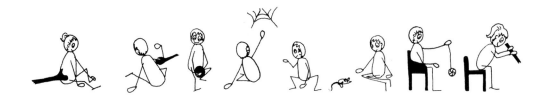

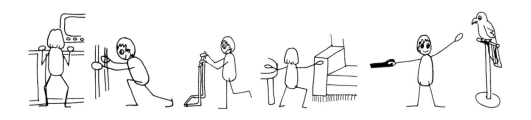

Physical ability assessment guide

Grading of ability

0 – No ability, no initiation
D – Initiates alone
C – Partial, laboured, unreliable or infrequent
B – Completes alone reliably but very abnormal performance
A – Completes reliably with near normal/normal performance
Maintains posture – 10 seconds
Locomotion – 10 steps
Stairs – 4 steps

Prone

0–3 months	Can be placed, head turns
	Raises head up
	Maintains head up
	On forearms, head, chest up
	Rises on to knees and forearms
3–6 months	Reaches forward with right arm (extended)
	Reaches forward with left arm (extended)
	Rolls over to right
	Rolls over to left
6–9 months	Creeps on abdomen
	Maintains on hands, elbows straight
	Rises on to hands and knees
	Maintains hands and knees
	Reaches forward with one hand, on hands posture
9–12 months	On hands and knees, lifts arm and opposite leg
	Pivots body using limbs to right
	Pivots body using limbs to left
	Crawls reciprocally
	Achieves sit from hands and knees
	Half-kneels with hand supports
	Rises to upright kneeling with hand supports
	Walks on hands and feet

12–24 months	Creeps on to table/couch
	Crawls upstairs
	Crawls downstairs backwards
	Kneels upright, hips straight, no support
	Half-kneels upright, no support
	Knee walks forwards
	Rises to stand, no support

Supine

0–3 months	Can be placed, head turns
	Head lag overcome slightly
	Reaches out along floor, to side
3–6 months	Head maintained in midline, symmetrical weight bears
	Hands together, symmetry
	Head raises, head lag overcome
	Reaches up, across body
	Bridges hips into extension, feet flat
6–9 months	Rolls over to right
	Rolls over to left
	Reaches, grasps foot
	Lying straight, arms down, head midline, turns
9–12 months	Rises to sitting through right side lying, alone
	Rises to sitting through left side lying, alone
	Pulls self to sitting

Sitting

0–3 months	Can be placed, head, trunk supported, flexes hips
	Vertical head control, trunk supported
	Leans on forearms or hands, trunk supported
3–6 months	Sits leaning on hands, no support to upper then lower trunk
	Sits in chair with back, sides or chest support

6–9 months	Sits with one hand support, uses other hand
	Saves self on hands forwards
	Sits arms free, alone
	Saves self to right side
	Saves self to left side
	Sits leaning forwards, re-erects alone
9–12 months	Sits, reaches across, to side, above head
	Sits and turns, reaches to right
	Sits and turns, reaches to left
	Side sits on right hip
	Side sits on left hip
	Changes to hands and knees
	Sits alone on regular chair
	Sits on chair, reaches in all directions
	Rises from sit to standing, holding on
	Sits and pivots on floor
	Sits and pivots on chair
	Bottom shuffles along floor
	Tilt reactions anterior-posterior
	Tilt reactions laterally
12–18 months	Seats self on low stool
	Rises from sit to stand, no holding
	Sits on high stool, legs dangling
	Squats at play
	Squat rises to stand and returns to squat
	Saves self if tipped backwards

Standing and walking

0–6 months	Weight bears, plantigrade feet, full then lower trunk support
	Steps, trunk supported
6–9 months	Stands, forearm leaning or holding on, pelvis supported
	Stands, holds on alone, hips may flex, feet flat
9–12 months	Pulls self to standing, holds on
	Stands, holds on, lifts right leg
	Stands, holds on, lifts left leg
	Cruises using two hands
	Stands, holds one hand, reaches in all directions

12–18 months	Stands alone
	Stands stoop and recover
	Walks, two hands held or grasps walker
	Walks, one hand help
	Walks alone
	Walks, carrying object
	Rises to stand from all positions, no support
	Walks backwards
	Walks upstairs, holds both sides, two feet per step
	Protective stagger reaction if pushed sideways
	Protective stagger reaction if pushed forward
	Protective stagger reaction if pushed backward
18–24 months	Stands, kicks ball
	Throws ball overhead
	Runs
	Walks, stops and turns (pivot)
	Walks upstairs, holding one rail, two feet per step
	Walks downstairs, both rails, two feet per step
2–3 years	Jumps in place
	Jumps off 6-inch step
	Pedals tricycle
	Broad jump (8 inches)
	Walks downstairs, on rail, alternate feet
	Walks upstairs, no hold, alternate feet
	Walks downstairs, no hold, alternate feet
3–4 years	Stands on preferred leg (5–10 seconds)
	Hops on preferred leg
	Heel-to-toe walk
	Catches bounced ball
	Uses large bat
4–5 years	Balances on one leg, 10 seconds
	Walks on narrow, straight line
	Walks between 8-inch parallels
	Walks on narrow plank/bench
	Steps over knee-high stick with right
	Steps over knee-high stick with left
	Backward, heel-to-toe walk

Note:

- Ages are in approximate sequence.
- Select items in each section (prone, supine, sitting, standing and walking) which have not yet been achieved as aims/objectives in a developmental therapy plan.
- Record items achieved with dates; use grading as outcomes/evaluations.
- All gross motor items from the Denver Developmental Screening Test are included and based on those ages (Frankenburg *et al.* 1992).

The Gross Motor Function Measure (Russell *et al.* 1989, 2002) is a validated measure which uses items in the above guide. Child and parent reports are needed for participation at home or in the community (see section 'Measures of daily activity and participation' in Chapter 8).

See Table 9.1 for development of hand function and eye–hand coordination (assessment guide).

Wheelchair use

Development of abilities – assessment outline:
Sits upright in wheelchair
Finds and grasps wheel on right side
Finds and grasps wheel on left side
Grasps both wheels simultaneously
Moves right wheel forward slightly (2 inches)
Moves left wheel forward slightly (2 inches)
Moves right wheel forward over 1 foot
Moves left wheel forward over 1 foot
Moves both wheels forward over 1 foot

Moves right wheel backward
Moves left wheel backward
Moves both wheels backward
Travels forward, brings wheelchair to a halt
Travels backward, brings wheelchair to a halt
Starts from stationary, turns wheelchair to right, 180°
Starts from stationary, turns wheelchair to left, 180°
Propels wheelchair round obstacles
Propels wheelchair between two objects forward
Propels wheelchair between two objects backward

- Increase distances and speed
- Explore child's own strategies

Transfers
Sitting, uses brake to halt wheelchair
Sitting, lifts leg rests out of way
Sit slides forward in seat pushing on armrests
Sit slides forward in seat using semipivot pelvis
Sit rises to stand on plantigrade feet, uses armrests or
Sit rises to stand, uses arms forward to grasp support
Sit transfers laterally to bed, to toilet, to chair
Sit slides along transfer board to new seat, uses hand
Sit transfers out of seat downward, to kneel or sit
Sit rises to stand using armrests or grasping support
Sit to stand, changes to new seat
Repeat any of the above in safe return to wheelchair

- Modify this list according to each child's own strategy and condition
- Therapist uses physical guidance and support to teach
- Demonstrate transfers to parents and carers so that they bend hips and knees correctly, and protect their own backs (see Fig. 9.179, rising)

Appendix 2: Equipment

Equipment lists and related information may be obtained from various voluntary organisations, parents of disabled children, Departments of Health, Social Services and Education in local authorities or other Government departments, and equipment lists from various medical equipment firms, toy manufacturers and education suppliers.

Consult organisations such as:

Association of Paediatric Chartered Physiotherapists, c/o Chartered Society of Physiotherapy, 14 Bedford Row, London WC1R 4ED. (www.apcp.org.uk)

Capability Scotland, Westerlea, 11 Ellersly Road, Edinburgh EH12 6HY. (www.capability-scotland.org.uk)

Disabled Living Foundation, 380/384 Harrow Road, London W9 2HU. (www.dlf.org.uk)

Halliwick Association of Swimming Therapy, c/o ADKC Centre, Whitstable House, Silchester Road, London W10 6SB. (www.halliwick.org.uk)

Headway – the brain injury association, 7 King Edward Court, King Edward Street, Nottingham NG1 1EW. (www.headway.org.uk)

KIDS – The disabled children's charity. Head Office, 49 Mecklenburgh Square, London WC1N 2NY. (www.kids.org.uk)

Mencap (Royal Mencap Society), 123 Golden Lane, London EC1Y 0RT. (www.mencap.org.uk)

National Association of Paediatric Occupational Therapists (Children, Young People & Families), c/o The College of Occupational Therapists, Specialist Section, 106–114 Borough High Street, London SE1 1LB. (www.cot.co.uk)

National Association of Swimming Clubs for the Handicapped, The Willows, Mayles Lane, Wickham, Hants PO17 5ND. (www.nasch.org.uk)

Play Matters (National Association of Toy and Leisure Libraries), 1A Harmood Street, London NW1 8DN. (www.natll.org.uk)

Riding for the Disabled Association, Norfolk House, 1a Tournament Court, Edgehill Drive, Warwick CV34 6LG. (www.rda.org.uk)

Royal College of Speech and Language Therapists, 2 White Hart Yard, London SE1 1NX. (Enquire for centres offering communication aids and advice.) (www.rcslt.org)

Royal National Institute for Deaf People (RNID), 19–23 Featherstone Street, London EC1Y 8SL. (www.rnid.org.uk)

Royal National Institute of Blind People (RNIB), 105 Judd Street, London WC1H 9NE. (www.rnib.org.uk)

Scope (for people with cerebral palsy), 6 Market Road, London N7 9PW. (www.scope.org.uk)

Sense (for deafblind people), 101 Pentonville Road, London N1 9LG. (www.sense.org.uk)

Basic equipment

Imaginative parents and therapists require a mat, chairs of different sizes, tables of different sizes and everyday objects in the home, especially in the kitchen, and also use of grass, sand, water, leaves and so on outside the house.

Additional equipment is selected *according to the children* and a therapist's assessment of them.

Postural management for day and night. Equipment includes lying, seating for chairs and wheelchairs, prone standers and upright standing frames. Wedges and other sponge rubber shapes are also used for correct positioning throughout the 24 hours.

Note: A manual handling assessment by an expert trainer is important for lifting patients, placing them in equipment and taking them out of equipment. There are also increasing numbers of designs on the market for safe manual handling such as electrical lifting apparatus, electric lifting mechanisms on standing frames, hoists, bathroom apparatus, electric wheelchairs and other equipment. *Contact should be made with each therapist's professional association for further information.* See booklet *Paediatric Manual Handling – Guidelines for Paediatric Physiotherapists*, Association of Paediatric Chartered Physiotherapists, UK.

Lying equipment among others are the Chailey lying frame for supine or prone, the Goldsmith Symmetrical Body Support 'Symmetrisleep' for rest and night positioning, and the 'Dreama' modular mattress designed by Jenx Ltd, Sheffield. This night-positioning mattress allows for support pads to be placed and locked almost anywhere for correcting individual postures of a child or older person in supine, prone or side lying. Side-lying boards/equipment used during the day with positioning of body and abducted legs and both arms forward are available from various manufacturers.

Wedges, other sponge rubber shapes or firm cushions.

Sponge rubber rolls of different diameters. Cover wedges, shapes, rolls with waterproof and washable material. Diameters of rolls are small for prone lying, chest support, to take weight on elbows or hands; take weight on knees, or sit astride. Large diameters for tilt reactions, arm saving reactions; lower to standing; standing arm support on roll, stepping push roll along.

Large inflatable balls including beach balls may be used instead of rolls. Therapy balls of large diameter such as 44 inches (1100 mm) and 32 inches (800 mm). Small beach balls of various sizes.

Seating. Various designs are available. See the section 'Development of sitting' in Chapter 9. This includes special chairs or adaptive seating; adjustable corner seat or floor seat with tray fitment and simple chairs with non-slip seats, backs and sides (removable) of different sizes to fit children. The slatted chair (Petö) is also useful for training various motor tasks as well as sitting. There are a variety of toilet seats, potties, hoist seats, car seats, bath seats, portable shower seats on wheels on the market.

Variable height tables should be obtained whenever possible. Cut-out tables should also be adjustable. Tables which tilt to different angles are available.

Crawlers. A canvas sling, under the child's abdomen and supports on casters, is essentially the basic principle used in crawlers when indicated. Many adjustments may be required to prevent *shooting* into abnormal extension or arms pushing into the area beneath the child's abdomen. Prone scooter boards or platforms on wheels, wedges on wheels (casters) or toy creations such as the dolphin on casters are also used by some children for crawling on hands only, on knees only or on hands and knees.

Apparatus for supported standing. Various standing frames are available. The child can also show ability to stand and hold parallel or vertical bars; backs of chairs or stationary walking aids (see Chapter 9).

Note: Standing aids do not train standing unless the aid is vertical with the line of gravity going from the child's head (ear) down to just behind his ankle. Adjust the foot pieces or straps to obtain the correct alignment, with symmetry and feet held at right angles.

Prone-standing frame attached at a forward angle to a table for schoolwork or hand activities corrects abnormal postures of the legs, keeps the trunk straight and stimulates head control and arm function. Periods of passive stretching of tight (spastic) muscles and joints are given to prevent deformities. Some prone standers are adjustable to become upright standers. Prone 20–30° incline is advisable.

Walking aids. There is a great variety and they should be carefully selected (see Chapter 9).

- *With trunk support* given by a padded support to chest or by chest slings attached overhead.
- *Without trunk support.* A four-point walker which can be pushed with grasp on the sides of the child or grasp in front of the child. Toy walkers or doll's prams are very popular. Large soft toys on wheels, large trucks, large toy boxes on casters and similar normal toys should be stable, weighted and checked for size according to the child. Pushing stable children's or adult's chairs which slide easily but not too quickly as well as boxes on skis and other simple aids also train walking. The slatted back walker is also useful.

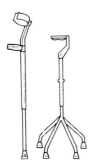

Figure A2.1 Walking aids. Usually managed from ages 5 to 6 years.

Note: Check that wheels on walkers are correct for the child. If they 'run away', preventing correct postures and establishment of the child's own control of his balance, use the walkers with crutch tips at each of the four points, ski sliders or other modifications. Crutches, elbow crutches, quadripods, tripods and thick-based sticks are used for *selected* children (Fig. A2.1). Frequently, progress is made from crutches to sticks. Check length, hand grasps and stability. Some sticks may be linked together with a centrepiece for initial stability.

Note: All walking aids should be checked for height so that the child does not grasp them with abnormal shoulder hunching, excessive flexion of the elbows and radial deviation of wrists. If grasp is not possible without these abnormalities, try a walking aid which requires pushing with flat hands and straight elbows, or use a chair.

Parallel bars. These should be adjustable in height, sometimes in width. Hand slides are used if the child cannot grasp and release to use the parallel bars. A chair at the end of the bars may be used for training standing up from sitting. Eversion boards, footprints and abduction boards have been placed between the bars when needed.

Appliances for correct posture in standing, weight bearing and trunk control:

- *Knee gaiters* or polythene knee moulds, plaster back-slabs to keep knees straight (Fig. A2.2).
- *Elbow gaiters* which keep elbows straight for correct arm push and grasp of walkers and other poles in other functions (Fig. A2.3).

Boots may:

(1) Be padded at the tongue to fit well around the ankle.

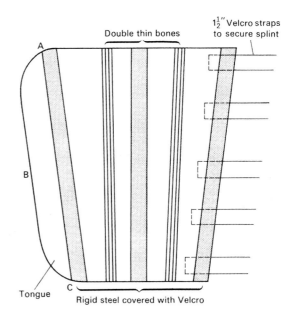

Figure A2.2 Leg gaiter made of white coutil. It is wrapped around the leg bringing Velcro straps over the front side of 'B' ($1'' \approx 25$ mm).

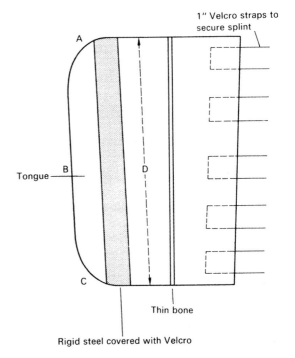

Figure A2.3 Arm splint made of white coutil. Wrap splint around arm bringing Velcro straps over side B.

(2) Have a strap to cross the front of the ankle to press heel well down.

(3) Have an inside mould at the inside arch to control valgus.

(4) Have an external heel extension on the inner side of the sole to prevent pronation (valgus) of the foot; on the outer side of the sole to prevent supination (varus).

(5) Have a raise on the heel, with a flare on the inner side for valgus; outer side for varus.

(6) Boots may be worn with special orthoses.

(7) Boot may have a sole raised to provoke forward weight shift to step, or to stretch heel cords. Sometimes just removal of the heels and thick soles stops toe walking in a mild spastic child.

(8) Boots or shoes may have a weighted base to add stability for, say, ataxic children.

(9) Stiffening on the boot leather may be given on the inside or outside to stop the foot rolling over into either pronation or supination, respectively. Heel cups on their own or with moulded extension to correct all foot arches may be needed.

(10) Toes of boots often have to be protected with thick rubbers, plastic coatings or metal to avoid the frequent wearing of the leather in *toe walkers* or *crawlers* who are just beginning to walk.

(11) Crawling children or non-walkers have boots and shoes to keep their feet warm, without any modifications. Booties or *trainers* stay on their feet better. Crawling is not possible in below-knee orthoses.

Note: Putting on and off shoes and boots is facilitated by the use of laces down to the toes as in Piedro shoes. Toes can then be held flat during application of boots. Velcro instead of laces makes it possible for some children to put their own shoes on and off. A tab on the back of the boot helps the child to pull on his boot.

There are various special trainers for children with cerebral palsy.

Stairs with banisters can be part of the physiotherapy department. Stairs should vary in height.

Ramps, uneven ground, various floor surfaces should be available for training walking.

Mirrors to floor level may be a help in training sitting, standing and walking.

Aids to activities of daily living

There are many different aids. Consult occupational therapists.

Feeding

Dycem mat, long-handled spoons, spoons of different sizes, metal and unbreakable polythene/bone spoons, rubberzote and other handles, dishes with and without sides. Suction rubbers to hold bowl on table. Bibs. Cups; non-slip, weighted, cup-and-straw, baby mugs with non-spill aids and training lids with small opening. Mugs with two handles or one handle which are easy to grasp.

Dressing

Velcro. Zips and special designs. Detachable fronts for children who drool or mess. Large buttons, hooks or other fastenings.

Bathing

Non-slip mat in bath, small bath within large bath. Special bath seats and safety neck supports. Liquid bath cleansers to avoid soaping when there are difficulties.

Toilet

See sections on chairs and sitting in Chapter 9. Many more are available.

Sleeping bags, cots, baby toys, etc.

As for normal babies.

Prams, pushchairs and baby buggies

As for normal children, but check postures more carefully. Special inserts for pushchairs and buggies which correct posture are available on the market.

Wheelchairs

A variety is available. References should be made to manufacturers of medical equipment, departments of health and voluntary organisations as lists of wheelchairs and their designs change and improve (see list of organisations and local seating clinics). The principles of correct seating discussed in section 'Development of sitting' in Chapter 9 are applied to the child in wheelchairs with the added considerations:

(1) Can he propel the chair himself or must it be pushed? Can he transfer?
(2) Facilities of the child's home for containing a wheelchair – stairs, doorways, sizes of rooms, use of table heights available, etc.
(3) Is the wheelchair useful indoors, outdoors or both?
(4) Can the wheelchair 'grow' with the child. What modifications?
(5) Can the wheelchair be transported, stored, put on public transport?

Special aids in the classroom

Typewriters; electronic aids to communication (augmented communication aids and also called communication systems). Advice and professional skills can be obtained from communication advice centres. Contact: Communication Matters (also known as ISAAC (UK)), c/o The ACE Centre, 92 Windmill Road, Oxford OX3 7DR (www.communicationmatters.org.uk). Various aids such as page-turners, pencil holders, page and book holders, various clips for drawing/writing paper and special low-vision aids are among many classroom aids offered by manufacturers of medical and educational equipment in their lists. Occupational therapists and speech and language therapists should be consulted (see addresses in list above).

Aids to mobility

Aids other than walkers, crawlers and wheelchairs such as go-karts, powered chariots; tricycles with adaptations. Hand-propelled tricycles and other special tricycles. Corner seat on casters. A variety of mobility toys is in development by engineers, research workers, parents, therapists and toy manufacturers. See adventure playground organisations, for example KIDS, Play Matters and the Disabled Living Foundation, in address list above.

Many toys and mobility aids are now operated by a variety of switches for severely impaired people. Enquire to College of Occupational Therapists (address above) and voluntary organisations about these electronic devices.

General

Helmets to protect the child's head if he falls frequently. Toy catalogues. Toy libraries' catalogues for appropriate toys. Gym apparatus (balls, hoops, ropes, climbing apparatus). Playground apparatus, playthings and equipment. Rocking boards, rocking toys, swings with supports and straps, slides, climbing frames.

Note: Treatment tables in physiotherapy should be high for some physiotherapy techniques and low for training the child to get off the treatment table into standing.

References

AACPDM (2004) *Methodology to Develop Systematic Reviews of Treatment Interventions (Revision 1.1)*. (http://www.aacpdm.org/resources/systematicReviewsMethodology.pdf)

Adler, S.S., Beckers, D. & Buck, M. (2008) *PNF in Practice: An Illustrated Guide*. 3rd edn. Springer, Heidelberg.

Ahl, L.E., Johansson, E., Granat, T. & Carlberg, E.B. (2005) Functional therapy for children with cerebral palsy: an ecological approach. *Dev. Med. Child Neurol.*, **47**, 613–619.

Akeson, W.H., Amiel, D., Abel, M.F., Garfin, S.R. & Woo, S.L. (1987) Effects of immobilization on joints. *Clinical Orthopaedics and Related Research*, **219**, 28–37.

Albright, A.L. & Neville, B. (2000) Pharmacological management of spasticity. In *The Management of Spasticity Associated with the Cerebral Palsies in Children and Adolescents* (eds A.L. Albright & B. Neville), pp. 121–133. Churchill Communications, Secaucus.

Amiel-Tison, C. & Grenier, A. (1986) *Neurological Assessment during the First Year of Life*. Oxford University Press, New York.

Andersson, C. & Mattsson, E. (2001) Adults with cerebral palsy: a survey describing problems, needs, and resources, with special emphasis on locomotion. *Dev. Med. Child Neurol.*, **43**, 76–82.

Andersson, C., Grooten, W., Hellsten, M., Kaping, K. & Mattsson, E. (2003) Adults with cerebral palsy: walking ability after progressive strength training. *Dev. Med. Child Neurol.*, **45**, 220–228.

Anttila, H., Autti-Ramo, I., Suoranta, J., Makela, M. & Malmivaara, A. (2008) Effectiveness of physical therapy interventions for children with cerebral palsy: a systematic review. *BMC Pediatrics*, 8, 14.

APCP (2002) *Paediatric Physiotherapy Guidance for Good Practice*. Available from Association of Paediatric Chartered Physiotherapists, London. (www.apcp.org.uk)

APCP (2005) *Paediatric Outcome Measurements*. Available from Association of Paediatric Chartered Physiotherapists, London. (www.apcp.org.uk)

APCP (2007) *Information to Guide Good Practice for Physiotherapist Working with Children*. Available from Association of Paediatric Chartered Physiotherapists, London. (www.apcp.org.uk)

APCP (2008) *The Use of Botulinum Toxin in Children with Neurological Conditions*. Available from Association of Paediatric Chartered Physiotherapists, London. (www.apcp.org.uk)

Aubert, E.J. (2008) Motor development in the normal child. In *Pediatric Physical Therapy*, 4th edn (ed. J.S. Tecklin), pp. 17–65. Lippincott Williams & Wilkins, Philadelphia.

Ayres, A.J. (1979) *Sensory Integration and the Child*. Western Psychological Services, Los Angeles.

Bailey, D.B. & Simeonsson, R.J. (1988) *Family Assessment in Early Intervention*. Merrill, Columbus, Ohio.

Bairstow, P., Cochrane, R. & Hur, J. (1993) Shortened version. *Evaluation of Conductive Education for Children with Cerebral Palsy (Final Report)*. HMSO, London.

Bairstow, P., Cochrane, R. & Rusk, I. (1991) Selection of children with cerebral palsy for conductive education. *Dev. Med. Child Neurol.*, **33**, 984.

Baker, R., Jasinski, M., Maciag-Tymecka, I., *et al.* (2002) Botulinum toxin treatment of spasticity in diplegic cerebral palsy: a randomized, double-blind, placebo-controlled, dose-ranging study. *Dev. Med. Child Neurol.*, **44**, 666–675.

Bardsley, D.G.I. (1993) Seating. In *Elements of Paediatric Physiotherapy* (ed. P. Eckersley), pp. 411–421. Churchill Livingstone, Edinburgh.

Bartlett, D. & Birmingham, T. (2003) Validity and reliability of the Pediatric Reach Test. *Pediatr. Phys. Ther.*, **15**, 84–92.

Bartlett, D.J. & Palisano, R.J. (2000) A multivariate model of determinants of motor change for children with cerebral palsy. *Phys. Ther.*, **80**, 598–614.

Bartlett, D.J. & Palisano, R.J. (2002) Physical therapists' perceptions of factors influencing the acquisition of motor abilities of children with cerebral palsy: implications for clinical reasoning. *Phys. Ther.*, **82**, 237–248.

Bartlett, D. & Purdie, B. (2005) Testing of the spinal alignment and range of motion measure: a discriminative measure of posture and flexibility for children with cerebral palsy. *Dev. Med. Child Neurol.*, **47**, 739–743.

Bax, M. (2001) Adolescence and after. *Dev. Med. Child Neurol.*, **43**, 435.

Bax, M. & Brown, K.J. (2004) The spectrum of disorders known as cerebral palsy. In *Management of the Motor Disorders of Children with Cerebral Palsy (2nd edition). Clinics in Developmental Medicine. No. 161* (eds D. Scrutton,

D. Damiano & M. Mayston), pp. 9–21. Mac Keith Press, London.

Bayley, N.A. (2005) *The Bayley Scales of Infant and Toddler Development*, 3rd edn. The Psychological Corporation, San Antonio.

Beach, R.C. (1988) Conductive education for motor disorders: new hope or false hope. *Arch. Dis. Child.*, **63**, 211.

Beckung, E., Carlsson, G., Carlsdotter, S. & Uvebrant, P. (2007) The natural history of gross motor development in children with cerebral palsy aged 1 to 15 years. *Dev. Med. Child Neurol.*, **49**, 751–756.

Beckung, E. & Hagberg, G. (2002) Neuroimpairments, activity limitations, and participation restrictions in children with cerebral palsy. *Dev. Med. Child Neurol.*, **44**, 309–316.

Belenkii, V.Y., Gurfinkel, V.S. & Paltsev, Y.I. (1967) Elements of control of voluntary movements. *Biophysics*, **12**, 135.

Bertoti, D.B. (1986) Effect of short leg casting on ambulation in children with cerebral palsy. *Phys. Ther.*, **66**, 1522–1529.

Bidabe, L. & Lollar, J.M. (1990) *MOVE/Mobility Opportunities Via Education*. MOVE International, Bakersfield.

Bjornson, K., Hays, R., Graubert, C., *et al.* (2007) Botulinum toxin for spasticity in children with cerebral palsy: a comprehensive evaluation. *Pediatrics*, **120**, 49–58.

Bjornson, K.F., Belza, B., Kartin, D., Logsdon, R., McLauglin, J. & Thompson, E.A. (2008) The relationship of physical activity to health status and quality of life in cerebral palsy. *Pediatr. Phys. Ther.*, **20**, 247–253.

Blackmore, A.M., Boettcher-Hunt, E., Jordan, M. & Chan, M.D.Y. (2007) A systematic review of the effects of casting on equinus in children with cerebral palsy: an evidence report of the AACPDM. *Dev. Med. Child Neurol.*, **49**, 781–790.

Blackmore, A.M., Garbellini, S.A., Buttigieg, P. & Wells, J. (2006) A systematic review of the effects of soft splinting on upper limb function in people with cerebral palsy. An AACPDM Evidence Report. (http://www.aacpdm.org/resources/treatmentOutcomeSoftsplintingreview.pdf)

Blair, E., Ballantyne, J., Horsman, S. & Chauvel, P. (1995) A studys of a dynamic proximal stability splint in the management of children with cerebral palsy. *Dev. Med. Child Neurol.*, **37**, 544–554.

Blanche, E., Botticelli, T. & Holloway, M. (eds) (1995) *Combining Neurodevelopmental and Sensory Integration Principles: An Approach to Physical Therapy*. Psychological Corporation, New York.

Blauw-Hospers, C.H. & Hadders-Algra, M. (2005) A systematic review of the effects of early intervention on motor development. *Dev. Med. Child Neurol.*, **47**, 421–432.

Blundell, S.W., Shepherd, R.B., Dean, C.M., *et al.* (2003) Functional strength training in cerebral palsy: a pilot study of a group circuit training class for children aged 4–8 years. *Clin. Rehabil.*, **17**, 48–57.

Bobath, B. (1965) *Abnormal Postural Reflex Activity Caused by Brain Lesions*. Heinemann, London.

Bobath, B. (1971) Motor development, its effect on general development and application to the treatment of cerebral palsy. *Physiotherapy*, **57**, 526.

Bobath, B. & Bobath, K. (1975) *Motor Development in the Different Types of Cerebral Palsy*. Heinemann, London.

Bobath, K. (1971) The normal postural reflex mechanism and its deviation in children with cerebral palsy. *Physiotherapy*, **57**, 515.

Bobath, K. (1980) *A Neurophysiological Basis for the Treatment of Cerebral Palsy*. Clin. Dev. Med. No. 75, SIMP, Heinemann Medical, London.

Bobath, K. & Bobath, B. (1972) Cerebral palsy, part 1, and the neurodevelopmental approach to treatment, part 2. In *Physical Therapy Services in the Developmental Disabilities* (eds P.H. Pearson & C.E. Williams). C.C. Thomas, Springfield, Illinois.

Bobath, K. & Bobath, B. (1984) The neuro-developmental treatment. In *Management of the Motor Disorders of Children with Cerebral Palsy* (ed. D. Scrutton), p. 6. SIMP, Blackwell Scientific Publications, Oxford.

Bodkin, A.W., Baxter, R.S. & Heriza, C.B. (2003) Treadmill training for an infant born preterm with a grade III intraventricular hemorrhage. *Phys. Ther.*, **83**, 1107–1118.

Bohannon, R.W. & Smith, M.B. (1987) Interrater reliability of a modified Ashworth scale of muscle spasticity. *Phys. Ther.*, **67**, 206–207.

Bottos, M., Feliciangeli, A., Sciuto, L., Gericke, C. & Vianello, A. (2001) Functional status in adults with cerebral palsy and its implications for treatment of children. *Dev. Med. Child Neurol.*, **43**, 516–528.

Bottos, M. & Gericke, C. (2003) Ambulatory capacity in cerebral palsy: prognostic criteria and consequences for intervention. *Dev. Med. Child Neurol.*, **45**, 786–790.

Bower, E. & Ashburn, A. (1998) Principles of physiotherapy assessment and outcome measures. In *Neurological Physiotherapy* (ed. M. Stokes), pp. 43–55. Mosby, London.

Bower, E. & McLellan, D.L. (1992) Effect of increased exposure to physiotherapy on skill acquisition of children with cerebral palsy. *Dev. Med. Child Neurol.*, **34**, 25.

Bower, E., McLellan, D.L., Arney, J. & Campbell, M.J. (1996) A randomised controlled trial of different intensities of physiotherapy and different goal-setting procedures in 44 children with cerebral palsy. *Dev. Med. Child Neurol.*, **38**, 226–237.

Bower, E., Michell, D., Burnett, M., Campbell, M.J. & McLellan, D.L. (2001) Randomized controlled trial of physiotherapy in 56 children with cerebral palsy followed for 18 months. *Dev. Med. Child Neurol.*, **43**, 4–15.

Boyce, C., Gowland, C., Rosenbaum, P.L. *et al.* (1995) The gross motor performance measure: validity and responsivity of a measure of quality of movement. *Phys. Ther.*, **75**, 603.

Boyd, R.N. (2004) A physiotherapy perspective on assessment and outcome measurement of children with cerebral palsy. In *Management of the Motor Disorders of Children with Cerebral Palsy. Clinics in Developmental Medicine No. 161* (eds D. Scrutton, D. Damiano & M. Mayston), pp. 52–66. Mac Keith Press, London.

Boyd, R.N., Dobson, F., Parrott, J., *et al.* (2001a) The effect of botulinum toxin type A and a variable hip abduction orthosis on gross motor function: a randomized controlled trial. *Eur. J. Neurol.*, **8**(Suppl. 5), 109–119.

Boyd, R.N. & Graham, H.K. (1999) Objective measurement of clinical findings in the use of botulinum toxin type A for the management of children with cerebral palsy. *Eur. J. Neurol.*, **6** (suppl. 4), S23–S35.

Boyd, R.N., Morris, M.E. & Graham, H.K. (2001b) Management of upper limb dysfunction in children with cerebral palsy: a systematic review. *Eur. J. Neurol.*, **8** (Suppl. 5), 150–166.

Brauer, S., Burns, Y. & Galley, P. (1999) Lateral reach: a clinical measure of medio-lateral postural stability. *Physiother. Res. Int.*, **4**, 81–88.

Brazelton, T. (1976) Case finding, screening, diagnosis and tracking. Discussants' comments. In *Intervention Strategies for High Risk Infants and Children* (ed. T.D. Tjossem). University Park Press, Baltimore.

Brown, G.T. & Burns, S.A. (2001) The efficacy of NDT in paediatrics: a systematic review. *Brit. J. Occup. Ther.*, **64**, 235–244.

Brown, J.K. (1985) Positional deformity in children with cerebral palsy. *Physiotherapy Practice*, **1**, 37–41.

Brunnstrom, S. (1970) *Movement Therapy in Hemiplegia – A Neurophysiological Approach*. Harper & Row, New York.

Burns, Y.R. & MacDonald, J. (eds) (1996) *Physiotherapy and the Growing Child*. Saunders, London.

Butler, C. & Darrah, J. (2001) Effects of neurodevelopmental treatment (NDT) for cerebral palsy: an AACPDM evidence report. *Dev. Med. Child Neurol.*, **43**, 778–790.

Butler, P., Engelbrecht, M., Major, R.E., Tait, J.H., Stallard, J. & Patrick, J.H. (1984) Physiological cost index of walking for normal children and its use as an indicator of physical handicap. *Dev. Med. Child Neurol.*, **26**, 607–612.

Butler, P.B. (1998) A preliminary report on the effectiveness of trunk targeting in achieving independent sitting balance in children with cerebral palsy. *Clin. Rehabil.*, **12**, 281–293.

Butler, P.B. & Major, R.E. (1992) The learning of motor control: biomechanical considerations. *Physiotherapy*, **78**, 1–6.

Butler, P.B., Thompson, N. & Major, R.E. (1992) Improvement in walking performance of children with cerebral palsy (preliminary results). *Dev. Med. Child Neurol.*, **34**, 567.

Campbell, S.K. (1999) The infant at risk for developmental disability. In *Decision Making in Pediatric Neurologic Physical Therapy* (ed. S.K. Campbell), pp. 260–332. Churchill Livingstone, New York.

Campbell, S.K. (2006) Are models of disability useful in real cases? Pediatric care examples realized in research, clinical practice, and education. *Phys. Ther.*, **86**, 881–887.

Campbell, S.K., Kolobe, T.H.A., Osten, E.T., Lenke, M. & Girolami, G.L. (1995) Construct validity of the test of infant motor performance. *Phys. Ther.*, **75**, 585–596.

Campbell, S.K., Vander Linden, D.W. & Palisano, R.J. (eds) (2006) *Physical Therapy for Children*, 3rd edn. Elsevier, Philadelphia.

Cantrell, E.G. (1997) Adult cerebral palsy. In *Rehabilitation of the Physically Disabled Adult*, 2nd edn (eds C.J. Goodwill, M.A. Chamberlain & C. Evans), pp. 295–313. Stanley Thornes, Cheltenham.

Capute, A.J., Palmer, F.B., Shapiro, B.K., Wachtel, R.C., Ross, A. & Accordo, P.J. (1984) Primitive reflex profile: a quantitation of primitive reflexes in infancy. *Dev. Med. Child Neurol.*, **26**, 375.

Carlberg, E.B. & Hadders-Algra, M. (2008) Postural control in sitting children with cerebral palsy. In *Postural Control: A Key Issue in Developmental Disorders. Clinics in Developmental Medicine No. 179* (eds M. Hadders-Algra & E.B. Carlberg), pp. 74–96. Mac Keith Press, London.

Carlsen, P.N. (1975) Comparison of two occupational therapy approaches for treating the young cerebral-palsied child. *Am. J. Occup. Ther.*, **29**, 267.

Carmick, J. (1993) Clinical use of neuromuscular electrical stimulation for children with cerebral palsy. Part I: Lower extremity & Part II: Upper extremity. *Phys. Ther.*, **73**, 505 & 514.

Carr, J.H. & Shepherd, R.B. (1987) A motor learning model for rehabilitation. In *Movement Science: Foundations for Physical Therapy in Rehabilitation* (eds J.H. Carr & R.B. Shepherd), p. 31. Aspen, Rockville, Maryland.

Carr, J.H. & Shepherd, R.B. (2003) *Neurological Rehabilitation: Optimizing Motor Performance*, 2nd edn. Butterworth Heinemann, Oxford.

Case-Smith, J. (ed.) (1993) *Pediatric Occupational Therapy and Early Intervention*. Andover Medical, Boston.

Caulton, J.M., Ward, K.A., Alsop, C.W., Dunn, G., Adams, J.E. & Mughal, M.Z. (2004) A randomised controlled trial of standing programme on bone mineral density in non-ambulant children with cerebral palsy. *Arch. Dis. Child.*, **89**, 131–135.

Chappell, F. & Williams, B. (2002) Rates and reasons for non-adherence to home physiotherapy in paediatrics: pilot study. *Physiotherapy*, **88**, 138–147.

Charles, J. & Gordon, A.M. (2005) A critical review of constraint-induced movement therapy and forced use in children with hemiplegia. *Neural. Plast.*, **12**, 245–261.

Charles, J.R., Wolf, S.L., Schneider, J.A. & Gordon, A.M. (2006) Efficacy of a child-friendly form of constraint-induced movement therapy in hemiplegic cerebral palsy: a randomized control trial. *Dev. Med. Child Neurol.*, **48**, 635–642.

Cherng, R.-J., Liu, C-F., Lau, T-W. & Hong, R-B. (2007) Effect of treadmill training with body weight support on gait and gross motor function in children with spastic cerebral palsy. *Am. J. Phys. Med. Rehabil.*, **86**, 548–555.

Chiou, I.L. & Burnett, C.N. (1985) Values of activities of daily living. *Phys. Ther.*, **65**, 901.

Cioni, G., Ferrari, F. & Prechtl, H.F.R. (1989) Posture and spontaneous motility in fullterm infants. *Early Human Dev.*, **18**, 247.

Cioni, G., Ferrari, F. & Prechtl, H.F.R. (1992) Early motor assessment in brain-damaged preterm infants. In *Movement Disorders in Children* (eds H. Forssberg & H. Hirschfeld), p. 72–79. Karger, Basel.

Collet, J-P., Vanasse, M., Marois, P., *et al.* (2001) Hyperbaric oxygen for children with cerebral palsy: a randomised multicentre trial. *The Lancet*, **357**, 582–586.

Collins, F. (2007) The JCM moonlite sleep system: assisting in the provision of 24-hour postural support. *Int. J. Ther. Rehabil.* **14** (7), 36–40.

Collis, E. (1947) *A Way of Life for the Handicapped Child.* Faber & Faber, London.

Collis, E., Collis, R., Dunham, W., Hilliard, L.T. & Lawson, D. (1956) *The Infantile Cerebral Palsies.* Heinemann, London.

Comeaux, P., Patterson, N., Rubin, M. & Meiner, R. (1997) Effect of neuromuscular electrical stimulation during gait in children with cerebral palsy. *Pediatr. Phys. Ther.,* **9**, 103–109.

Cooper, J., Moodley, M. & Reynell, J. (1978) *Helping Language Development.* Edward Arnold, London.

Cordo, P.J. & Nashner, L.M. (1982) Properties of postural adjustments associated with rapid arm movements. *J. Neurophysiol.,* **47**, 287.

Corry, I.S., Cosgrove, A.P., Duffy, C.M., McNeill, S., Taylor, T.C. & Graham, H.K. (1998) Botulinum toxin A compared with stretching casts in the treatment of spastic equinus: a randomised prospective trial. *J. Pediatr. Orthop.,* **18**, 304–311.

Corry, I.S., Cosgrove, A.P., Walsh, E.G., McClean, D. & Graham, H.K. (1997) Botulinum toxin A in the hemiplegic upper limb: A double-blind trial. *Dev. Med. Child Neurol.,* **39**, 185–193.

Cosgrove, A. (2000) Orthopaedic surgery in spastic cerebral palsy. In *The Management of Spasticity Associated with the Cerebral Palsies in Children and Adolescents* (eds A.L. Albright & B. Neville), pp. 75–92. Churchill Communications, Secaucus.

Cosgrove, A.P., Corry, I.S. & Graham, H.K. (1994) Botulinum toxin in the management of the lower limb in cerebral palsy. *Dev. Med. Child Neurol.,* **36**, 386–396.

Cottalorda, J., Gautheron, V., Metton, G., Charmet, E. & Chavrier, Y. (2000) Toe-walking in children younger than six years with cerebral palsy. The contribution of serial corrective casts. *J. Bone Joint Surg. Br.,* **82**, 541–544.

Cottam, P. & Sutton, A. (1988) *Conductive Education: A System for Overcoming Motor Disorder.* Croom Helm, London.

Cotton, E. (1970) Integration of treatment and education in cerebral palsy. *Physiotherapy,* **56** (4), 143.

Cotton, E. (1974) Improvement in motor function with the use of conductive education. *Dev. Med. Child Neurol.,* **16**, 637.

Cotton, E. (1975) *Conductive Education and Cerebral Palsy.* The Spastics Society, London.

Cotton, E. (1980) *The Basic Motor Pattern.* The Spastics Society, London.

Cotton, E. (1984) Integration of disciplines in the treatment and education of children with cerebral palsy. In *Paediatric Developmental Therapy* (ed S. Levitt), pp. 246–258. Blackwell Scientific Publications, Oxford.

Craft, M.J., Lakin, J.A., Oppliger, R.A., Clancy, G.M. & Vanderlinden, D.W. (1990) Siblings as change agents for promoting the functional status of children with cerebral palsy. *Dev. Med. Child Neurol.,* **32**, 1049–1057.

Cratty, B.J. (1970) *Perceptual and Motor Development in Infants and Children.* Macmillan, London.

Crompton, J., Galea, M.P. & Phillips, B. (2007) Hand-held dynamometry for muscle strength measurement in children with cerebral palsy. *Dev. Med. Child Neurol.,* **49**, 106–111.

Crothers, B. & Paine, R.S. (1959) *The Natural History of Cerebral Palsy.* Reprinted in 1988 as *Classics in Developmental Medicine No 2.* Mac Keith Press, London.

Cummins, R.A. (1988) *The Neurologically Impaired Child: Doman-Delacato Techniques Reappraised.* Croom Helm, London.

Dale, N. (1996) *Working with Families of Children with Special Needs.* Routledge, London.

Damiano, D. (2004) Physiotherapy management in cerebral palsy: moving beyond philosophies. In *Management of the Motor Disorders of Children with Cerebral Palsy. Clinics in Developmental Medicine No. 161* (eds D. Scrutton, D. Damiano & M. Mayston), pp. 161–169. Mac Keith Press, London.

Damiano, D. (2007) Strengthening exercises. In *Physical Therapy of Cerebral Palsy* (ed. F. Miller), pp. 346–348. Springer, New York.

Damiano, D.L. & Abel, M.F. (1998) Functional outcomes of strength training in spastic cerebral palsy. *Arch. Phys. Med. Rehabil.,* **79**, 119–125.

Damiano, D.L., Kelly, L.E. & Vaughan, C.L. (1995a) Effects of a quadriceps femoris strengthening program on crouch gait in children with cerebral palsy. *Physical Therapy,* **75**, 658–667.

Damiano, D.L., Vaughan, C.L. & Abel, M.F. (1995b) Muscle response to heavy resistance exercise in children with spastic cerebral palsy. *Dev. Med. Child Neurol.,* **37**, 731–739.

Damiano, D.L., Dodd, K. & Taylor, N.F. (2002a) Should we be testing and training muscle strength in cerebral palsy? *Dev. Med. Child Neurol.,* **44**, 68–72.

Damiano, D.L., Quinlivan, J.M., Owen, B.F., Payne, P., Nelson, K.C. & Abel, M.F. (2002b) What does the Ashworth scale really measure and are instrumented measures more valid and precise? *Dev. Med. Child Neurol.,* **44**, 112–118.

Daniels, N., Gopsill, C., Armstrong, J., Pinnington, L. & Ward C. (2004) *An Evaluation of Standing Frames for 8 to 14 Years Olds (MHRA 04159).* Department of Health, London.

Darrah, J., Watkins, B., Chen., L. & Bonin, C. (2004) Conductive education intervention for children with cerebral palsy: an AACPDM evidence report. *Dev. Med. Child Neurol.,* **46**, 187–203.

Darrah, J., Wessel, J., Nearingburg, P. & O'Connor, M. (1999) Evaluation of a community fitness program for adolescents with cerebral palsy. *Pediatr. Phys. Ther.,* **11**, 18–23.

d'Avignon, M., Noren, L. & Arman, T. (1981) Early physiotherapy ad modum Vojta or Bobath in infants with suspected neuromotor disturbance. *Neuropediatrics,* **12**, 232–241.

Davis, E., Davies, B., Wolfe, R., Raadsveld, R., Heine, B., Thomason, P., Dobson, F. & Graham, H.K. (2009) A randomized controlled trial of the impact of therapeutic horse riding on the quality of life, health, and function of children with cerebral palsy. *Dev. Med. Child Neurol.*, **51**, 111–119.

Day, S.M., Wu, Y.W., Strauss, D.J., Shavelle, R.M. & Reynolds, R.J. (2007) Change in ambulatory ability of adolescents and young adults with cerebral palsy. *Dev. Med. Child Neurol.*, **49**, 647–653.

De Groot, L. (1993) *Posture and Motility in Preterm Infants: A Clinical Approach.* VU University Press, Amsterdam.

De Groot, L. (2000) Posture and motility in preterm infants. *Dev. Med. Child Neurol.*, **41**, 65–68.

DeLuca, S.C., Echols, K., Ramey, S.L. & Taub, E. (2003) Pediatric constraint-induced movement therapy for a young child with cerebral palsy: two episodes of care. *Phys.Ther.*, **83**, 1003–1013.

DeMatteo, C., Law, M., Russell, D., Pollock, N., Rosenbaum, P. & Walter, S. (1993) The reliability and validity of the quality of upper extremity skills test. *Phys. Occup. Ther. Pediatr.*, **13** (2), 1–18.

Department of Health and Department for Education and Skills (2004) *National Service Framework for Children, Young People and Maternity Services: Disabled Children and Young People and Those with Complex Health Needs.* HMSO, London.

Desloovere, K., Molenaers, G., Feys, H., Huenaerts, C., Callewaert, B. & Walle P. (2006) Do dynamic and static clinical measurements correlate with gait analysis parameters in children with cerebral palsy? *Gait & Posture*, **24**, 302–313.

De Souza, L.H. (1997) Physiotherapy. In *Rehabilitation of the Physically Disabled Adult* (eds C.J. Goodwill, M.A. Chamberlain & C. Evans), pp. 560–575. Stanley Thornes, Cheltenham.

Dietz, V. (1992) Spasticity: exaggerated reflexes or movement disorder? In *Movement Disorders in Children* (eds H. Forssberg & H. Hirschfeld), p. 225–233. Karger, Basel.

Dietz, V. & Berger, W. (1983) Normal and impaired regulation of muscle stiffness in gait: a new hypothesis about muscle hypertonia. *Exp. Neurol.*, **79**, 680.

Dietz, V. & Berger, W. (1995) Cerebral palsy and muscle transformation. *Dev. Med. Child Neurol.*, **37**, 180–184.

Dobson, F., Morris, M.E., Baker, R. & Graham, H.K. (2007) Gait classification in children with cerebral palsy: a systematic review. *Gait & Posture*, **25**, 140–152.

Dodd, K.J. & Foley, S. (2007) Partial body-weight-supported treadmill training can improve walking in children with cerebral palsy: a clinical controlled trial. *Dev. Med. Child Neurol.*, **49**, 101–105.

Dodd, K.J., Taylor, N.F. & Graham, H.K. (2003) A randomized clinical trial of strength training in young people with cerebral palsy. *Dev. Med. Child Neurol.*, **45**, 652–657.

Doman, R.J., Spitz, E.R., Zucman, E., Delacato, C.H. & Doman, G. (1960) Children with severe brain injuries: neurological organization in terms of mobility. *JAMA*, **174**, 257–262.

Donahoe, B., Turner, D. & Worrell, T. (1994) The use of functional reach as a measurement of balance in boys and girls without disabilities ages 5 to 15 years. *Pediatr. Phys. Ther.*, **6**, 189–193.

Drillien, C.M. & Drummond, M.B. (eds) (1977) *Neurodevelopmental Problems in Early Childhood: Assessment and Management.* Blackwell Scientific, Oxford.

Drillien, C.M. & Drummond, M.B. (1983) *Developmental Screening and the Child with Special Needs.* Heinemann, London.

Dumas, H.M., O'Neil, M.E. & Fragala, M.A. (2001) Expert consensus on physical therapist intervention after botulinum toxin A injection for children with cerebral palsy. *Pediatr. Phys. Ther.*, **13**, 122–132.

Durham, S., Eve, L., Stevens, C. & Ewins, D. (2004) Effect of functional electrical stimulation on asymmetries in gait of children with hemiplegic cerebral palsy. *Physiotherapy*, **90**, 82–90.

Eames, N.W.A., Baker, R., Hill, N., Graham, K., Taylor, T. & Cosgrove, A. (1999) The effect of botulinum toxin A on gastrocnemius length: magnitude and duration of response. *Dev. Med. Child Neurol.*, **41**, 226–232.

Eckersley, P.M. (ed.) (1993) *Elements of Paediatric Physiotherapy.* Churchill Livingstone, Edinburgh.

Edwards, S., Partridge, C.J. & Mee, R. (1990) Treatment schedules for research: a model for physiotherapy. *Physiotherapy*, **76**, 605.

Einspieler, C., Prechtl, H.F.R., Bos, A.F., Ferrari, F. & Cioni, G. (eds) (2005) *Prechtl's Method on the Qualitative Assessment of General Movements in Preterm, Term and Young Infants. Clinics in Developmental Medicine No. 167.* Mac Keith Press, London.

Eliasson, A-C. & Burtner, P.A. (eds) (2008) *Improving Hand Function in Children with Cerebral Palsy. Clinics in Developmental Medicine No. 178.* Mac Keith Press, London.

Eliasson, A-C., Krumlinde-Sundholm, L., Rosblad, B., *et al.* (2006) The manual ability classification system (MACS) for children with cerebral palsy: scale development and evidence of validity and reliability. *Dev. Med. Child Neurol.*, **48**, 549–554. (www.macs.nu)

Ellenberg, J.H. & Nelson, K.B. (1981) Early recognition of infants at high risk for cerebral palsy: examination at age four months. *Dev. Med. Child Neurol.*, **23**, 705.

Engsberg, J.R., Ross, S.A. & Collins, D.R. (2006) Increasing ankle strength to improve gait and function in children with cerebral palsy: a pilot study. *Pediatr. Phys. Ther.*, **18**, 266–275.

Farber, S.D. (1982) A multisensory approach to neurorehabilitation. In *Neurorehabilitation: A Multisensory Approach* (ed. S.D. Farber). Saunders, Philadelphia.

Farmer, S.E., Butler, P.B. & Major, R.E. (1999) Targeted training for crouch posture in cerebral palsy. *Physiotherapy*, **85**, 242–247.

Fay, T. (1954a) Rehabilitation of patients with spastic paralysis. *J. Intern. Coll. Surgeons*, **22**, 200.

Fay, T. (1954b) Use of pathological and unlocking reflexes in the rehabilitation of spastics. *Am. J. Phys. Med.*, **33** (6), 347.

Featherstone, H. (1981) *A Difference in the Family.* Basic Books, New York.

Fehlings, D., Rang, M., Glazier, J. & Steele, C. (2001) Botulinum toxin type A injections in the spastic upper extremity of children with hemiplegia: child characteristics that predict a positive outcome. *Eur. J. Neurol.*, **8** (suppl 5), 145–149.

Feldenkrais, M. (1980) *Awareness through Movement*. Penguin Books, London.

Figueiredo, E.M., Ferreira, G.B., Maia Moreira, R.C., Kirkwood, R.N. & Fetters, L. (2008) Efficacy of ankle-foot orthoses on gait of children with cerebral palsy: systematic review of literature. *Pediatr. Phys. Ther.*, **20**, 207–223.

Finnie, N. (1997) *Handling the Young Cerebral Palsied Child at Home*, 3rd edn. Butterworth-Heinemann, Oxford.

Fisher, A.G., Murray, E. & Bundy, A. (1991) *Sensory Integration: Theory and practice*. Davis, Philadelphia.

Florence, J.M., Pandya, S., King, W.M., *et al.* (1992) Intrarater reliability of manual muscle test (Medical Research Council scale) grades in Duchenne's muscular dystrophy. *Phys. Ther.*, **72**, 115–122.

Foley, J. (1977) Cerebral palsy – physical aspects. In *Neurodevelopmental Problems in Early Childhood: Assessment and Management* (eds C.M. Drillien & M.B. Drummond), pp. 269–282. Blackwell Scientific Publications, Oxford.

Foley, J. (1983) The athetoid syndrome. *J. Neurol. Neurosurg. Psychiatry*, **46**, 289.

Foley, J. (1998) *Human Postural Reactions*. Available from Association of Paediatric Chartered Physiotherapists, London. (www.apcp.org.uk)

Folio, M.R. & Fewell, R.R. (2000) *Peabody Developmental Motor Scales*, 2nd edn. Therapy Skill Builders, San Antonio.

Forssberg, H. (1985) Ontogeny of human locomotor control I. Infant stepping, supported locomotion and transition to independent locomotion. *Exp. Brain Res.*, **57**, 480.

Forssberg, H. & Hirschfeld, H. (eds) (1992) *Movement Disorders in Children*. Karger, Basel.

Fosang, A.L., Galea, M.P., McCoy, A.T., Reddihough, D.S. & Story, I. (2003) Measures of muscle and joint performance in the lower limb of children with cerebral palsy. *Dev. Med. Child Neurol.*, **45**, 664–670.

Fox, A.M. (1975) *They Get This Training But They Don't Really Know How You Feel: Transcripts of Interviews with Parents of Handicapped Children*. Institute of Child Health, London.

Fragala, M.A., Goodgold, S. & Dumas, H.M. (2003) Effects of lower extremity passive stretching: pilot study of children and youth with severe limitations in self-mobility. *Pediatr. Phys. Ther.*, **15**, 167–175.

Fraiberg, S. (1977) *Insights from the Blind*. Human Horizon Series. Souvenir Press (Educational and Academic), London.

Franjoine, M.R., Gunther, J.S. & Taylor, M.J. (2003) Pediatric Balance Scale: a modified version of the Berg Balance Scale for the school-age child with mild to moderate motor impairment. *Pediatr. Phys. Ther.*, **15**, 114–128.

Frankenburg, W.K., Dodds, J., Archer, P., Shapiro, H. & Bresnick. B. (1992) The Denver II: a major revision and restandardization of the Denver developmental screening Test. *Pediatrics*, **89**, 91–97.

Friedman, A., Diamond, M., Johnston, M.V. & Daffner, C. (2000) Effects of botulinum toxin A on upper limb spasticity in children with cerebral palsy. *Am. J. Phys. Med. Rehabil.*, **79**, 53–59.

Fry, N.R., Gough, M. & Shortland, A.P. (2004) Three-dimensional realisation of muscle morphology and architecture using ultrasound. *Gait & Posture*, **20**, 177–182.

Gage, J.R. (1991) *Gait Analysis in Cerebral Palsy. Clinics in Developmental Medicine No. 121*. Mac Keith Press, London.

Gage, J.R. (ed.) (2009) *The Treatment of Gait Problems in Cerebral Palsy. Clinics in Developmental Medicine No. 182–183*. Mac Keith Press, London.

Gentile, A.M. (1987) Skill acquisition: action, movement and neuromotor processes. In *Movement Science: Foundations for Physical Therapy in Rehabilitation* (eds J.H. Carr & R.B. Shepherd), p. 93. Aspen, Rockville, Maryland.

Gericke, T. (2006) Postural management for children with cerebral palsy: consensus statement. *Dev. Med. Child Neurol.*, **48**, 244.

Gesell, A. (1971) *The First Five Years of Life*. Harper & Row, New York.

Giuliani, C.A. (1992) Dorsal rhizotomy as a treatment for improving function in children with cerebral palsy. In *Movement Disorders in Children* (eds H. Forssberg & H. Hirschfeld), p. 247–254. Karger, Basel.

Glanzman, A.M., Kim, H., Swaminathan, K. & Beck, T. (2004) Efficacy of botulinum toxin A, serial casting, and combined treatment for spastic equinus: a retrospective study. *Dev. Med. Child Neurol.*, **46**, 807–811.

Goldkamp, O. (1984) Treatment effectiveness in cerebral palsy. *Arch. Phys. Med. Rehab.*, **65**, 232.

Goldschmied, E. (1975) Playing with babies. In *Creative Therapy* (ed. S. Jennings), pp. 52–67. Pitman, London.

Goldsmith, E., Golding, R.M., Garstang, R. & MacRae, A. (1992) A technique to measure windswept deformity. *Physiotherapy*, **78**, 235–242.

Goldsmith, S. (2000) The Mansfield project: postural care at night within a community setting: a feedback study. *Physiotherapy*, **86**, 528–534.

Goodman, M., Rothberg, A.D. & Jacklin, L.A. (1991) 6 year follow up of early physiotherapy intervention in very low birthweight infants. In *Proceedings of the World Confederation of Physical Therapy Congress*, p. 1211. WCPT, London.

Gordon, A.M., Charles, J. & Wolf, S.L. (2005) Methods of constraint-induced movement therapy for children with hemiplegic cerebral palsy: development of a child-friendly intervention for improving upper-extremity function. *Arch. Phys. Med. Rehabil.*, **86**, 837–844.

Gordon, A.M. & Duff, S.V. (1999) Relation between clinical measures and fine manipulative control in children with hemiplegic cerebral palsy. *Dev. Med. Child Neurol.*, **41**, 586–591.

Gordon, J. (1987) Assumptions underlying physical therapy intervention: Theoretical and historical perspectives. In *Movement Science: Foundations for Physical Therapy in Rehabilitation* (eds J.H. Carr & R.B. Shepherd), p. 1. Aspen, Rockville, Maryland.

Gorter, J.W., Ketelaar, M., Rosenbaum, P., Helders, P.J.M. & Palisano, R. (2009) Use of the GMFCS in infants with CP: the need for reclassification at age 2 years or older. *Dev. Med. Child Neurol.*, **51**, 46–52.

Gorter, J.W., Rosenbaum, P.L., Hanna, S.E., *et al.* (2004) Limb distribution, motor impairment, and functional classification of cerebral palsy. *Dev. Med. Child Neurol.*, **46**, 461–467.

Gough, M. (2009) Continuous postural management and the prevention of deformity in children with cerebral palsy: an appraisal. *Dev. Med. Child Neurol.*, **51**, 105–110.

Gough, M., Fairhurst, C. & Shortland, A.P. (2005) Botulinum toxin and cerebral palsy: time for reflection? *Dev. Med. Child Neurol.*, **47**, 709–712.

Graham, H.K. (2004) Mechanisms of deformity. In *Management of the Motor Disorders of Children with Cerebral Palsy. Clinics in Developmental Medicine No. 161* (eds D. Scrutton, D. Damiano & M. Mayston), pp. 105–129. Mac Keith Press, London.

Graham, H.K., Aoki, K.R, Autti-Ramo, I., *et al.* (2000) Recommendations for the use of botulinum toxin type A in the management of cerebral palsy. *Gait & Posture*, **11**, 67–79.

Green, E.M., Mulcahy, C.M. & Pountney, T.E. (1995) An investigation into the development of early postural control. *Dev. Med. Child Neurol.*, **37**, 437–448.

Greenhalgh, T. (2006) *How to Read a Paper: The Basics of Evidence-Based Medicine*, 3rd edn. Blackwell, Oxford.

Greenhalgh, T. & Taylor, R. (1997) How to read a paper: papers that go beyond numbers (qualitative research). *BMJ*, **315**, 740–743.

Greer, J.G. & Wethered, C.E. (1984) Learned helplessness: a piece of the burnout puzzle. *Exceptional Children*, **50**, 524.

Grenier, A. (1988) Prevention of early deformations of the hip in brain damaged neonates. *Annales Pediatrica*, **35**, 423–427.

Griffiths, M. & Clegg, M. (1988) *Cerebral Palsy: Problems and Practice*, Chapter 3. Souvenir Press, London.

Gudjonsdottir, B. & Mercer, V.S. (1997) Hip and spine in children with cerebral palsy: musculoskeletal development and clinical implications. *Pediatr. Phys. Ther.*, **9**, 179–185.

Haas, B.M. & Crow, J.L. (1995) Towards a clinical measurement of spasticity? *Physiotherapy*, **81**, 474–479.

Hadders-Algra, M. (2000) The neuronal group selection theory: promising principles for understanding and treating developmental motor disorders. *Dev. Med. Child Neurol.* **42**, 707–715.

Hadders-Algra, M. (2001) Early brain damage and the development of motor behavior in children: clues for therapeutic intervention? *Neural Plasticity*, **8**, 31–49.

Hadders-Algra, M., Brogren, E. & Forssberg, H. (1996) Training affects the development of postural adjustments in sitting infants. *J. Physiol.* **493**, 289–298.

Hadders-Algra, M. & Carlberg, E.B. (eds) (2008) *Postural Control: A Key Issue in Developmental Disorders. Clinics in Developmental Medicine No. 179*. Mac Keith Press, London.

Hagbarth, K.-E. & Eklund, G. (1969) The muscle vibrator – a useful tool in neurological therapeutic work. *Scan. J. Rehab. Med.*, **1**, 26.

Hagberg, B., Hagberg, G., Olow, I. & von Wendt, L. (1996) The changing panorama of cerebral palsy in Sweden. The birth year period 1987–90. *Acta Paediatr. Scand.*, **85**, 954–960.

Haley, S.M., Coster, W.J., Ludlow, L.H., Haltiwanger, J. & Andrellos, P. (1992) *The Pediatric Evaluation of Disability Inventory: Development Standardization and Administration Manual.* New England Medical Center, Boston.

Hall, D.M.B. (1984) *The Child with a Handicap.* Blackwell Scientific Publications, Oxford.

Hanna, S.E., Bartlett, D.J., Rivard, L.M. & Russell, D.J. (2008) Reference curves for the Gross Motor Function Measure: percentiles for clinical description and tracking over time among children with cerebral palsy. *Phys. Ther.*, **88**, 596–607.

Hanna, S.E., Rosenbaum, P.L., Bartlett, D.J., *et al.* (2009) Stability and decline in gross motor function among children and youth with cerebral palsy aged 2 to 21 years. *Dev. Med. Child Neurol.*, **51**, 295–302.

Hankinson, J. & Morton, R.E. (2002) Use of a lying hip abduction system in children with bilateral cerebral palsy. *Dev. Med. Child Neurol.*, **44**, 177–180.

Hanzlik, J. (1990) Nonverbal interaction patterns of mothers and their infants with cerebral palsy. *Educ. Train. Mental Retard.*, **25**, 333.

Hardy, P., Collet, J-P., Goldberg, J., *et al.* (2002) Neuropsychological effects of hyperbaric oxygen therapy in cerebral palsy. *Dev. Med. Child Neurol.*, **44**, 436–446.

Hari, M. & Akos, K. (1988) *Conductive Education.* Tavistock/Routledge, London.

Hari, M. & Tillemans, T. (1984) Conductive education. In *Management of the Motor Disorders of Children with Cerebral Palsy* (ed. D. Scrutton), p. 19. SIMP, Blackwell Scientific Publications, Oxford.

Harryman, S.E. (1992) Lower extremity surgery for children with cerebral palsy: physical therapy management. *Phys. Ther.*, **72**, 16–24.

Hartveld, A. & Hegarty, J. (1996) Frequent weightshift practice with computerised feedback by cerebral palsied children – four single-case experiments. *Physiotherapy*, **82**, 573–580.

Harvey, A., Robin, J., Morris, M.E., Graham, H.K. & Baker, R. (2008) A systematic review of measures of activity limitation for children with cerebral palsy. *Dev. Med. Child Neurol.*, **50**, 190–198.

Hazlewood, M.E., Brown, J.K., Rowe, P.J. & Salter, P.M. (1994) The use of therapeutic electrical stimulation in the treatment of hemiplegic cerebral palsy. *Dev. Med. Child Neurol.*, **36**, 661–673.

Held, R. (1965) Plasticity in sensory motor systems. *Sci. Am.*, **213** (5), 84.

Hicks, C.L., von Baeyer, C.L., Spafford, P., van Korlaar, I. & Goodenough, B. (2001) The faces pain scale – revised: toward a common metric in pediatric pain measurement. *Pain*, **93**, 173–183.

Hicks, C.M. (2004) *Research Methods for Clinical Therapists: Applied Project Design and Analysis*, 4th edn. Churchill Livingstone, Edinburgh.

Himmelmann, K., Beckung, E., Hagberg, G. & Uvebrant, P. (2006) Gross and fine motor function and accompanying impairments in cerebral palsy. *Dev. Med. Child Neurol.*, **48**, 417–423.

Himmelmann, K., Hagberg, G., Beckung, E., Hagberg, B. & Uvebrant, P. (2005) The changing panorama of cerebral palsy in Sweden. IX. Prevalence and origin in the birth-year period 1995–1998. *Acta Paediatr.* **94**, 287–294.

Hinojosa, J. (1990) How mothers of pre-school children with cerebral palsy perceive occupational and physical therapists and their influence on family life. *Occup. Ther. J. Res.*, **10**, 144.

Hiroshima, K. & Ono, K. (1979) Correlation between muscle shortening and derangement of the hip joint with spastic cerebral palsy. *Clin. Orthopaed. Rel. Res.*, **144**, 186–193.

Hirschfeld, H. (1992) Postural control: acquisition and integration during development. In *Movement Disorders in Children* (eds H. Forssberg & H. Hirschfeld), p. 199. Karger, Basel.

Hodgkinson, I., Jindrich, M.L., Duhaut, P., Vadot, J.P., Metton, G. & Berard, C. (2001) Hip pain in 234 non-ambulatory adolescents and young adults with cerebral palsy: a cross-sectional multicentre study. *Dev. Med. Child Neurol.*, **43**, 806–808.

von Hofsten, C. (1992) Development of manual actions from a perceptual perspective. In *Movement Disorders in Children* (eds H. Forssberg & H. Hirschfeld), p. 113. Karger, Basel.

von Hofsten, C. & Ronnqvist, L. (1988) Preparation for grasping an object: a developmental study. *J. Exp. Psychol.*, **4**, 610.

von Hofsten, C. & Rosblad, B. (1988) The integration of sensory information in the development of precise manual pointing. *Neuropsychologia*, **20**, 461.

Holt, K.S. (ed.) (1975) *Movement and Child Development*. Heinemann – Spastics International Medical Publications, London.

Holt, K.S. Jones, R.B. & Wilson, R. (1974) Gait analysis by means of a multiple sequential camera. *Dev. Med. Child Neurol.*, **16**, 742.

Hopkins, B. & Westra, T. (1989) Maternal expectations of their infants' development: some cultural differences. *Dev. Med. Child Neurol.*, **31**, 384–390.

Horak, F.B. (1992) Motor control models underlying neurologic rehabilitation of posture in children. In *Movement Disorders in Children* (eds H. Forssberg & H. Hirschfeld), pp. 21–30. Karger, Basel.

Horn, E.M., Warren, S.F. & Jones, H.A. (1995) An experimental analysis of a neurobehavioral motor intervention. *Dev. Med. Child Neurol.*, **37**, 697–714.

Horstmann, H.M. & Bleck, E.E. (2007) *Orthopaedic Management in Cerebral Palsy (2nd Edition). Clinics in Developmental Medicine No. 173–174*. Mac Keith Press, London.

Howle, J.M. (2002) *Neuro-Developmental Treatment Approach: Theoretical Foundations and Principles of Clinical Practice*. Neuro-Developmental Treatment Association, Laguna Beach.

Hufschmidt, A. & Mauritz, K-H. (1985) Chronic transformation of muscle in spasticity: a peripheral contribution to increased tone. *J. Neurol. Neurosurg. Psychiatry*, **48**, 676–685.

Hunt, A., Goldman, A., Seers, K., *et al.* (2004) Clinical validation of the paediatric pain profile. *Dev. Med. Child Neurol.*, **46**, 9–18.

Huntley, M. (1996) *The Griffiths Mental Development Scales – Revised: Birth to 2 Years*. Hogrefe, Oxford.

Hurvitz, E.A., Leonard, C., Ayyangar, R. & Nelson, V.S. (2003) Complementary and alternative medicine use in families of children with cerebral palsy. *Dev. Med. Child Neurol.*, **45**, 364–370.

Hylton, N. (1989) Postural and functional impact of dynamic AFOs and FOs in a paediatric population. *J. Prosthet. Orthot.*, **2**, 40–53.

Hylton, N. & Allen, C. (1997) The development and use of SPIO lycra compression bracing in children with neuromotor deficits. *Pediatr. Rehabil.*, **1**, 109–116.

Illingworth, R.S. (1983) *The Development of the Infant and Young Child, Normal and Abnormal*, 8th edn. Churchill Livingstone, Edinburgh.

Jahnsen, R., Aamodt, G. & Rosenbaum, P. (2006) Gross motor function classification system used in adults with cerebral palsy: agreement of self-reported versus professional rating. *Dev. Med. Child Neurol.*, **48**, 734–738.

Jahnsen, R., Villien, L., Stanghelle, J.K. & Holm, I. (2003) Fatigue in adults with cerebral palsy in Norway compared with the general population. *Dev. Med. Child Neurol.* **45**, 296–303.

Jan, J.E., Freeman, R.D. & Scott, E.P. (1977) *Visual Impairment in Children and Adolescents*. Grune & Stratton, New York.

Jansen, L.M.C., Ketelaar, M. & Vermeer, A. (2003) Parental experience of participation in physical therapy for children with physical disabilities. *Dev. Med. Child Neurol.*, **45**, 58–69.

Jefferson, R.J. (2004) Botulinum toxin in the management of cerebral palsy. *Dev. Med. Child Neurol.*, **46**, 491–499.

Jones, M. (1993) Serial splinting in hemiplegic cerebral palsy. In *Elements of Paediatric Physiotherapy* (ed. P.M. Eckersley), p. 364. Churchill Livingstone, Edinburgh.

Jones, R.B. (1975) The Vojta method of treatment of cerebral palsy. *Physiotherapy*, **61**, 112.

Jonsdottir, J., Fetters, L. & Kluzik, J. (1997) Effects of physical therapy on postural control in children with cerebral palsy. *Pediatr. Phys. Ther.*, **9**, 68–75.

Kabat, H. (1961) Proprioceptive facilitation in therapeutic exercise. In *Therapeutic Exercise* (ed. S. Licht), 2nd edn, Chapter 13. Licht, New Haven, Connecticut.

Kabat, H., McLeod, M. & Holt, C. (1959) The practical application of proprioceptive neuromuscular facilitation. *Physiotherapy*, **45**, 87.

Kamm, K., Thelen, E. & Jensen, J.L. (1990) A dynamical systems approach to motor development. *Phys. Ther.*, **70**, 763–775.

Kanda, T., Yuge, M., Yamori, Y., Suzuki, J. & Fukase, H. (1984) Early physiotherapy in the treatment of spastic diplegia. *Dev. Med. Child Neurol.*, **26**, 438–444.

Katona, F. (1989) Clinical neurodevelopmental diagnosis and treatment. In *Challenges to Developmental Paradigms: Implications for Theory, Assessment and Treatment.* (eds P.R. Zelazo & R.G. Barr), pp. 167–187. Lawrence Erlbaum, London.

Katz, R.T. & Rymer, W.Z. (1989) Spastic hypertonia: mechanisms and measurement. *Arch. Phys. Med. Rehabil.* **70**, 144–155.

Kazdin, E. (1982) *Single-case Research Designs.* Oxford University Press, London.

Kelly, M. & Darrah, J. (2005) Aquatic exercise for children with cerebral palsy. *Dev. Med. Child Neurol.*, **47**, 838–842.

Kembhavi, G., Darrah, J., Magill-Evans, J & Loomis, J. (2002) Using the Berg balance scale to distinguish balance abilities in children with cerebral palsy. *Pediatr. Phys. Ther.* **14**, 92–99.

Kerr, C., McDowell, B., Cosgrove, A., Walsh, D., Bradbury, I. & McDonough, S. (2006) Electrical stimulation in cerebral palsy: a randomized controlled trial. *Dev. Med. Child Neurol.*, **48**, 870–876.

Kerr, C., McDowell, B. & McDonough, S. (2004) Electrical stimulation in cerebral palsy: a review of effects on strength and motor function. *Dev. Med. Child Neurol.*, **46**, 205–213.

Kerr, C., McDowell, B. & McDonough, S. (2007) The relationship between gross motor function and participation restriction in children with cerebral palsy: an exploratory analysis. *Child Care Health Dev.*, **33**, 22–27.

Ketelaar, M., Vermeer, A., & Helders, P.J.M. (1998) Functional motor abilities of children with cerebral palsy: a systematic literature review of assessment measures. *Clin. Rehabil.*, **12**, 369–380.

Kidd, G., Lawes, N. & Musa, I. (1992) *Understanding Neuromuscular Plasticity: A Basis for Clinical Rehabilitation.* Edward Arnold, London.

King, G., King, S., Rosenbaum, P. & Goffin, R. (1999) Family-centred caregiving and well-being of parents of children with disabilities: linking process with outcome. *J. Pediatr. Psychol.*, **24**, 41–52.

King, G.A., Rosenbaum, P.L. & King, S.M. (1997) Evaluating family-centred service using a measure of parents' perceptions. *Child Care Health Dev.*, **23**, 47–62.

Kinsman, R., Verity, R. & Walker, J.A. (1988) A conductive education approach for adults with neurological dysfunction. *Physiotherapy*, **74**, 277–280.

Kitzinger, M. (1980) Planning management of feeding in the visually handicapped child. *Child Care Health Dev.*, 6, 291.

Knapp, D.R., Jr & Cortes, H. (2002) Untreated hip dislocation in cerebral palsy. *J. Pediatr. Orthop.*, **22**, 668–671.

Knott, M. & Voss, D.E. (1968) *Proprioceptive Neuromuscular Facilitation. Patterns and Techniques*, 2nd edn. Harper & Row, New York.

Knowles, M. (1984) *The Adult Learner: A Neglected Species*, 3rd edn. Gulf, Houston.

Knox, V. (2002) Evaluation of the sitting assessment test for Children with neuromotor dysfunction as a measurement tool in cerebral palsy: case study. *Physiotherapy*, **88**, 534–541.

Kogan, K., Tyler, N. & Turner, P. (1974) The process of interpersonal adaptation between mothers and their cerebral palsied children. *Dev. Med. Child Neurol.*, **16**, 518.

Koman, L.A., Brashear, A., Rosenfeld, S., *et al.* (2001) Botulinum toxin type A neuromuscular blockade in the treatment of equinus foot deformity in cerebral palsy: a multicenter, open-label clinical trial. *Pediatrics*, **108**, 1062–1071.

Kong, E. (1987) The importance of early treatment. In *Early Detection and Management of Cerebral Palsy* (eds H. Galjaard, H.F.R. Prechtl & M. Velickovic), p. 107. Martinus Nijhoff, Dordrecht.

Kraus de Camargo, O., Storck, M. & Bode, H. (1998) Video-based documentation and rating system of the motor behaviour of handicapped children treated with physiotherapy – a new outcome measure. *Pediatr. Rehabil.*, **2**, 21–26.

Krumlinde-Sundholm, L., Holmefur, M., Kottorp, A. & Eliasson, A-C. (2007) The assisting hand assessment: current evidence of validity, reliability, and responsiveness to change. *Dev. Med. Child Neurol.*, **49**, 259–264.

Lannin, N., Scheinberg, A. & Clark, K. (2006) AACPDM systematic review of the effectiveness of therapy for children with cerebral palsy after botulinum toxin A injections. *Dev. Med. Child Neurol.*, **48**, 533–539.

Lannin, N.A., Novak, I. & Cusick, A. (2007) A systematic review of upper extremity casting for children and adults with central nervous system motor disorders. *Clin. Rehabil.*, **21**, 963–976.

Larsson, M. (2000) Organizing habilitation services: team structures and family participation. *Child Care Health Dev.*, **26**, 501–514.

Latham, C. (1984) Communicating with children. In *Paediatric Developmental Therapy* (ed. S. Levitt), pp. 53–62. Blackwell Scientific Publications, Oxford.

Law, M., Baptiste, S., Carswell, A., *et al.* (1998) *Canadian Occupational Performance Measure*, 3rd edn. CAOT, Ottawa. (www.caot.ca)

Law, M., Darrah, J., Pollock, N., *et al.* (2007) Focus on function – a randomized controlled trial comparing two rehabilitation interventions for young children with cerebral palsy. *BMC Pediatrics*, **7**, 31.

Leach, M. (1993) *Activities for People with a Multiple Disability*. The Spastics Society, London.

Lee, D.N. & Aronson, E. (1974) Visual proprioceptive control of standing in human infants. *Percept. Psychophysiol.*, **15**, 529.

Lee, M.G. (2004) *Co-ordination Difficulties: Practical Ways Forward*. David Fulton, London.

Lee, T.S., Sullivan, G. & Lansbury, G. (2006) Physiotherapists' perceptions of clients from culturally diverse backgrounds. *Physiotherapy*, **92**, 166–170.

Leonard, C.T., Hirschfeld, H. & Forssberg, H. (1988) Gait acquisition and reflex abnormalities in normal children and children with cerebral palsy. In *Posture and Gait: Development, Adaptation and Modulation* (eds B. Amblard, A. Berthoz & F. Clarac), p. 33. Elsevier, Amsterdam.

Leonard, C.T., Hirschfeld, H. & Forssberg, H. (1991) The development of independent walking in children with cerebral palsy. *Dev. Med. Child Neurol.*, **33**, 567.

Lesny, I., Stehlik, A., Tomasek, J., Tomankova, A. & Havlicek, I. (1993) Sensory disorders in cerebral palsy: two-point discrimination. *Dev. Med. Child Neurol.*, 35, 402–405.

Levine, R.A., Rosenbaum, A.E., Waltz, J.M. & Scheinberg, L.C. (1970) Cervical spondylosis and dyskinesias. *Neurology*, 29, 1194–1199.

Levitt, S. (1962) *Physiotherapy in Cerebral Palsy*. Thomas, Springfield, Illinois.

Levitt, S. (1966) Proprioceptive neuromuscular facilitation techniques in cerebral palsy. *Physiotherapy*, 52, 46.

Levitt, S. (1969) The treatment of cerebral palsy and proprioceptive neuromuscular facilitation techniques. In *On the Treatment of Spastic Pareses*. Institute Neurology, Stockholm. [Also in *Sjukgymnasten*, 1968, 27, 3].

Levitt, S. (1970a) Principles of treatment in cerebral palsy. *Fysioterapeuten*, 10.

Levitt, S. (1970b) Adaptation of PNF for cerebral palsy. In *Proceedings of the World Confederation of Physical Therapy Congress, Amsterdam*. WCPT, London.

Levitt, S. (1974) Common factors in the different systems of treatment in cerebral palsy. *CDI Cahiers*, No. 59, Masson et Cie, Paris.

Levitt, S. (1975) A study of the gross motor skills of cerebral palsied children in an adventure playground for handicapped children. *Child Care Health Dev.*, 1, 29–43.

Levitt, S. (1976) Stimulation of movement: a review of therapeutic techniques. In *Early Management of Handicapping Disorders* (eds T.E. Oppé & F.P. Woodford). IRMMH. Associated Scientific Publishers, Amsterdam, reprinted from *Movement and Child Development* (ed. K.S. Holt). Heinemann – Spastics International Medical Publications, London.

Levitt, S. (1977) *Treatment of Cerebral Palsy and Motor Delay*. Blackwell Scientific Publications, Oxford.

Levitt, S. (1982) Movement training. In *Profound Mental Handicap* (ed. D. Norris), pp. 65–74. Costello, Tunbridge Wells.

Levitt, S. (ed.) (1984) *Paediatric Developmental Therapy*. Blackwell Scientific Publications, Oxford.

Levitt, S. (1986) Handling the child with paediatric developmental disability. *Physiotherapy*, 72, 161.

Levitt, S. (1987) Therapy for the motor disorders. In *Early Detection and Management of Cerebral Palsy* (eds H. Galjaard, H.F.R. Prechtl & M. Velickovic), p. 113. Martinus Nijhoff, Dordrecht.

Levitt, S. (1991a) International therapy workshops. In Proceedings of the 11th International Congress of the WCPT, p. 283. WCPT, London.

Levitt, S. (1991b) Family-centred physiotherapy. In Proceedings of the 11th International Congress of the WCPT, pp. 1236–1238. WCPT, London.

Levitt, S. (1994) *Basic Abilities – A Whole Approach*. Souvenir Press, London.

Levitt, S. (1999) The collaborative learning approach in community based rehabilitation. In *Cross-cultural Rehabilitation*. (ed. R.L. Leavitt), pp. 151–161. Saunders, London.

Levitt, S. & Goldschmied, E. (1990) As we teach, so we treat. *Physiotherapy Theory & Practice*, 6, 227.

Levitt, S. & Miller, C. (1973) The interrelationships of speech therapy and physiotherapy in children with neurodevelopmental disorders. *Dev. Med. Child Neurol.*, 15, 2.

Liao, H-F., Jeng, S-F., Lai, J-S., Cheng, C-K. & Hu, M-H. (1997) The relation between standing balance and walking function in children with spastic diplegic cerebral palsy. *Dev. Med. Child Neurol.*, 39, 106–112.

Lieber, R.L. & Friden, J. (2002) Spasticity causes a fundamental rearrangement of muscle–joint interaction. *Muscle Nerve*, 25, 265–270.

Lin, J-P. (2000) The pathophysiology of spasticity and dystonia. In *The Management of Spasticity Associated with the Cerebral Palsies in Children and Adolescents* (eds A.L. Albright & B. Neville), pp. 11–38. Churchill Communications, Secaucus.

Lin, J-P. (2004) The assessment and management of hypertonus in cerebral palsy: a physiological atlas ('road map'). In *Management of the Motor Disorders of Children with Cerebral Palsy. Clinics in Developmental Medicine No 161* (eds D. Scrutton, D. Damiano & M. Mayston), pp. 85–104. Mac Keith Press, London.

Logan, L., Byers-Hinley, K. & Ciccone, C. (1990) Anterior vs posterior walkers for children with cerebral palsy: a gait analysis study. *Dev. Med. Child Neurol.*, 32, 1044.

Long, T. & Toscano, K. (2002) *Handbook of Pediatric Physical Therapy*, 2nd edn, pp. 162–164. Lippincott Williams & Wilkins, Philadelphia.

Luiz, D., Barnard, A., Knosen, N., *et al.* (2006) *Griffiths Mental Development Scales – Extended Revised: 2 to 8 Years*. Hogrefe, Oxford.

Maathuis, K.G., van der Schans, C.P., van Iperen, A., Rietman, H.S. & Geertzen, J.H. (2005) Gait in children with cerebral palsy: observer reliability of physician rating scale and Edinburgh visual gait analysis interval testing scale. *J. Pediatr. Orthop.*, 25, 268–272.

MacKean, G.L., Thurson, W.E. & Scott, C.M. (2005) Bridging the divide between families and health professionals: perspectives on family-centred care. *Health Expectations*, 8, 74–85.

Mackey, A.H., Lobb, G.L., Walt, S.E. & Stott, N.S. (2003) Reliability and validity of the observational gait scale in children with spastic diplegia. *Dev. Med. Child Neurol.*, 45, 4–11.

Mackie, P.C., Jessen, E.C. & Jarvis, S.N. (1998) The lifestyle assessment questionnaire: an instrument to measure the impact of disability on the lives of children with cerebral palsy and their families. *Child Care Health Dev.*, 24, 473–486.

MacPhail, H.E. & Kramer, J.F. (1995) Effect of isokinetic strength-training on functional ability and walking efficiency in adolescents with cerebral palsy. *Dev. Med. Child Neurol.*, 37, 763–775.

Maloney, F.P., Mirrett, P., Brooks, C. & Johannes, K. (1978) Use of the goal attainment scale in the treatment and ongoing evaluation of neurologically handicapped children. *Am. J. Occup. Ther.*, 32, 505–510.

Marsden, C.D., Merton, P.A. & Merton, H.B. (1981) Human postural responses. *Brain*, **104**, 513.

Marshall, S., Teasell, R., Bayona, N., *et al.* (2007) Motor impairment rehabilitation post acquired brain injury. *Brain Injury*, **21**, 133–160.

Martin, J. (1981) The Halliwick method. *Physiotherapy*, **67**, 288–291.

Martin, J.P. (1965) Tilting reactions and disorders of the basal ganglia. *Brain*, **88**, 855.

Martin, J.P. (1967) *The Basal Ganglia and Posture*. Pitman Medical Publications, London.

Martin, S.E., Marshall, I. & Douglas, N.J. (1995) The effect of posture on airway caliber with the sleep apnea/hypopnea syndrome. *Am. J. Respir. Care Med.*, **152**, 721–724.

Mayston, M. (2004) Physiotherapy management in cerebral palsy: and update on treatment approaches. In *Management of the Motor Disorders of Children with Cerebral Palsy. Clinics in Developmental Medicine No. 161* (eds D. Scrutton, D. Damiano & M. Mayston), pp. 147–160. Mac Keith Press, London.

Mayston, M. (2008) Editorial: Bobath concept: Bobath@50: mid-life crisis – What of the future? *Physiother. Res. Int.*, **13**, 131–136.

Mayston, M.J. (1992) The Bobath concept – evolution and application. In *Movement Disorders in Children* (eds H. Forssberg & H. Hirschfeld), pp. 1–6. Karger, Basel.

McBurney, H., Taylor, N.F., Dodd, K.J. & Graham, H.K. (2003) A qualitative analysis of the benefits of strength training for young people with cerebral palsy. *Dev. Med. Child Neurol.*, **45**, 658.

McClenaghan, B.A., Thombs, L. & Milner, M. (1992) Effects of seat surface inclination on postural stability and function of the upper extremity of children with cerebral palsy. *Dev. Med. Child Neurol.*, **34**, 40.

McConachie, H. (1986) Parents' contribution to the education of their child. In *The Education of Children with Severe Learning Difficulties: Bridging the Gap between Theory and Practice* (eds J. Coupe & J. Porter), p. 253. Croom Helm, London.

McCormick, A., Brien, M., Plourde, J., Wood, E., Rosenbaum, P. & McLean, J. (2007) Stability of the gross motor function classification system in adults with cerebral palsy. *Dev. Med. Child Neurol.*, **49**, 265–269.

McDonald, R., Surtees, R. & Wirz, S. (2003) A comparison between parents' and therapists' views of their child's individual seating systems. *Int. J. Rehabil. Res.*, **3**, 235–243.

McDowell, B.C., Hewitt, V., Nurse, A., Weston, T. & Baker, R. (2000) The variability of goniometric measurements in ambulatory children with spastic cerebral palsy. *Gait & Posture*, **12**, 114–121.

McDowell, B.C., Kerr, C., Parkes, J. & Cosgrove, A. (2005) Validity of a 1 minute walk test for children with cerebral palsy. *Dev. Med. Child Neurol.*, **47**, 744–748.

McGrath, P.J., Rosmus, C., Canfield, C., Campbell, M.A. & Hennigar, A.W. (1998) Behaviours caregivers use to determine pain in non-verbal, cognitively impaired individuals. *Dev. Med. Child Neurol.*, **40**, 340–343.

McGraw, M. (1989) *The Neuromuscular Maturation of the Human Infant*. Clinics in Dev. Med. Mac Keith Press, London.

McKinlay, I.A. (1989) Therapy for cerebral palsy. *Seminars Orthopaed.*, **4**, 220.

McKinlay, I.A., Hyde, E. & Gordon, N.S. (1980) Baclofen: a team approach to drug evaluation of spasticity in childhood. In *Baclofen: A Broader Spectrum of Activity*, p. 26. A supplement to *Scott. Med. J.*

McLaughlin, J.F. (2000) Selective dorsal rhizotomy. In *The Management of Spasticity Associated with the Cerebral Palsies in Children and Adolescents* (eds A.L. Albright & B. Neville), pp. 107–119. Churchill Communications, Secaucus.

McLaughlin, J.F., Bjornson, K.F., Astley, S.J., *et al.* (1998) Selective dorsal rhizotomy: efficacy and safety in an investigator-masked randomized clinical trial. *Dev. Med. Child Neurol.*, **40**, 220–232.

McLellan, D.L. (1977) Co-contraction and stretch reflexes in spasticity during treatment with baclofen. *J. Neurol. Neurosurg. Psychiatry*, **40**, 30–38.

McLellan, L. (1984) Therapeutic possibilities in cerebral palsy: a neurologist's view. In *Management of the Motor Disorders of Children with Cerebral Palsy* (ed. D. Scrutton), p. 96. SIMP, Blackwell Scientific Publications, Oxford.

McMulkin, M.L., Gulliford, J.J., Williamson, R.V. & Ferguson, R.L (2000) Correlation of static to dynamic measures of lower extremity range of motion in cerebral palsy and control populations. *J. Pediatr. Orthopedics*, **20**, 366–369.

McNee, A.E., Shortland, A.P., Eve, L.C., Robinson, R.O. & Gough, M. (2004) Lower limb extensor moments in children with spastic diplegic cerebral palsy. *Gait & Posture*, **20**, 171–176.

McNee, A.E., Will, E., Lin, J-P., Eve, L.C., Gough, M., Morrissey, M.C. & Shortland, A.P. (2007) The effect of serial casting on gait in children with cerebral palsy: preliminary results from a crossover trial. *Gait & Posture*, **25**, 463–468.

Miedaner, J. (1990) An evaluation of weight-bearing forces at various angles for children with cerebral palsy. *Pediatr. Phys. Ther.*, **2**, 215.

Miller, F. (2007) *Physical Therapy of Cerebral Palsy*. Springer, New York.

Molnar, G.E. & Gordon, S.U. (1976) Cerebral palsy: predictive value of selected clinical signs for early prognostication of motor function. *Arch. Phys. Med. Rehabil.*, **57**, 153–158.

Montgomery, P.C. (1998) Predicting potential for ambulation in children with cerebral palsy. *Pediatr. Phys. Ther.*, **10**, 148–155.

Morris, C. (2002) A review of the efficacy of lower-limb orthoses used for cerebral palsy. *Dev. Med. Child Neurol.*, **44**, 205–211.

Morris, C. & Dias, L. (eds) (2007) *Paediatric Orthotics. Clinics in Developmental Medicine No. 175*. Mac Keith Press, London.

Morris, C., Kurinczuk, J.J., Fitzpatrick, R. & Rosenbaum, P.L. (2006) Who best to make the assessment? Professionals' and families' classifications of gross motor function in cerebral palsy are highly consistent. *Arch. Dis. Child.*, **91**, 675–679.

Morris, K. (1996) Physiotherapy management of the neonate and infant – developmental problems. In *Physiotherapy and the Growing Child.* (eds Y.R. Burns & J. MacDonald), pp. 343–357. Saunders, London.

Morton, R., Benton, S., Bower, E., *et al.* (1999) Multidisciplinary appraisal of the British Institute for Brain Injured Children, Somerset, UK. *Dev. Med. Child Neurol.*, **41**, 211–212.

Mosely, A.M. (1997) The effect of casting combined with stretching on passive ankle dorsiflexion in adults with traumatic brain injuries. *Phys. Ther.*, **77**, 240.

MOVE Europe (2001) *Mobility Opportunities via Education.* Available from MOVE Europe, Unit C, London.

Msall, M.E., DiGaudio, K., Rogers, B.T., *et al.* (1994) The functional independence measure for children (WeeFIM): conceptual basis and pilot use in children with developmental disabilities. *Clin. Pediatr.*, **33**, 421–430.

Mulcahy, C.M., Pountney, T.E., Nelham, R.L., Green, E.M. & Billington, G.D. (1988) Adaptive seating for motor handicap: problems, a solution, assessment and prescription. *Br. J. Occup. Ther.*, **51**, 347.

Mulder, T. (1985) *The Learning of Motor Control Following Brain Damage: Experimental and Clinical Studies.* Swets & Zeitlinger, Lisse.

Mulder, T. (1991) A process oriented model of human motor behavior: implications for rehabilitation medicine. *Phy. Ther.*, **71**, 157.

Mulder, T. & Hochstenbach, J. (2002) Motor control and learning: Implications for neurological rehabilitation. In *Handbook of Neurological Rehabilitation*, 2nd edn (eds R.J. Greenwood, T.M. McMillan, M.P. Barnes & C.D. Ward), pp. 143–157. Psychology Press, London.

Mulder, T. & Hulstijn, W. (1988) From movement to action: the learning of motor control following brain damage. In *Complex Human Movement Behavior* (eds O.G. Meijer & K. Roth), p. 247. Elsevier, Amsterdam.

Murphy, K., Molnar, G. & Lankasky, K. (1995) Medical and functional status of adults with cerebral palsy. *Dev. Med. Child Neurol.*, **37**, 1075–1084.

Mutlu A., Krosschell, K. & Spira, D.G. (2009) Treadmill training with partial body-weight support in children with cerebral palsy: a systematic review. *Dev. Med. Child Neurol.*, **51**, 268–275.

Myhr, U. & von Wendt, L. (1990) Reducing spasticity and enhancing postural control for the creation of a functional sitting position in children with cerebral palsy: a pilot study. *Physiotherapy Theory & Practice*, **6**, 65.

Myhr, U., von Wendt, L., Norrlin, S. & Radell, U. (1995) Five-year follow-up of functional sitting position in children with cerebral palsy. *Dev. Med. Child Neurol.*, **37**, 587–596.

Nashner, L.M., Shumway-Cook, A. & Marin, O. (1983) Stance posture in select groups of children with cerebral palsy: deficits in sensory organisation and muscular condition. *Exp. Brain Res.*, **49**, 393.

Nathan, P. (1969) Annotation: treatment of spasticity with peri-neural injections of phenol. *Dev. Med. Child Neurol.*, **11**, 384.

Neistadt, M.E. (1994) Perceptual retraining for adults with diffuse brain injury. *Am. J. Occup. Ther.*, **48**, 877.

Nelson, K.B. & Ellenberg, J.H. (1982) Children who 'outgrew' cerebral palsy. *Pediatrics*, **69**, 529.

Neville, B. (2000) Introduction. In *The Management of Spasticity Associated with the Cerebral Palsies in Children and Adolescents* (eds A.L. Albright & B. Neville), pp. 1–10. Churchill Communications, Secaucus.

Neville, B. & Goodman, R. (eds) (2001) *Congenital Hemiplegia. Clinics in Developmental Medicine No. 150.* Mac Keith Press, London.

Newson, E. (1976) Parents as a resource in diagnosis and assessment. In *Early Management of Handicapping Disorders* (eds T.E. Oppé & F.P. Woodford), p. 105. Associated Scientific Publishers, Amsterdam.

Nichols, D.S. & Case-Smith, J. (1996) Reliability and validity of the pediatric evaluation of disability inventory. *Pediatr. Phys. Ther.*, **8**, 15.

Nicholson, J.H., Morton, R.E., Attfield, S. & Rennie, D. (2001) Assessment of upper-limb function and movement in children with cerebral palsy wearing lycra garments. *Dev. Med. Child Neurol.*, **43**, 384–391.

Niznik, T.M., Turner, D. & Worrell, T.W. (1995) Functional reach as a measurement of balance for children with lower extremity spasicity. *Phys. Occup. Ther. Pediatr.*, **15** (3), 1–16.

Norén, L. & Franzén, G. (1982) An evaluation of 7 postural reactions selected by Vojta in 25 healthy infants. *Neuropediatrics*, **12**, 308.

Novacheck, T.F., Stout, J.L. & Tervo, R. (2000) Reliability and validity of the Gillette functional assessment questionnaire as an outcome measure in children with walking disabilities. *J. Pediatr. Orthop.*, **20**, 75–81.

Nwaobi, O.M. (1987) Seating orientations and upper extremity function in children with cerebral palsy. *Phys. Ther.*, **67**, 1209.

Nwaobi, O.M., Brubaker, C., *et al.* (1983) Electromyographic investigation of extensor activity in cerebral palsy children in different seating positions. *Dev. Med. Child Neurol.*, **25**, 175.

Odman, P., Krevers, B. & Oberg, B. (2007) Parents' perceptions of the quality of two intensive training programmes for children with cerebral palsy. *Dev. Med. Child Neurol.*, **49**, 93–100.

Odman, P. & Oberg, B. (2005) Effectiveness of intensive training for children with cerebral palsy – a comparison between child and youth rehabilitation and conductive education. *J. Rehabil. Med.*, **37**, 263–270.

Ohata, K., Tsuboyama, T., Haruta, T., Ichihashi, N., Kato, T. & Nakamura, T. (2008) Relation between muscle thickness, spasticity, and activity limitations in children and adolescents with cerebral palsy. *Dev. Med. Child Neurol.*, **50**, 152–156.

Ohata, K., Tsuboyama, T., Ichihashi, N. & Minami, S. (2006) Measurement of muscle thickness as quantitative muscle evaluation for adults with severe cerebral palsy. *Phys. Ther.*, 86, 1231–1239.

Olow, I. (1986) Children with cerebral palsy. In *Neurologically Handicapped Children: Treatment and Management* (eds N.S. Gordon & I.A. McKinlay), p. 60. Blackwell Scientific Publications, Oxford.

O'Neil, M.E., Fragala, M.A. & Dumas, H.M. (2003) Physical therapy intervention for children with cerebral palsy who receive botulinum toxin A injections. *Pediatr. Phys. Ther.*, 15, 204–215.

Oppenheim, W.L., Staudt, L.A. & Peacock, J.W. (1992) The rationale for rhizotomy. In *The Diplegic Child* (ed. M.D. Sussman), p. 271. American Academy of Orthopedic Surgeons, Rosemont.

Ostensjo, S., Carlberg, E.B. & Vollestad, N.K. (2003) Everyday functioning in young children with cerebral palsy: functional skills, caregiver assistance, and modifications of the environment. *Dev. Med. Child Neurol.*, 45, 603–612.

Ostensjo, S., Carlberg, E.B. & Vollestad, N.K. (2004) Motor impairments in young children with cerebral palsy: relationship to gross motor function and everyday activities. *Dev. Med. Child Neurol.*, 46, 580–589.

Ottenbacher, K.J. (1986) *Evaluating Clinical Change: Strategies for Occupational and Physical Therapists.* Williams & Wilkins, Baltimore.

Paine, R.S. (1962) On the treatment of cerebral palsy – the outcome of 177 patients, 74 totally untreated. *Pediatrics*, 29, 605.

Palisano, R., Rosenbaum, P., Walter, S., Russell, D., Wood, E. & Galuppi, B. (1997) The development and reliability of a system to classify gross motor function in children with cerebral palsy. *Dev. Med. Child Neurol.*, 39, 214–223.

Palisano, R.J., Rosenbaum, P., Bartlett, D. & Livingston, M.H. (2008) Content validity of the expanded and revised gross motor function classification system. *Dev. Med. Child Neurol.*, 50, 744–750.

Palmer, F.B., Shapiro, B.K., Wachtel, R.C., *et al.* (1988) The effects of physical therapy on cerebral palsy. *N. Engl. J. Med.*, 318, 803.

Pandyan, A.D., Johnson, G.R., Price, C.I., Curless, R.H., Barnes, M.P. & Rodgers, H. (1999) A review of the properties and limitations of the Ashworth and modified Ashworth scales as measures of spasticity. *Clin. Rehabil.*, 13, 373–383.

Parette, H.P. & Hourcade, J.J. (1984) A review of therapeutic intervention research on gross and fine motor progress in young children with cerebral palsy. *Am. J. Occup. Ther.*, 38, 462.

Parker, D.F., Carriere, L., Hebestreit, H., Salsberg, A. & Bar-Or, O. (1993) Muscle performance and gross motor function of children with spastic cerebral palsy. *Dev. Med. Child Neurol.*, 35, 17–23.

Patton, M.Q. (1980) *Qualitative Evaluation Methods.* Sage, Beverly Hills.

Paus, T., Zijdenbos, A., Worsley, K., *et al.* (1999) Structural maturation of neural pathways in children and adolescents: in vivo study. *Science*, 283, 1908–1911.

Peacock, W.J. & Staudt, L.A. (1991) Functional outcomes following selective posterior rhizotomy in children with cerebral palsy. *J. Neurosurg.*, 74, 380–385.

Pearson, P.H. & Williams, C.E. (eds) (1972) *Physical Therapy Services in the Developmental Disabilities.* Thomas, Springfield, Illinois.

Pederson, E. (1969) *Spasticity, Mechanism, Measurement, Management.* Thomas, Springfield, Illinois.

Phelps, W.M. (1949) Description and differentiation of types of cerebral palsy. *Nerv. Child*, 8, 107.

Phelps, W.M. (1952) The role of physical therapy in cerebral palsy and bracing in the cerebral palsies. In *Orthopaedic Appliances Atlas 1* (ed. J.W. Edwards), pp. 251–522. Illinois University Press, Ann Arbor.

Phelps, W.M. (1959) Prevention of acquired dislocation of the hip in cerebral palsy. *J. Bone Joint Surg. Am.*, 41, 440–448.

Phillips, W.E. & Audet, M. (1990) Use of serial casting in the management of knee joint contractures in an adolescent with cerebral palsy. *Phys. Ther.*, 70, 521–523.

Piggot, J., Hocking, C. & Paterson, J. (2003) Parental adjustment to having a child with cerebral palsy and participation in home therapy programs. *Phys. Occup. Ther. Pediatr.* 23 (4), 5–29.

Pimm, P. (1992) Physiological burn-out and functional skill loss in cerebral palsy. *Interlink*, 4 (3), 18–20.

Pin, T., Dyke, P. & Chan, M. (2006) The effectiveness of passive stretching in children with cerebral palsy. *Dev. Med. Child Neurol.*, 48, 855–862.

Piper, M.C. & Darrah, J. (1994) *Motor Assessment of the Developing Infant.* Saunders, Philadelphia.

Pirpiris M, Wilkinson A., Rodda J., *et al.* (2003) Walking speed in children and young adults with neuromuscular disease: comparison between two assessment methods. *J Pediatr. Orthop.* 23, 302–307.

Plum, P. & Molhave, A. (1956) Clinical analysis of static and dynamic patterns in cerebral palsy with a view to active correction. *Arch. Phys. Med.*, 37, 8.

Polak, F., Clift, M. & Clift, L. (2008) *Buyers' Guide: Night Time Postural Management Equipment for Children (CEP 08030).* Centre for Evidence-based Purchasing, London. (www.pasa.nhs.uk/cep)

Pountney, T.E. & Green, E.M. (2006) Hip dislocation in cerebral palsy. *BMJ*, 332, 772–775.

Pountney, T.E., Mulcahy, C.M., Clarke, S.M & Green, E.M. (2004) *The Chailey Approach to Postural Management*, 2nd edn. Active Design, Birmingham.

Prechtl, H.F.R. (2001) General movement assessment as a method of developmental neurology: new paradigms and consequences. *Dev. Med. Child Neurol.*, 43, 836–842.

Presland, J.L. (1982) *Paths to Mobility in 'Special Care'*, pp. 19, 35–8. British Institute of Mental Handicap, Kidderminster.

Price, E., Thylefors, I. & von Wendt, L. (1991) The role of the physiotherapist in the Swedish paediatric rehabilitation teams. In *Proceedings of the World Confederation of Physical Therapy Congress, London*, p. 1187. WCPT, London.

Radtka, S., Skinner, S.R., Dixon, D.M. & Johanson, M.E. (1997) A comparison of gait with solid, dynamic and no ankle-foot orthoses in children with spastic cerebral palsy. *Phys. Ther.*, 77, 395–409.

Randall, M., Carlin, J.B., Chondros, P. & Reddihough, D. (2001) Reliability of the Melbourne assessment of unilateral upper limb function. *Dev. Med. Child Neurol*, 43, 761–767.

Read, H.S., Hazlewood, M.E., Hillman, S.J., Prescott, R.J. & Robb, J.E. (2003) Edinburgh visual gait score for use in cerebral palsy. *J. Pediatr. Orthop.*, 23, 296–301.

Reddihough, D., King, J., Coleman, G. & Catanese, T. (1998) Efficacy of programmes based on conductive education for young children with cerebral palsy. *Dev. Med. Child Neurol.*, 40, 763–770.

Reid, D.T. (1995) Development and preliminary validation of an instrument to assess quality of sitting of children with neuromotor dysfunction. *Phys. Occup. Ther. Pediatr.*, 15 (1), 53–82.

Reid, D.T. (1996) The effects of the saddle seat on seated postural control and upper extremity movement in children with cerebral palsy. *Dev. Med. Child Neurol.*, 38, 805–815.

Reid, D.T. (1997) *The SACND: A Standardised Protocol for Describing Postural Control.* Therapy Skill Builders, San Antonio.

Reimers, J. (1990) Functional changes in the antagonists after lengthening of the agonists in cerebral palsy. I. Triceps surae lengthening. *Clin. Orthop. Relat. Res.*, 253, 30–34.

Rennie, D.J., Attfield, S.F., Morton, R.E., Polak, F.J. & Nicholson, J. (2000) An evaluation of lycra garments in the lower limb using 3-D gait analysis and functional assessment (PEDI). *Gait & Posture*, 12, 1–6.

Reynell, J. & Zinkin, P. (1975) New procedures for the developmental assessment of young children with severe visual handicaps. *Child Care Health Dev.*, 1, 61.

Riddoch, J. & Lennon, S. (1991) Evaluation of practice: the single case study approach. *Physiotherapy Theory & Practice*, 7, 3.

Robson, P. (1970) Shuffling, hitching, scooting or sliding: some observations in 30 otherwise normal children. *Dev. Med. Child Neurol.*, 12, 608.

Rogers, C.R. (1983) *Freedom to Learn for the 80s.* Merrill, Columbus, Ohio.

Rogers, C.R. (2003) *Client-Centered Therapy: Its Current Practice, Implications and Theory.* Constable & Robinson, London.

Rood, M.S. (1962) Use of sensory receptors to activate, facilitate and inhibit motor response, automatic and somatic, in developmental sequence. In *Approaches to the Treatment of Patients with Neuromuscular Dysfunction* (ed. C. Sattely). *Third International Congress of World Federation of Occupational Therapists*, pp. 26–37.

Rosblad, B. & von Hofsten, C. (1992) Perceptual control of manual pointing in children with motor impairments. *Physiotherapy Theory & Practice*, 8, 223.

Rosenbaum, P. (2004) Families and service providers: forging effective connections, and why it matters. In *Management of the Motor Disorders of Children with Cerebral Palsy.*

Clinics in Developmental Medicine No 161 (eds D. Scrutton, D. Damiano & M. Mayston), pp. 22–31. Mac Keith Press, London.

Rosenbaum, P., King, S., King, G., Law, M. & Evans, J. (1998) Family-centred services: a conceptual framework and research review. *Phys. Occup. Ther. Pediatr.*, 18 (1), 1–20.

Rosenbaum, P.L., Walter, S.D., Hanna, S.E., *et al.* (2002) Prognosis for gross motor function in cerebral palsy: creation of motor development curves. *JAMA*, 288, 1357–1363.

Rosenbloom, L. (1995) Diagnosis and management of cerebral palsy. *Arch. Dis. Child.*, 72, 350–354.

Ross, K. & Thomson, D. (1993) An evaluation of parents' involvement in the management of their cerebral palsy children. *Physiotherapy*, 79, 561.

Ross, S.A. & Engsberg, J.R. (2002) Relation between spasticity and strength in individuals with spastic diplegic cerebral palsy. *Dev. Med. Child Neurol.*, 44, 148–157.

Ross, S.A. & Engsberg, J.R. (2007) Relationships between spasticity, strength, gait, and the GMFM-66 in persons with spastic diplegia cerebral palsy. *Arch. Phys. Med. Rehabil.*, 88, 1114–1120.

Rothwell, J.C., Traub, M.M., Day, B.L., *et al.* (1982) Manual performance in a deafferented man. *Brain*, 105, 515.

Rushworth (1961) Posture and righting reflexes. *Cerebral Palsy Bulletin*, 3, 535.

Russell, A. & Cotton, E. (eds) (1994) *The Peto System and its Evolution in Britain.* Acorn Foundation, London.

Russell, D.J., Avery, L.M., Rosenbaum, P.L., Raina, P.S., Walter, S.D. & Palisano, R.J. (2000) Improved scaling of the gross motor function measure for children with cerebral palsy: evidence of reliability and validity. *Phys. Ther.*, 80, 873–885.

Russell, D.J., Rosenbaum, P.L., Avery, L.M. & Lane, M. (2002) *Gross Motor Function Measure (GMFM-66 and GMFM-88) User's Manual. Clinics in Developmental Medicine No. 159.* Mac Keith Press, London.

Russell, D.J., Rosenbaum, P.L., Cadman, D.T., Gowland, C., Hardy, S. & Jarvis, S. (1989) The gross motor function measure: a means to evaluate the effects of physical therapy. *Dev. Med. Child Neurol.*, 31, 341–352.

Sackett, D.L., Rosenberg, W.M.C., Gray, J.A.M., Haynes, R.B. & Richardson, W.S. (1996) Evidence based medicine: what it is and what it isn't. *BMJ*, 312, 71–72.

Sackett, D.L., Straus, S.E., Richardson, W.S., Rosenberg, W. & Haynes, R.B. (2001) *Evidence-Based Medicine: How to Practice and Teach EBM*, 2nd edn. Churchill Livingstone, Edinburgh.

Sahrmann, S.A. & Norton, B.J. (1977) The relationship of voluntary movement to spasticity in the upper motor neurone syndrome. *Ann. Neurol.*, 2, 460–465.

Samilson, R.L. (ed.) (1975) *Orthopaedic Aspects of Cerebral Palsy.* Heinemann – Spastics International Medical Publications, London.

Sanger, T.D., Delgado, M.R., Gaebler-Spira, D., *et al.* (2003) Classification and definition of disorders causing hypertonia in childhood. *Pediatrics*, 111, e89–97.

Schindl, M.R., Forstner, C., Kern, H. & Hesse, S. (2000) Treadmill training with partial body weight support in non-ambulatory patients with cerebral palsy. *Arch. Phys. Med. Rehabil.*, **81**, 301–306.

Scholtes, V.A.B., Becher, J.G., Beelen, A. & Lankhorst, G.J. (2006) Clinical assessment of spasticity in children with cerebral palsy: a critical review of available instruments. *Dev. Med. Child Neurol.*, **48**, 64–73.

Scrutton, D. (1978) Developmental deformity and the profoundly retarded child. In *Care of the Handicapped Child. Clinics in Developmental Medicine* (ed. J. Apley), pp. 83–91. Mac Keith Press, London.

Scrutton, D. (ed.) (1984) *Management of the Motor Disorders of Children with Cerebral Palsy*. SIMP, Blackwell Scientific Publications, Oxford.

Scrutton, D. & Baird, G. (1997) Surveillance measures of the hips of children with bilateral cerebral palsy. *Arch. Dis. Child.*, **76**, 381–384.

Scrutton, D., Baird, G. & Smeeton, N. (2001) Hip dysplasia in bilateral cerebral palsy: incidence and natural history in children aged 18 months to 5 years. *Dev. Med. Child Neurol.*, **43**, 586–600.

Seglow, D. (1984) A pattern of early intervention. In *Paediatric Developmental Therapy* (ed. S. Levitt), pp. 76–87. Blackwell Scientific Publications, Oxford.

Seligman, M.E.P. (1992) *Helplessness: On Development, Depression and Death*. Freeman, San Francisco.

Shepherd, R.B. (1995) *Physiotherapy in Paediatrics*, 3rd edn. Butterworth-Heinemann, Oxford.

Sheridan, M.D. (1975) *The Developmental Progress of Infants and Young Children*, 3rd edn. HMSO, London.

Sheridan, M.D. (1977) Development and assessment of vision and hearing. In *Neurodevelopmental Problems in Early Childhood: Assessment and Management* (eds C.N. Drillien & M.B. Drummond) pp. 150–167. Blackwell Scientific Publications, Oxford.

Sheridan, M.D., Sharma, A. & Cockerill, H. (2008) *From Birth to Five Years: Children's Developmental Progress*, 3rd edn. Routledge, London.

Shortland, A.P., Harris, C.A., Gough, M., *et al.* (2002) Architecture of the medial gastrocnemius in children with spastic diplegia. *Dev. Med. Child Neurol.*, **44**, 158–163.

Shumway-Cook, A., Hutchinson, S., Kartin, D., Price, R. & Woollacott, M. (2003) Effect of balance training on recovery of stability in children with cerebral palsy. *Dev. Med. Child Neurol.*, **45**, 591–602.

Shumway-Cook, A. & Woollacott, M.H. (2001) *Motor Control: Theory and Practical Applications*, 2nd edn. Lippincott Williams & Wilkins, Baltimore.

Siebes, R.C., Wijnroks, L. & Vermeer, A. (2002) Qualitative analysis of therapeutic motor intervention programmes for children with cerebral palsy: an update. *Dev. Med. Child Neurol.*, **44**, 593–603.

Simeonsson, R.J. & McHale, S.M. (1981) Review: research on handicapped children: sibling relationships. *Child Care Health Dev.*, **7**, 153.

Simpson, D.M., Gracies, J.M., Graham, H.K., *et al.* (2008) Assessment: botulinum neurotoxin for the treatment of spasticity (an evidence-based review): report of the Therapeutics and Technology Assessment Subcommittee of the American Academy of Neurology. *Neurology*, **70**, 1691–1698.

Slawek, J. & Klimont, L. (2003) Functional improvement in cerebral palsy patients treated with botulinum toxin A injections – preliminary results. *Eur. J. Neurol.*, **10**, 313–317.

Slominski, A.H. (1984) Winthrop Phelps and the Children's Rehabilitation Institute. In *Management of the Motor Disorders of Children with Cerebral Palsy* (ed. D. Scrutton), p. 59. SIMP, Blackwell Scientific Publications, Oxford.

Sluijs, E.M., van der Zee, J. & Kok, G.J. (1993) Differences between physical therapists in attention paid to patient education. *Physiotherapy Theory and Practice*, **9** (2), 103–118.

Snider, L., Korner-Bitensky, N., Kammann, C., Warner, S. & Saleh, M. (2007) Horseback riding as therapy for children with cerebral palsy: is there evidence of its effectiveness? *Phys. Occup. Ther. Pediatr.*, **27** (2), 5–23.

Soames, R. (2003) *Joint Motion: Clinical Measurement and Evaluation*. Churchill Livingstone, Edinburgh.

Solomons, G. & Solomons, H.C. (1975) Motor development in Yucatecan infants. *Dev. Med. Child Neurol.*, **17**, 41–46.

Sonksen, P. (1979) Sound and the visually handicapped baby. *Child Care Health Dev.*, **5**, 413.

Sonksen, P., Levitt, S. & Kitzinger, M. (1984) Identification of constraints acting on motor development in young visually disabled children and principles of remediation. *Child Care Health Dev.*, **10**, 273.

Sowell, E.R., Trauner, D.A., Gamst, A. & Jernigan, T.L. (2002) Development of cortical and subcortical brain structures in childhood and adolescence: a structural MRI study. *Dev. Med. Child Neurol.*, **44**, 14–16.

Sparrow, S. & Zigler, E. (1978) Evaluation of a patterning treatment for retarded children. *Pediatrics*, **62**, 137.

Speth, L.A., Leffers, P., Janssen-Potten, Y.J. & Vles, J.S. (2005) Botulinum toxin A and upper limb functional skills in hemiparetic cerebral palsy: a randomized trial in children receiving intensive therapy. *Dev. Med. Child Neurol.*, **47**, 468–473.

Spittle, A.J., Orton, J., Doyle, L.W. & Boyd, R. (2007) Early developmental intervention programs post hospital discharge to prevent motor and cognitive impairments in preterm infants. *Cochrane Database Syst. Rev.*, CD005495.

Sporns, O. & Edelman, G.M. (1993) Solving Bernstein's problem: a proposal for the development of coordinated movement by selection. *Child Development*, **64**, 690–981.

Stanley, F.J., Blair, E. & Alberman, E. (eds) (2000) *Cerebral Palsies: Epidemiology and Causal Pathways. Clinics in Developmental Medicine No. 151*. Mac Keith Press, London.

Stavness, C. (2006) The effect of positioning for children with cerebral palsy on upper-extremity function: a review of the evidence. *Phys. Occup. Ther. Pediatr.*, **26** (3), 39–53.

Steel, S. (1993) Individual learning programmes. In *Elements of Paediatric Physiotherapy* (ed. P.M. Eckersley), p. 369. Churchill Livingstone, Edinburgh.

Steenbeek, D., Ketelaar, M., Galama, K. & Gorter, J.W. (2008) Goal Attainment Scaling in paediatric rehabilitation:

a report on the clinical training of an interdisciplinary team. *Child Care Health Dev.*, 34, 521–529.

Steenbergen, B. & Gordon, A.M. (2006) Activity limitation in hemiplegic cerebral palsy: evidence for disorders in motor planning. *Dev. Med. Child Neurol.*, 48, 780–783.

Steinbok, P., Reiner, A. & Kestle, J.R.W. (1997b) Therapeutic electrical stimulation following selective posterior rhizotomy in children with spastic diplegic cerebral palsy: a randomized clinical trial. *Dev. Med. Child Neurol.*, 39, 515–520.

Steinbok, P., Reiner, A.M., Beauchamp, R., Armstrong, R.W. & Cochrane, D.D. (1997a) A randomized clinical trial to compare selective posterior rhizotomy plus physiotherapy with physiotherapy alone in children with spastic diplegic cerebral palsy. *Dev. Med. Child Neurol.*, 39, 178–184.

Sterba, J.A. (2007) Does horseback riding therapy or therapist-directed hippotherapy rehabilitate children with cerebral palsy? *Dev. Med. Child Neurol.*, 49, 68–73.

Stern, D.N. (1985) *The Interpersonal World of the Infant.* Basic Books, New York.

Stewart, P.C. & McQuilton, G. (1987) Straddle seating for the cerebral palsied child. *Br. J. Occup. Ther.*, 50, 136.

Stockmeyer, S.A. (1967) The Rood approach. *Am. J. Phys. Med.*, 46 (1), 900.

Stockmeyer, S.A. (1972) A sensorimotor approach to treatment. In *Physical Therapy Services in the Developmental Disabilities* (eds P.H. Pearson & C.E. Williams), Chapter 4. Thomas, Springfield, Illinois.

Stone, S. (1991) Qualitative research methods for physiotherapists. *Physiotherapy*, 77, 449–452.

Stott, N.S. & Piedrahita, L. (2004) Effects of surgical adductor releases for hip subluxation in cerebral palsy: an AACPDM evidence report. *Dev. Med. Child Neurol.*, 46, 628–645.

Strauss, D., Brooks, J., Rosenbloom, L. & Shavelle, R. (2008) Life expectancy in cerebral palsy: an update. *Dev. Med. Child Neurol.*, 50, 487–493.

Strauss, D., Ojdana, K., Shavelle, R. & Rosenbloom, L. (2004) Decline in function and life expectancy of older persons with cerebral palsy. *NeuroRehabilitation*, 19, 69–78.

Stroh, K., Robinson, T. & Proctor, A. (2008) *Every Child Can Learn.* Sage, London.

Stuberg, W.A. (1992) Considerations related to weight-bearing programs in children with developmental disabilities. *Phys. Ther.*, 72, 35–40.

Stuberg, W.A., Fuchs, R.H. & Miedaner, J.A. (1988) Reliability of goniometric measurements of children with cerebral palsy. *Dev. Med. Child Neurol.*, 30, 657.

Sugden, D.A. (1992) Postural control: developmental effects of visual and mechanical perturbations. *Physiotherapy Theory & Practice*, 8, 165.

Sussman, M.D. (ed.) (1992) *The Diplegic Child.* American Academy of Orthopedic Surgeons, Rosemont.

Sykanda, A.M. & Levitt, S. (1982) The physiotherapist in the developmental management of the visually impaired child. *Child Care Health Dev.*, 8, 261.

Tabary, J.C., Tardieu, C., Tardieu, G. & Goldspink, G. (1972) Physiological and structural changes in the cat's soleus muscles due to immobilisation at different lengths by plaster casts. *J. Physiol. (Lond.)*, 224, 231.

Tabary, J.-C., Tardieu, C., Tardieu, G. & Tabary, C. (1981) Experimental rapid sarcomere loss with concomitant hypo-extensibility. *Muscle Nerve*, 4, 198–203.

Tardieu, C., Huet de la Tour, E., Bret, M.D., *et al.* (1982) Muscle hypoextensibility in children with cerebral palsy. *Arch. Phys. Med. Rehab.*, 63, 97.

Tardieu, C., Lespargot, A., Tabary, C. & Bret, M.D. (1988) For how long must the soleus muscle be stretched each day to prevent contracture? *Dev. Med. Child Neurol.*, 30, 3–10.

Tardieu, G., Shentoub, S. & Delarue, R. (1954) A la recherche d'une technique de mesure de la spasticite. *Rev. Neurol.* 91, 143–144.

Tarran, E.C. (1981) Parents' views of medical and social work services for families with young cerebral-palsied children. *Dev. Med. Child Neurol.*, 23, 173.

Tatlow, A. (2005) *Conductive Education for Children and Adolescents with Cerebral Palsy.* The Spastics Association of Hong Kong, Hong Kong.

Taub, E. (1980) Somatosensory deafferentation research with monkeys: implications for rehabilitation medicine. In *Behavioral Psychology in Rehabilitation Medicine: Clinical implications* (ed. L.P. Ince), p. 371. Williams & Wilkins, Baltimore.

Taub, E., Ramey, S.L., DeLuca, S. & Echols, K. (2004) Efficacy of constraint-induced movement therapy for children with cerebral palsy with asymmetric motor impairment. *Pediatrics*, 113, 305–312.

Taylor, N.F., Dodd, K.J. & Graham, H.K. (2004) Test–retest reliability of hand-held dynamometric strength testing in young people with cerebral palsy. *Arch. Phys. Med. Rehabil.*, 85, 77–80.

Tecklin, J.S. (ed) (2008) *Pediatric Physical Therapy*, 4th edn. Lippincott Williams & Wilkins, Philadelphia.

Tedroff, K., Knutson, L.M. & Soderberg, G.L. (2006) Synergistic muscle activation during maximum voluntary contractions in children with and without spastic cerebral palsy. *Dev. Med. Child Neurol.*, 48, 789–796.

Terjesen, T., Lange, J.E. & Steen, H. (2000) Treatment of scoliosis with spinal bracing in quadriplegic cerebral palsy. *Dev. Med. Child Neurol.*, 42, 448–454.

Thelen, E. (1992) Development of locomotion from a dynamic systems approach. In *Movement Disorders in Children* (eds H. Forssberg & H. Hirschfeld), pp. 169–173. Karger, Basel.

Thelen, E., Kelso, J.A.S. & Fogel, A. (1987) Self-organizing motor systems and infant motor development. *Developmental Review*, 7, 39–65.

Thelen, E., Ulrich, B.D. & Jensen, J.L. (1989) The developmental origins of locomotion. In *Development of Posture and Gait across the Life Span* (eds M.H. Woollacott & A. Shumway-Cook), p. 25. University of South Carolina Press, Columbia.

Thomas, A.P., Bax, M.C.O. & Smyth, D.P.L. (1989) *The Health and Social Needs of Young Adults with Physical Disabilities.* Mac Keith Press, Blackwell Scientific Publications, Oxford.

Thomson, G. (2005) *Children with Severe Disabilities and the MOVE Curriculum*. East River Press, Chester, NY.

Thylefors, I., Price, E., Persson, T.O. & von Wendt, L. (2000) Teamwork in Swedish neuropaediatric habilitation. *Child Care Health Dev.*, **26**, 515–532.

Tieman, B.L., Palisano, R.J., Gracely, E.J. & Rosenbaum, P.L. (2004) Gross motor capability and performance of mobility in children with cerebral palsy: a comparison across home, school, and outdoors/community settings. *Phys. Ther.*, **84**, 419–429.

Tirosh, E. & Rabino, S. (1989) Physiotherapy in children with cerebral palsy: evidence for its efficacy. *Am. J. Dis. Child*, **143**, 552.

Titchener, J. (1983) A preliminary evaluation of conductive education. *Physiotherapy*, **69**, 313–315.

Tizard, J.P.M., Paine, R.S. & Crothers, B. (1954) Disturbances of sensation in children with hemiplegia. *J. Amer. Med. Assoc.*, **155**, 628–632.

Touwen, B.C.L. (1978) Variability and stereotypy in normal and deviant development. In *Care of the Handicapped Child* (ed. J. Apley), p. 99. SIMP, Heinemann, London.

Touwen, B.C.L. (1987) The significance of neonatal neurological diagnosis. In *Early Detection and Management of Cerebral Palsy* (eds H. Galjaard, H.F.R. Prechtl & M. Velickovic), p. 69. Martinus Nijhoff, Dordrecht.

Trefler, E., Hanks, S., Huggins, P., *et al.* (1978) A modular seating system for cerebral-palsied children. *Dev. Med. Child Neurol.*, **20**, 199.

Tremblay, F., Malouin, F., Richards, C.L. & Dumas, F. (1990) Effects of prolonged muscle stretch on reflex and voluntary muscle activation in children with spastic cerebral palsy. *Scand. J. Rehabil. Med.*, **22**, 171–180.

Turker, R.J. & Lee, R. (2000) Adductor tenotomies in children with quadriplegic cerebral palsy: Longer term follow-up. *J. Pediatr. Orthoped.*, **20**, 370–374.

Twitchell, T.E. (1961) The nature of the motor deficit in double athetosis. *Arch. Phys. Med.*, **42**, 63.

Ubhi, T., Bhakta, B.B., Ives, H.L., Allgar, V. & Roussounis, S.H. (2000) Randomised double blind placebo controlled trial of the effect of botulinum toxin on walking in cerebral palsy. *Arch. Dis. Child.*, **83**, 481–487.

Umphred, D. (1984) An integrated approach to treatment of the pediatric neurologic patient. In *Pediatric Neurologic Physical Therapy* (ed. S.K. Campbell), Chapter 3. Churchill Livingstone, New York.

Umphred, D.A. (2000) *Neurological Rehabilitation*, 4th edn. Mosby, St Louis.

Van Vliet, P. (ed.) (1992) Special issue: issues in the training of postural control. *Physiotherapy Theory & Practice*, **8** (3).

Varni, J.W., Burwinkle, T.M., Berrin, S.J., *et al.* (2006) The PedsQL in pediatric cerebral palsy: reliability, validity, and sensitivity of the generic core scales and cerebral palsy module. *Dev. Med. Child Neurol.*, **48**, 442–449.

Varni, J.W., Burwinkle, T.M., Sherman, S.A., *et al.* (2005) Health-related quality of life of children and adolescents with cerebral palsy: hearing the voices of children. *Dev. Med. Child Neurol.*, **47**, 592–597.

Visser, J.E. & Bloem, B.R. (2005) Role of the basal ganglia in balance control. *Neural Plast.*, **12**, 161–174.

Vogtle, L., Morris, D. & Denton, B. (1998) An aquatic programme for adults with cerebral palsy living in group homes. *Phys. Ther. Case Reports*, **1**, 250–259.

Vojta, V. (1984) The basic elements of treatment according to Vojta. In *Management of the Motor Disorders of Children with Cerebral Palsy* (ed. D. Scrutton), p. 75. SIMP, Blackwell Scientific Publications, Oxford.

Vojta, V. (1989) *Die Cerebralen Bewegungsstorungen im Sauglingsalter*, 5th edn. Ferdinand Enke Verlag, Stuttgart.

Von Aufschnaiter, D. (1992) Vojta: a neurophysiological treatment. In *Movement Disorders in Children* (eds H. Forssberg & H. Hirschfeld), pp. 7–15. Karger, Basel.

Voorman, J.M., Dallmeijer, A.J., Knol, D.L., Lankhorst, G.J. & Becher, J.G. (2007) Prospective longitudinal study of gross motor function in children with cerebral palsy. *Arch. Phys. Med. Rehabil.*, **88**, 871–876.

Voss, D.E. (1972) Proprioceptive neuromuscular facilitation. In *Physical Therapy Services in the Developmental Disabilities* (eds P.H. Pearson & C.E. Williams), Chapter 5. Thomas, Springfield, Illinois.

Voss, D.E., Jonta, M. & Meyers, B. (1985) *Proprioceptive Neuromuscular Facilitation Patterns and Techniques*, 3rd edn. Harper & Row, New York.

Wallen, M., O'Flaherty, S.J. & Waugh, M.C. (2007) Functional outcomes of intramuscular botulinum toxin type A and occupational therapy in the upper limbs of children with cerebral palsy: a randomized controlled trial. *Arch. Phys. Med. Rehabil.*, **88**, 1–10.

van der Weel, F.R., van der Meer, A.L. & Lee, D.N. (1991) Effect of task on movement control in cerebral palsy: implications for assessment and therapy. *Dev. Med. Child Neurol.*, **33**, 419–426.

von Wendt, L., Ekenberg, L., Dagis, D. & Janlert, U. (1984) A parent-centred approach to physiotherapy for their handicapped children. *Dev. Med. Child Neurol.*, **26**, 445.

Whalley Hammell, K. & Carpenter, C. (eds) (2004) *Qualitative Research in Evidence-Based Rehabilitation*. Churchill Livingstone, Edinburgh.

White, H., Jenkins, J., Neace, W.P., Tylkowski, C. & Walker, J. (2002) Clinically prescribed orthoses demonstrate an increase in velocity of gait in children with cerebral palsy: a retrospective study. *Dev. Med. Child Neurol.*, **44**, 227–232.

WHO (2001) *International Classification of Functioning, Disability and Health (ICF)*. World Health Organization, Geneva.

Wiley, M.E. & Damiano, D.L. (1998) Lower-extremity strength profiles in spastic cerebral palsy. *Dev. Med. Child Neurol.*, **40**, 100–107.

Wilmshurst, S.W., Adams, K., Langton, C.M. & Mughal, M.Z. (1996) Mobility status and bone density in cerebral palsy. *Arch. Dis. Child.*, **75**, 164–165.

Wilner, L. (ed.) (1996) *Getting On with Cerebral Palsy: From Adolescence to Old Age*. Scope, London.

Winnicott, D.W. (1964) *The Child, the Family and the Outside World*. Penguin Books, London.

Winstein, C.J. & Schmidt, R.A. (1990) Reduced frequency of knowledge of results enhances motor skill learning. *J. Exp. Psychol. Learn. Memory*, **16**, 677.

Winstein, C.J., Gardner, E.R., McNeal D.R., *et al.* (1989) Standing balance training: effect on balance and locomotion in hemiparetic adults. *Arch. Phys. Med. Rehabil.*, **70**, 755–762.

Winstein, C.J. & Schmidt, R.A. (1989) Sensorimotor feedback. In *Human Skills*, 2nd edn (ed. D.H. Holding), p. 17. Wiley, Chichester.

Winstock, A. (2005) *Eating and Drinking Difficulties in Children: A Guide for Practitioners*. Speechmark, Bicester.

Wong, D. & Baker, C. (1988) Pain in children: comparison of assessment scales. *Pediatric Nursing*, **14**, 9–17.

Wood, E. & Rosenbaum, P. (2000) The gross motor function classification system for cerebral palsy: a study of reliability and stability over time. *Dev. Med. Child Neurol.*, **42**, 292–296.

Woollacott, M., Shumway-Cook, A., Hutchinson, S., Ciol, M., Price, R. & Kartin, D. (2005) Effect of balance training on muscle activity used in recovery of stability in children with cerebral palsy: a pilot study. *Dev. Med. Child Neurol.*, **47**, 455–461.

Wright, F.V., Sheil, E., Drake, J., Wedge, J.H. & Naumann, S. (1998) Evaluation of selective dorsal rhizotomy for the reduction of spasticity in cerebral palsy: a randomized controlled trial. *Dev. Med. Child Neurol.*, **40**, 239–247.

Wright, T. & Nicholson, J. (1973) Physiotherapy for the spastic child: an evaluation. *Dev. Med. Child Neurol.*, **15**, 146–163.

Wu, Y.W., Day, S.M., Strauss, D.J. & Shavelle, R.M. (2004) Prognosis for ambulation in cerebral palsy: a population-based study. *Pediatrics*, **114**, 1264–1271.

Yasukawa, A. (1990) Upper extremity casting: adjunct treatment for a child with cerebral palsy hemiplegia. *Am. J. Occup. Ther.*, **44**, 840–846.

Yekutiel, M., Jariwala, M. & Stretch, P. (1994) Sensory deficit in the hands of children with cerebral palsy: a new look at assessment and prevalence. *Dev. Med. Child Neurol.*, **36**, 619–624.

Young, N.L., Wright, J.G., Lam, T.P., Rajaratnam, K., Stephens, D. & Wedge, J.H. (1998) Windswept hip deformity in spastic quadriplegic cerebral palsy. *Pediatr. Phys. Ther.*, **10**, 94–100.

Young, R.R. & Wiegner, A.W. (1987) Spasticity. *Clin. Orthopaed. Rel. Res.*, **219**, 50.

Zacharkow, D. (1988) *Posture, Sitting, Standing, Chair Design and Exercise*. Thomas, Springfield, Illinois.

Zinkin, P. (1979) The effect of visual handicap on early development. In *Visual Handicap in Children* (eds V. Smith & J. Keen), p. 132. Spastics Int. Med. Publ., London.

Index

Note: Italicised letters after page numbers refer to figures and tables.

guidelines for therapists in, 76
learning methods in, 77–8
  behaviours, 77
  emotions, 77–8
learning principles, 76
options for therapists, 78
practice and experience, 84–5
promoting attention in, 79
prone position, 261–2
rewards, 84
task analysis in, 81
tasks for adults, 78
verbal guidance in, 83–4
motor growth curves, 108–9
motor patterns, basic, 67
motor training, 76–85, 125–9
  age of child and techniques, 127–8
  aims and methods, 125–6
  applications of techniques, 128–9
  in daily life activities, 126
  developmental levels, 126–7
  diagnosis and techniques, 128
  general plan of developmental programme, 127
  onset and techniques, 127–8
  related procedures, 126
mouth actions, 268
MOVE Europe programme, 113–21
movement patterns, 37
  training of, 73
movement superimposed on co-contraction, 64
muscle education and braces
  braces, 35
  calipers, 35
  modalities, 34–5
  muscle education, 35–6
  specific diagnostic classification of child, 34
muscles, strength of, 67–8, 103
musculoskeletal deformities, 72, 89, 275–305

naso-gastric tube, 269
National Association of Paediatric Occupational Therapists, 317
National Association of Swimming Clubs for the Handicapped, 317
National Association of Toy and Leisure Libraries, 317
neck deformities, 303–4
neck righting, 118*t*
negative supporting, 118*t*
neurodevelopmental treatment (NDT), 39–40, 53
neurofacilitation treatment, 74–5
neuromotor development, 38

neuromuscular electrical stimulation, 43–4
neuronal group selection theory, 48–9
neuroplasticity, 47–8
Neurosensory and Motor Developmental Assessment for Infants and Young Children, 112
night-splint ankle–foot orthoses, 226
non-motor impairments, 12
normal child development, 3–4
nystagmus, 10

Observational Gait Scale, 112–13
occupational therapy, 13, 42, 66, 87, 96, 114, 125, 259, 262, 272, 320
older person with cerebral palsy, 86–94
  aims of therapy, 86
  collaborative learning approach, 86–7
    adolescent distancing from parents, 86–7
    confidentiality, 87
    sense of control, 86
    sensitive listening to individuals, 86
  cosmetic appearance, 93
  deformities, 90–91
  development of community mobility, 93
  health lifestyle, 92
  issues of concern in, 88–9
    discrimination, 89
    early and minor deterioration, 88–9
    fatigue, 88
    increased musculoskeletal deformities, 89
    new environments, 89
    pain, 88
    services for older people, 89
    urinary problems, 89
  knowledge about condition, 93–4
  measures, 94
  motor abilities, 89–90
  motor developmental assumptions, 90
  role of physiotherapist and occupational therapist, 87
  self-care activities, 89–90
  self-care training, 93
  studies of function, 87–8
  therapeutic motor activities, 94
ontogenetic developmental sequence, 40, 67
optical reflex, 119*t*
orthoses, arm, 91, 303–4. *See also* hand function
orthoses, lower limb, 209, 224–7
  types of, 224–7. *See also* splints
    ankle–foot orthoses, 224–7
    hip abduction with trunk brace (SWASH), 224, 227*f*
    knee gaiters, 224
orthoses, trunk (body), 44, 183, 189, 304